TEACHING

PSYCHOTHERAPEUTIC

MEDICINE

LONDON

GEOFFREY CUMBERLEGE

OXFORD UNIVERSITY PRESS

TEACHING
PSYCHOTHERAPEUTIC
MEDICINE

AN EXPERIMENTAL COURSE
FOR GENERAL PHYSICIANS

GIVEN BY

WALTER BAUER, M.D.   M. RALPH KAUFMAN, M.D.

DOUGLAS D. BOND, M.D.   JOHN M. MURRAY, M.D.

HENRY W. BROSIN, M.D.   THOMAS A. C. RENNIE, M.D.

DONALD W. HASTINGS, M.D.   JOHN ROMANO, M.D.

HAROLD G. WOLFF, M.D.

EDITED BY HELEN LELAND WITMER, PH.D.
INTRODUCTORY CHAPTER BY GEDDES SMITH

NEW YORK · 1947

THE COMMONWEALTH FUND

PUBLISHED BY THE COMMONWEALTH FUND

41 EAST 57TH STREET, NEW YORK 22, N.Y.

───────

PRINTED IN THE UNITED STATES OF AMERICA

BY E. L. HILDRETH & COMPANY, INC.

Foreword

THIS book has been drawn from automatic recordings of lectures and discussions heard at the pilot course in Psychotherapy in General Practice given at the University of Minnesota in April 1946. Verbatim records of extemporaneous speech always need editing to become easily readable. These records have been edited, but the speakers have generally refrained from recasting their material in the polite forms of written English. Had they done so, or had they elaborated their exposition at the many points where such elaboration would be necessary in a textbook, this record would have lost its flavor and its value as an exhibit of teaching method. It is offered here not as a manual of psychotherapeutic medicine but as the protocol of an experiment in postgraduate medical education.

Much of the introductory chapter has been published in pamphlet form under the title Psychotherapy in General Medicine: Report of an Experimental Postgraduate Course (New York, The Commonwealth Fund, 1946).

Contents

Introductory: The Course

GEDDES SMITH

THERE has been growing uneasiness among thoughtful teachers of medicine about the fragmentation of medical knowledge and the failure of medicine, as commonly practiced, to deal helpfully with a very large group of very real troubles brought to the doctor by unhappy patients. To quote Dr. David P. Barr, physician-in-chief of the New York Hospital:

In every outpatient department and in every practitioner's office there are many patients whose complaints are troublesome and chronic, whose diagnoses are often in doubt, and whose treatment is less than satisfactory. They are in general people who are emotionally maladjusted and ill-fitted to cope with the stress of daily life. They include those who without organic defect are anxious, depressed, and insecure to a degree that they consider themselves ill and more or less incapacitated. Among them are many who have been diagnosed as migraine, peptic ulcer, ulcerative colitis, and hypertension. Some of them may be found in the nose and throat clinic, complaining of vasomotor rhinitis, laryngitis, and other conditions indicative of inflamed and over-secreting mucous membranes. . . . Their complaints are numerous and insistent. They try the patience of their physicians who seldom have sufficient time to examine and analyze the background of their insecurity.

These are patients whom the physician has always with him, but it took the war and its psychiatric casualties to spotlight their need. The impetus for the particular experiment with which this volume is concerned came from a group of military and naval psychiatrists and medical educators who met at Hershey, Pennsylvania, in February 1945, under the auspices of the National Committee for Mental Hygiene and the Commonwealth Fund, to discuss the needs of veterans with psychoneurotic reactions.* This group agreed that care of such patients must be given primarily by general physicians, and recommended that

* *Medicine and the Neuroses: Report of the Hershey Conference on Psychiatric Rehabilitation.* New York, The National Committee for Mental Hygiene, 1945.

a pilot course, or courses, be set up at the postgraduate level to explore the possibilities of educating men in practice for this responsibility. The Commonwealth Fund undertook to provide such an experimental course and called into consultation, to plan it, a number of psychiatrists with relevant teaching experience, led by Dr. Thomas A. C. Rennie, Associate Professor of Psychiatry, Cornell University Medical College, and Dr. John M. Murray, who had organized and directed the psychiatric training program of the Army Air Forces at Fort Logan, Colorado.* After careful preparation the course was given in the first two weeks of April 1946, in cooperation with the Division of Postgraduate Education of the University of Minnesota.

This postgraduate course was an attempt, on a small scale, to get the most pertinent parts of basic psychiatric thinking into general medicine. It relied, at bottom, on three factors: the coherent presentation in simple terms of a few basic concepts, clinical practice under supervision, and abundant discussion of a very informal kind. Lectures dealt with the personality, its development, and its disorders; with the interplay of the emotions and physical function; with the physician-patient relationship; and with the elements of psychotherapy. For clinical teaching the University Hospital provided from its medical clinics patients with vague and often long-standing physical complaints. Discussion was encouraged by the formation of small teaching groups and was warmed by the friendly association of instructors and students, who lived together in the Center for Continuation Study, generously made available by the University.†

The student group was selected by the Division of Postgraduate Education in such a way as to provide a representative sample of general medicine as practiced in Minnesota and the neighboring states. Twenty-three of the twenty-five were general physicians or internists; most of the latter were in group practice. One was a pediatrician, one a dermatologist. Thirteen men were in their thirties, ten in their forties,

* Dr. John C. Whitehorn, Professor of Psychiatry at Johns Hopkins University School of Medicine, though he was unable to participate in the teaching, shared helpfully in the early planning of the course.

† This remarkable building, with dormitories, a cafeteria, a garage, classrooms, and an ample lounge all under one roof, has great advantages over the makeshift accommodations commonly available for postgraduate teaching.

two in their early fifties. Five were veterans who had spent the previous three months in postgraduate study at the University of Minnesota in preparation for a return to civilian practice. Two others were about to begin residencies. Of the other eighteen, three had practices in the Twin Cities, five others in cities of 25,000 or more, seven in cities of between 1,000 and 25,000, and three in towns of 1,000 or less. Students paid fees for board, lodging, and tuition at the rates usually charged at the Center.

The teaching staff was drawn chiefly from the ranks of the younger psychiatrists, most of them fresh from war service, who felt that psychiatry had something that could and must be shared with general medicine and recognized the urgent need of collaboration from general medicine in the care of the psychoneuroses. It included the following persons:

ELEANOR BARNES
> Information Secretary, New York City Committee on Mental Hygiene
> *Formerly* Chief Social Worker, New York University Clinics, New York University Medical School

WALTER BAUER, M.D.
> Associate Professor in Medicine, Harvard Medical School
> *Formerly* Colonel, M.C., Medical Consultant, Headquarters, 8th Service Command

DOUGLAS D. BOND, M.D.
> Professor of Psychiatry, Western Reserve University School of Medicine
> *Formerly* Major, M.C., Chief of the Neuropsychiatric Branch, Professional Service Division, Office of the Air Surgeon; Director of Psychiatry, 8th Air Force, Central Medical Establishment

HENRY W. BROSIN, M.D.†
> Professor of Psychiatry, University of Chicago School of Medicine
> *Formerly* Colonel, M.C., Neuropsychiatric Consultant, Headquarters, 3rd Service Command

DONALD W. HASTINGS, M.D.†
> Professor of Psychiatry, University of Minnesota Medical School
> *Formerly* Lieutenant Colonel, M.C., Chief of the Neuropsychiatric Branch, Professional Service Division, Office of the Air Surgeon; Chief Consultant in Psychiatry, 8th Air Force

† Present for the second week.

M. RALPH KAUFMAN, M.D.*

Psychiatrist, The Mount Sinai Hospital, New York

Formerly Colonel, M.C., Consultant Psychiatrist, Pacific Ocean Areas; Associate in Psychiatry, Harvard Medical School

JOHN M. MURRAY, M.D.

Professor of Clinical Psychiatry, Boston University School of Medicine; Chief of Psychiatric Section, New England Branch of the Veterans Administration

Formerly Colonel, M.C., Chief of the Neuropsychiatric Branch, Professional Service Division, Office of the Air Surgeon; Director, Aviation Psychiatry Training Program, and Psychiatric Consultant to Army Air Forces Personnel Distribution Command, Fort Logan, Colorado; Consultant in Psychiatry, Dartmouth College

THOMAS A. C. RENNIE, M.D.*

Associate Professor of Psychiatry, Cornell University Medical College; Director, Division on Rehabilitation, National Committee for Mental Hygiene

Formerly Associate in Psychiatry, Johns Hopkins School of Medicine

JOHN ROMANO, M.D.

Professor of Psychiatry, University of Rochester School of Medicine

Formerly Professor of Psychiatry, University of Cincinnati College of Medicine; Instructor in Medicine, Harvard Medical School; Associate in Medicine, Peter Bent Brigham Hospital

KATHARINE M. WICKMAN

Psychiatric Social Worker, Pediatric-Psychiatric Clinic, Babies Hospital, Columbia-Presbyterian Medical Center; Instructor, New York School of Social Work (Columbia University)

Formerly Psychiatric Social Worker, Institute for Child Guidance, New York

HAROLD G. WOLFF, M.D.†

Associate Professor of Medicine and Associate Professor of Psychiatry, Cornell University Medical College

DR. GEORGE N. AAGAARD, JR., Assistant Professor of Medicine, at Minnesota in charge of the medical outpatient department, made all arrangements for the clinical part of the course and selected patients for teaching purposes. Assisting in the clinical teaching was a group of psychiatrists on the staff of the University of Minnesota Medical School, as follows:

* Present for the first week.   † Present for the second week.

S. ALLAN CHALLMAN, M.D.
Clinical Assistant Professor of Neuropsychiatry
LILLIAN COTTRELL, M.D.
Assistant Professor of Neuropsychiatry
HAROLD B. HANSON, M.D.
Clinical Assistant Professor of Pediatrics and Neuropsychiatry
ROBERT G. HINCKLEY, M.D.
Associate Professor of Neuropsychiatry
REYNOLD A. JENSEN, M.D.
Associate Professor of Pediatrics and Neuropsychiatry
HYMAN S. LIPPMAN, M.D.
Clinical Associate Professor of Pediatrics and Neuropsychiatry
BURTRUM C. SCHIELE, M.D.
Associate Professor of Neuropsychiatry

The length of the course was dictated by practical considerations. Precedents at the Center for Continuation Study pointed to a week as the outer limit of courses for active practitioners. Some of the teaching group, despairing of covering the ground adequately, set three or four weeks as a minimum. Since only a short course seemed likely to set a pattern that could be generally followed and since it would be difficult to hold either students or instructors for longer than two weeks, that period was adopted as a workable compromise.

Two weeks is a short time in which to reorient men in medicine. The schedule was a full one. After some experimentation it took form as follows:

Monday through Friday
    8:30–10:20 Lecture, followed by discussion (entire student group)
  10:30–12:00 Section meetings devoted to discussion of clinical work (instructor and five students)
    1:00– 2:30 General seminar (entire student group) or section meetings
    3:00– 5:00 Supervised clinical work (one instructor and one assistant to each five students)
    8:00– 9:00 Films and special seminars as requested
Saturday
    8:30–12:00 Review, case presentations, and discussion

In planning this schedule the intent was that the morning lectures would lay the theoretical groundwork for the kind of medical care that the students were to learn; the afternoon seminars would provide opportunity for the presentation and discussion of methodology; and the clinic sessions, with the section meetings at which clinical procedures could be discussed in detail, would help the students to get and assimilate first-hand experience in the care of patients.

*

Clinical teaching is the crucial part of a course like this. The instructors felt that the meaning and methods of psychotherapy could not have been conveyed adequately by lectures and discussions alone. As one student remarked: "The lectures are fine, but the doctors in the clinic show you something you can't put into words." Unfortunately that part of the course which "you can't put into words" is inevitably missing from this book. Interviews between student-physicians and their patients could not be recorded verbatim without threatening or breaching the confidential relationship on which good therapy depends. The consensus among the instructors was that not even a one-way screen or other device for making an interview audible to unperceived auditors could be used without violating the patient's trust. Nor was it possible to record the hot-off-the-griddle discussions that took place as the student and instructor walked out of the consulting room, though these may well have been the crux of the verbal teaching that was done.

Some cases were reported at length in the closing sessions of the course, and these reports appear in the pages which follow. These retrospective presentations, however, lack the fire and urgency of the discussion of fresh clinical problems that took place in the small section meetings. Only a small fraction of this discussion could be recorded, and the excerpts printed here—as clinical footnotes to the lectures and seminar material—make no claim to being comprehensive or even representative. Perhaps they do show how clinical problems were attacked—problems such as every student in the course and every general physician who may read this book meets in his everyday practice. The purpose of the book would be defeated, however, if any reader got the impression that one can teach, or learn, psychotherapeutic medicine merely by talking about it.

In preliminary discussion some of the instructors had asked for patients illustrating various aspects of acute anxiety, including perhaps a few veterans, who might respond visibly to brief but reasonably intensive treatment. The general and special medical clinics of the university hospital held far less of such material than these instructors hoped to find, but more than made up for this lack by offering in large abundance cases of long-standing distress, more or less disabling, of the sort that Dr. Barr describes. Some of these patients had been known to the clinic for a long time; some had had varied medical and surgical treatment elsewhere: one woman had had eleven gynecological operations. They complained of pain in the stomach, abdomen, back, legs, and so on, flatulence, palpitation, nervousness, fatigue, sleeplessness, headache. About three-fourths were women; considerably more than half came from small towns or the open country; a few were in their teens, a few more were young adults, but many more were in their middle or later years. There were few textbook psychoneuroses, but many psychoneurotic people in the group; it was an excellent sample of the persistently unwell.

At the beginning of the course a few patients had been studied by one of the psychiatric social workers in the teaching group in the effort to clear the way for incisive therapy. As it became clear that the clinical work done in the course was more likely to demonstrate chronic psychoneurotic situations than acute anxiety, cases were taken about as they came and were put in the hands of the student-doctors as soon as a minimum physical work-up had been completed by the regular clinic staff.

Methods of supervision varied from one instructor to another; in general the student was left to make his own contact with the patient and was joined by the instructor only for a part of the interview. Some instructors spent much time with the students immediately after the patients left. The assignment of two persons, an instructor and an assistant, to each group of five students in the clinic was barely adequate for good supervision: some men got less than would have been desirable, particularly during the earlier part of the course, when two interviews were scheduled for each student each day.

The following table shows the distribution of the 279 visits made by the 121 patients seen by the student group:

Visits per patient	Number of patients	Total visits
1	40	40
2	36	72
3	20	60
4	20	80
5	4	20
7	1	7
	121	279

The interesting point here is that 37 per cent of the patients were seen three times or oftener in a total of ten clinic sessions.* The intensity of treatment varied, of course, with the student, the instructor, and the case. Some of the instructors were particularly adept in making teaching points after brief contacts with patients; others were interested in demonstrating the cumulative results of repeated interviews. The two students who saw the largest number of patients—eight and seven respectively—saw none of them more than twice. Most of the men had a somewhat more concentrated experience: three students saw six patients each, twelve saw five, eight saw three or four each.

Borrowing patients from a going outpatient service involved certain inconveniences and hazards. Though it was not easy to incorporate twenty-five visitors into the regular routines of a large teaching clinic, schedules were staggered and the operation went off more smoothly than might have been expected. The hazards related to the establishment of doctor-patient relationships which had to be broken so soon. The psychiatric social workers on the teaching staff helped in preparing patients for this brief experience and in tying up the loose ends when they were turned back to the permanent staff. The collaboration of members of the psychiatric staff of the University of Minnesota was another aid to continuity. This problem would have been more difficult had a greater number of acutely ill patients been seen.

* The clinic director estimated that not more than one return appointment out of every twenty-five was broken.

Naturally, no student made final disposition of any case. Those patients who had served their purpose for teaching, or with whom the student had gone as far as it seemed likely that he could go, were referred back to the medical clinic, with a final note in the record summing up the student's impression. Students were asked to keep separate notes of any data too personal to appear in the clinic record. Twenty-three patients in need of continued care at the psychiatric level were referred to specially assigned members of the psychiatric staff or to the psychiatric service of the department of pediatrics, and fuller information about them was transmitted, in most instances both verbally and in writing, to the person assuming responsibility.

The greatest weakness of the clinical teaching, from a theoretical standpoint, was the fact that the students did not work up their cases fully from the beginning. Ideally a general physician or internist should be taught by doing what he would do in good practice—taking a complete history, making a physical examination, and securing what laboratory or x-ray data he felt he needed, weighing one diagnostic indication against another until he reached a well-founded and well-balanced opinion as to the causes of the patient's condition. Because the psychotherapeutic use of the interview was an unfamiliar technique and because time was short, in most instances these students took their physical and laboratory data from the record, and related physical data gotten by other people to what they were getting for themselves on emotional issues. Had they been young and inexperienced, this might have skewed their thinking; but since nearly all of them were seasoned practitioners, long accustomed to conventional diagnostic procedures, there was little danger that they would skimp their physical medicine when they went back to their own offices. It was necessary, however, to challenge them from time to time to make sure that they kept the balance even, and at best the dichotomy was unfortunate.

In this situation the students and instructors leaned heavily on the internist who served as general medical consultant both in the seminar room and in the clinic. Dr. Bauer's wide knowledge of medicine enabled him to speak with authority on many problems raised by the medical history of the patient and to evaluate the patient's present condition in terms of accepted clinical considerations. His own interest and skill were broad enough to bridge the gap often left between somatic and psychological study of a given patient. It seems evident that if this gap is to be bridged, internists and psychiatrists should share in the teaching of psychotherapy for general practitioners under whatever auspices it is given.

The two psychiatric social workers attached to the teaching group also gave consultant service in the clinic and in discussion. Because most of the men in this course practiced in communities where skilled case work was not available to them, or was available only from public employees with many prior claims on their time, it would have been foolish to teach them to place much reliance on social work collaboration. Representatives of social service agencies in Minnesota were given an opportunity to tell them what facilities were at hand in that state. In occasional cases seen in the clinic where social work had been done in Minneapolis, or obviously needed to be done, the two consultants acquainted students with its methods. With experience and skill in analyzing the emotional patterns of parents and children, these women were often able to interpret such material as it presented itself in the clinical handling of patients enmeshed—as most patients are—in the complications of family life.

*

It was the purpose of this course to show people and their ailments in fresh perspective, so that the doctor's effort to help them might be at once more realistic and more effective. There had to be people—patients—in the picture, for only so could the forces that make up human personality and shape the doctor-patient relationship be demonstrated *in vivo*. But there had also to be a clear presentation of the concepts that defined this perspective. The course was designed to offer a rationale of medicine and an opportunity to feel, as well as understand, its worth. Students had to be prepared intellectually for a kind of medical practice they were not accustomed to, for unfamiliar ways of talking with and thinking about their patients.

The content and form of the course were discussed at length in preliminary conferences among members of the teaching staff, the University, and the Fund. In this process much proposed subject-matter melted away and some professional preoccupations were whittled down.

When the core of the teaching to be done became visible, it was seen to relate to the everyday practice of medicine. It differed from most conventional courses in either medicine or psychiatry chiefly in taking as its point of departure the emotional life, and particularly the interpersonal relations, of the patient. Pausing only for a general preview of the course in an introductory lecture, the teachers were to lay first before the students their concept of the doctor-patient relationship as the cornerstone of therapy. This was to be followed by an exposition of normal personality development. That may seem unduly theoretical for a two weeks' course in the care of emotionally handicapped patients, but there was sound reason for approaching psychotherapeutic medicine in this way. The major intellectual adjustment the students needed to make was to get the emotional life of the patient into a biological frame of reference along with the organic data they were accustomed to consider, to learn to think of hostility as something just as real, and just as pertinent to the clinical picture, as an enlarged heart. This point could be illustrated by clinical observation (and was, throughout the course) and documented by the results of physiological experimentation (and was, in lectures near the end of the two weeks). It needed to be made, however, in broad and basic terms: one way to do this was to show that the emotional life had coherence and continuity; that its growth and development paralleled physical growth and development; that it was subject to trauma and degeneration; and that like the behavior of the adrenals or the heart rate it was governed by the principle of homeostasis.

It was this principle which gave point to the next step in the exposition—the definition of psychoneurosis not as a collection of specific disorders but as a way of meeting life when it got difficult. This led in turn to the discussion of anxiety as a familiar human experience and as the common denominator of many kinds of emotional dysfunction. Not until later in the course—and never with much emphasis—was any systematic attempt made to classify the neuroses as diagnostic entities. Stress was laid on the broad considerations which made the patient understandable and on the simple things the general physician could do to relieve the patient's distress. Obviously the progression was from the normal to the pathological, from the general to the specific. With such a pattern it was not hard to keep the language of instruction simple and to avoid for the most part those diagnostic and terminological mazes which are unhappily associated with psychological medicine as it has often been taught.

Indeed the lectures were actually given at a simpler and often more colloquial level, and in broader terms, than had been anticipated in the preliminary conferences. Although the major strategy of the course was unchanged, schedules were freely altered as the instructors met from day to day to consider how things were going; in particular, time was taken from the large group seminars, at which techniques were to be discussed in general terms, to permit more small section meetings at which technical problems could be worked out in terms of specific cases. The lectures and the section meetings proved more successful vehicles for teaching than the group seminars. Discussion in the full group of twenty-five, and in the presence of a number of auditors not enrolled in the course, never quite satisfied either the students or the teachers, and the group seminars became in effect minor lectures given at a time of day when no one was quite as fresh as he had been at the morning session.* One instructor, after a week's experience, felt that an hour a day of straight didactic teaching was all that should be attempted. The best teaching was done in the section meetings, where give and take was easy and continual and where the significance of the clinical work was hammered out case by case.

Teaching methods, it will be seen, were fluid and informal. The over-all plan was to keep driving at the major points by statement and restatement with all the variety a diversified group of teachers could give them. In the lecture room the presence of a rather large group of instructors was an asset, for one reinforced another and there was repetition without monotony—indispensable to good teaching. If discussion lacked the contrapuntal quality that the freer expression of student opinion might have given, there was at least abundant development of the central theme.

* Partly for this reason no attempt has been made in this book to record student discussion in full. Only those parts which elicited new or important teaching points have, as a rule, been included.

Comments from several men suggested that the informality of the course (in which students and instructors were housed together, ate together, and palavered together at all hours) and the simplicity of presentation were important aids in the learning process. One man wrote that the faculty was "so nonprofessorial"; another, ". . . the fundamentals were presented without the use of many new terms. . . . I was pleased that the instructors did not at any time 'talk down' to the students." The teamwork on the part of the instructors, who as a matter of fact did subordinate their occasional differences of opinion in order to present an integrated concept of psychotherapy, was appreciated especially by men who knew that such agreement did not come about by chance.

As finally given, the program of didactic exercises was as follows:

Monday, April 1
    Morning: General Orientation
                Lecturer, Dr. Rennie
                Discussion leader, Dr. Bauer
    Afternoon: The Patient-Physician Relationship
                Leader, Dr. Kaufman
Tuesday, April 2
    Morning: Normal Personality Development
                Lecturer, Dr. Murray
    Afternoon: Section Meetings
    Evening: Showing of Film
                Combat Fatigue; Irritability*
                Discussion leader, Dr. Bond
Wednesday, April 3
    Morning: Normal Personality Development
                Lecturer, Dr. Murray
    Afternoon: Psychotherapy
                Leader, Dr. Romano
Thursday, April 4
    Morning: The Meaning of a Psychoneurosis
                Lecturer, Dr. Kaufman
    Afternoon: Section Meetings

  * This session was not recorded.

Friday, April 5
    Morning: The Meaning of a Psychoneurosis
            Lecturer, Dr. Kaufman
    Afternoon: Diagnosis of Psychoneurosis
            Leader, Dr. Romano
Saturday, April 6
    Morning: Summary by Dr. Rennie
Monday, April 8
    Morning: Anxiety
            Lecturer, Dr. Romano
    Afternoon: General Principles of Psychotherapy
            Leader, Dr. Murray
    Evening: Special Therapies
            Leader, Dr. Hastings
Tuesday, April 9
    Morning: Anxiety
            Lecturer, Dr. Romano
    Afternoon: Common Psychopathology
            Leader, Dr. Brosin
    Evening: Sex Education and Marriage Counseling*
            Leader, Dr. Murray
Wednesday, April 10
    Morning: Common Psychopathology
            Lecturer, Dr. Bond
    Afternoon: The Care of Veterans
            Leader, Dr. Hastings
Thursday, April 11, and Friday, April 12
    Morning: Life Situation, Emotions, and Disease
            Lecturer, Dr. Wolff
    Afternoon: Case Presentations
            Discussion led by Dr. Bauer and psychiatrists
Saturday, April 13
    Morning: Case Presentations, Discussion, and Summary

Some men felt and expressed an understandable desire for more time for reading and the assimilation of new material, but the group as a whole followed this concentrated instruction with surprising ease

* This session was not recorded.

and with unflagging attention. There were few vacant chairs at the beginning of any session; virtually none at the end. Only the three evening sessions drew definitely unfavorable comments. The students were so full of the subject that they spent hours at night talking with each other and with members of the teaching staff, and they much preferred this to formal exercises in the evening.

*

The course opened on Monday morning with a general introduction which covered a good deal of ground rather rapidly. At the section meetings which followed the men were briefed on the point of view with which they would meet patients in the afternoon and the methods they would use in talking with them. A history outline was presented and in some sections reviewed in detail.* The students were asked to *listen* to the patient, to give him a sense of undivided and unhurried attention, and specifically, in the clinic, to talk with patients for an hour instead of the ten or fifteen minutes they were accustomed to give in their offices. The first afternoon seminar was devoted to what proved to be one of the two or three most fertile concepts offered in the course —the patient-physician relationship.

With this technical and psychological preparation the students plunged into the handling of their own patients in the medical clinic, some with a considerable measure of ease and success, some with neither. Naturally they were not equally skillful in playing the role of listener or in guiding the conversation into areas where what the patient said threw light on the pattern of his troubles. Some clung to inadequate organic explanations of the patient's symptoms. Sometimes a man seeing his first patient would miss completely the import of what the patient told him. Sometimes the instructor, who usually came in just before the end of the hour, quickly brought out factors the student had missed. This was an instructive experience, and the second patient seen was likely to be better handled than the first. The most serious peda-

* Not much was heard of the history outline after its introduction. The tempo of the course was such that emphasis quickly fell on the give and take of actual treatment situations; it was tacitly recognized by both instructors and students that technical details must be assimilated later and at leisure.

gogical question which arose in retrospect was whether a better preparation could have been given the students for their first interview by demonstrating in addition to discussing interview techniques.

At the end of the first day the faculty group felt that instruction was getting rather ahead of schedule. One student had been heard to remark, "They're giving us an awful lot, but they've taken the hot air out of it." Some of the men at least were eager for more and talked right through the evening. At a corridor conference where the treatment of a twelve-year-old girl was under discussion, one student said, "Well, then, you talk her into eating." The instructor's answer was, "You don't talk her into it; you let her talk herself out of the reasons for not doing it"—and that summed up the lessons of the day.

On the second and third mornings a basis for understanding both the patient and the relationship between the patient and the doctor was laid in lectures on normal personality development. These drew upon the Freudian psychology in which most of the instructors had been trained and which gave unity to what they taught. But much abstruse matter had been cleared away from it, and only a few basic concepts remained. These were given in simple terms—the Freudian *id* became "old man river"—and illustrated in homely ways. Although it was not the intent of these lectures to discuss child psychology in terms of the pediatric and parental care of children, this application was quickly made by students in discussion.

From the idea that the emotional life has its own natural history, and that while the healthy individual progresses from one stage of emotional development to another he often slips back, it was easy for the students to pass to the idea that childhood patterns of dependence, with or without accompanying hostility, may recur in the relation between patient and physician. This reinforced what they had been told previously about that relationship. As a footnote to these considerations a motion picture illustrating some phases of hostility and its management, issued by the Navy for training purposes, was shown and discussed at an evening session.

It had been intended to follow these lectures by talks on the interview and on history-taking, but by this time the students were already

so deep in the problem of what to do with the patients they were meeting that the first of these seminars was given up for section meetings
and the second was replaced by a lecture which put psychotherapy—a
term which still carries for many physicians a hint of something esoteric
—on a simple footing. It sounded not very different from what a family physician might do without calling it psychotherapy, and in apparent recognition of this fact discussion turned quickly to what the doctor is accustomed to call the art of medicine.

In these first three days students took what was offered with an easy
acquiescence which somewhat surprised the instructors. In some, it developed later, this was a mask for confusion; they felt themselves at
sea. In others it was evidence of a greater preparedness for this range
of ideas than the teachers had hoped for. In either case it took time in
this unfamiliar situation for men to get enough confidence in themselves to challenge what was being given them and to speak out in open
session.

On the fourth day things came to a head. One general practitioner,
who had run into a dead end in his first interview with a patient,
pounded the table in section meeting and said, "What do I do now?"
In the large group a doctor asked whether after all it wasn't a good
idea to treat the psychoneurotic patient for the organic condition he
thought he had, even though the doctor knew better. A young student
asked pointedly for some generalizations. One section devoted its afternoon session to a frank discussion of the goals of the course. Some students were asking about psychoanalysis and whether insulin shock was
better than electrical shock. Another said, "I think we will be able to
take care of the presenting complaint, but we won't be able to cure the
patient." All of them wanted to know how far to go with patients. In
this section the instructor summed up by saying, "I think your general
handling of patients will be definitely better and that as a result, if you
maintain this point of view and approach, you will touch the lives of
very many people more constructively than you might otherwise have
done. If you get that out of the course, it is enough." All this discussion helped to clear the air, and when that same afternoon the man
who had pounded the table had the heart-warming experience of hear-

ing an elderly patient disburden herself of painful memories she had kept hidden for years, and saw the relief she got in doing so, his morale shot upward.

On this day and the next the morning lectures were on the meaning of a psychoneurosis. The nub of the argument was that psychoneurosis *has* meaning as a compromise solution of a conflict between different parts of the personality; that symptoms form part of a purposive pattern which represents the patient's reaction, in terms of his own life experience, to a situation which he finds unmanageable by other means. On the afternoon of the fifth day the discussion was implemented by suggestions for the systematic diagnosis of a psychoneurotic state, with emphasis on another cardinal point: that a valid diagnosis of psychoneurosis can be made only on positive evidence and not merely by exclusion of organic factors.

By Saturday of the first week, when the time came to sum up, many of the students, listening to patients, asking them clumsy but essentially pertinent questions, hearing them talk as some of them had never talked to a doctor before, had the excitement that comes from simultaneously knowing and feeling the dynamic quality of human relationship. As doctors they had come alive for their patients; their patients had come alive for them. Those men who had been unable to reach this point themselves had seen their instructors touch the springs of feeling in their patients and knew that the result was good. For their part, the instructors were exhilarated by a quicker response from the students than they had dared hope for. The week ended on a high note of shared enthusiasm.

Some of the students practiced in towns near enough to Minneapolis to go home for the week-end, and one of the older men came back on Monday eager to tell how, among the ten or eleven patients he had seen, three had given him opportunity to try out, with some success, the new techniques he had learned. Had the course ended at this point, the students would without doubt have carried back into their practices new ideas about the meaning and function of an interview with a patient, a new sense of their own worth to the patient, and a determination to put more time and more humanity into their contacts with patients. But their enthusiasm might well have lapsed as old difficulties began to reappear. They needed to be steadied and strengthened by a more realistic understanding of the possibilities and limitations of psychotherapy and its relation to physical medicine. This was the task of the second week.

As the week opened, two instructors had left, two new ones were introduced, and sections were reassigned. There was some loss of continuity and momentum as new instructors took over the supervision of cases; the rapport already established was important to the students. On the didactic side these changes were stimulating rather than disturbing; from the first all the instructors had participated freely in discussion and the addition of new points of view and new methods of presentation was interesting to the students. For example, a simple wavy line, drawn on the blackboard on Monday to illustrate the oscillations between adult and adolescent or childish levels which are to be looked for on occasion in all adults, figured in discussion throughout the week as the "Brosin curve" (see page 281). Yet the course had reached a point where heavy going was to be expected.

The first lectures of this week dealt with anxiety as the major source of psychoneurotic difficulties. The afternoon seminars accompanying these lectures were devoted to a continued discussion of psychotherapy and psychopathology, with somewhat more emphasis on the doctor's share in the relation between patient and physician, and a more detailed discussion of specific psychoneurotic mechanisms, than had been given before. At one of these sessions a tentative but deliberate attempt was made to focus discussion on the emotional status of the doctor himself as it influenced the interview situation. There were moments of tense silence which suggested that the students were stirred and were thinking seriously about themselves. Few were ready to talk freely to that point in such a setting, but some did so privately.

Evening sessions on Monday and Tuesday explored matters on which the students, greatly interested in problems of treatment, had asked for help. Such special therapies as electrical and insulin shock and sodium pentothal narcosynthesis were discussed as techniques which the doctor should be aware of but should not attempt to use himself. Attention was drawn also to the significant problem of the delirious patient as seen in the general hospital and in practice. Sex education and marriage counseling were discussed in terms of demands frequently made upon the general practitioner, but the students were cautioned that the cure of deep-seated problems of sexual dysfunction was something they should not attempt. This was a course in psychotherapeutic medicine, not psychiatry, and though the dividing line was not always drawn sharply, it was never forgotten.

The morning lecture on the ninth day of the course also dealt with areas where it is the general practitioner's function to know what is going on but not to take responsibility for treatment. This discussion of common psychopathology was keyed, nevertheless, to the doctor's familiar experience. Just as normal reactions to illness had been used as the starting point for the discussion of anxiety, so normal grief was considered as a baseline for the recognition and understanding of severe depressions. The burden of this lecture was to leave the students with a few essential warnings as to what not to do with patients in these categories.

This was followed by a seminar devoted to the care of veterans. Though two sessions had originally been set apart for the discussion of war psychoneuroses, this topic aroused only lukewarm interest. Throughout the course those instructors who had been active in the armed forces had drawn freely on their experience to illustrate psychoneurotic mechanisms and methods of treatment, and while the students were always greatly interested in these case stories, they seemed to feel little need, in thinking about their own practice, to set the psychoneurotic veteran apart from their other patients.

The formal didactic exercises were completed with two lectures on physiological functioning as affected by the emotions. These gave experimental evidence, obtained by the quantitative methods of the physiological laboratory, that emotional states were linked with fluctuations in gastric, cardiac, vascular, and respiratory function. This group of students, chosen in the first place as good doctors, had by now accepted on clinical evidence the validity of the emotions as a factor in the patient's disease. They did not need laboratory confirmation of the fact that inner conflict may be accompanied by measurable changes in vascular tone in the skin, gastric mucosa, or turbinates; but as physicians trained to value quantitative methods in medicine, they felt more comfortable about the underlying thesis of the course in the face of data of this sort.

In the clinic some students found themselves bumping along the hard road of reality. After two or three interviews with the same patient many of them were, as one instructor put it, stuck. The new patients who came in were more and more like the discouraging cases at home. The students began to wonder what they would do with such people in their own offices when there was nobody to turn to for help. Patients with proven physical lesions *and* emotional handicaps challenged the doctors' ability to hold the two aspects of medicine in balance. Patients already on the road to definite psychoses and other patients whose difficulties called aloud for skilled psychiatric care seemed to whittle down the opportunities for the general practitioner. It was at this point that previous plans for the closing sessions of the week were laid aside and it was decided to devote three seminars to case presentations before the entire group, with the student-doctor outlining his findings, the psychiatrist-instructor tracing the emotional pattern, and Dr. Bauer, as consultant in internal medicine, relating the organic findings to the over-all medical picture. These did much to put the whole course into perspective.

*

For the instructors this course was a rewarding experience. They were young men, men with strong convictions. They believed that psychiatry was concerned with personal relationships, depended for its therapeutic value on personal relationships, and should be taught accordingly. They welcomed an opportunity to show how creative this point of view could be in a teaching situation free of the rigidities of the conventional curriculum. They believed, moreover, that people handicapped by psychoneuroses are not now being adequately helped by American physicians. They felt the burden of finding out how to better this situation. Realizing the sharp limitations on what psychiatrists could do alone, they were encouraged by discovering that men in general practice could learn so much and so readily about ways of helping psychoneurotic patients. After this course it seemed quite unnecessary to take counsel with the pessimists and write off the present generation of men in practice as too old to learn the psychotherapy they had never been taught. The physicians present at Minneapolis, at least, were both eager and quick to learn. From this point of view the instructors felt the course to be a success.

This general feeling of satisfaction was tempered by a realistic appraisal of what could and could not be done in two weeks. The over-all purpose of the course was, as one instructor put it, to sensitize doctors to emotional problems in their medical practice. This, the instructors felt, was accomplished. When this general statement was broken down, degrees of accomplishment became clearer. In retrospect specific goals were defined somewhat as follows:

1. To give the doctor a feeling of the dynamic qualities and the value of the doctor-patient relationship.
2. To introduce him to broad patterns of human motivation and to the common causes and backgrounds of emotional disturbance.
3. To lead him to think in terms of the relation between emotional disturbance and illness.
4. To teach him easily understandable methods of therapy so that he can treat a share of such illness.
5. To give him some knowledge of more malignant conditions so that he may refer them to specialists.

The first of these objectives was unquestionably reached; rather by identification with the instructor, perhaps, than by an intellectual process. This was a point at which feeling was quite as important as understanding, perhaps more so.

The second objective was achieved in general terms. No firm grasp of any comprehensive theory of human behavior is to be had in two weeks, but at least the students were led to see emotional phenomena in a biological rather than a moral or mechanical perspective. Their own knowledge of people and abundant illustrations drawn from the instructors' experience as parents and therapists documented the theory.

The third objective was reached, at least in principle. This kind of thinking was accepted by some students only after a real struggle to reconcile it with the mechanistic etiology in which they had been trained. In a longer course, with more clinical experience, students might be able to work out the relation between emotional disturbance and illness in specific cases for themselves. Here they had to take it mostly on faith.

The fourth objective—the learning of therapeutic methods—is one in which the limitations of a two weeks' course are most evident. Few or none of the men learned to see therapeutic possibilities clearly or to formulate treatment plans. Perhaps the most that could be expected was that they should learn to do no harm—whether by overexamination, hasty diagnosis, or ill-advised treatment—and to give the patient the relief that comes from talking out his troubles. This, the instructors thought, was accomplished, and growing experience would gradually increase the doctors' ability to carry treatment further.

The fifth objective, too, was one that could be only partly reached. The intelligent selection of cases for treatment at varying levels of intensity requires a skill quite beyond the reach of men so briefly trained. It was possible to warn the students against dangerous ways of handling severely ill patients, and in general to caution them against attempting to deal with unconscious material. Most of these doctors were not without experience in dealing with psychotic patients. Their maturity and common sense were, in the opinion of the instructors, reasonable insurance against serious clinical errors.

The rapport between students and instructors was vital to the learning process. The evident hunger of the students for knowledge in this area of medicine was its substrate. The instructors brought to the task of teaching the same sort of skills they were accustomed to use in establishing rapport with patients. They endeavored to teach, as one said, "with warmth, conviction, and enthusiasm, at an intimate but not frightening level." They were themselves learning how to do a job for which there were few precedents. The students shared the experimental flavor of the experience. The stuff they worked on—instructors and students together—was the stuff of life itself.

*

Although the didactic material was concentrated, and some men freely admitted that (especially in the early part) they found it difficult because of their own lack of preparation, the consensus among the students was that the content of the course was clear and of practical value. Some men found it illuminating in terms of previous reading of their own; some men took it as a useful guide to future reading. It seems reasonable to believe that nearly all of them grasped the essential points —the significance of the doctor-patient relationship; the interplay of emotion, physiological function, and disease; the need for comprehensive diagnosis and therapy; and the usefulness of the interview in both. Most of the men learned, in the lecture room and clinic, to approach patients more helpfully, to take a better history, and to use rapport consciously as a resource in treatment.

Near the end of the course the student-physicians were asked to comment on it in writing.* What they wrote documented what they had been saying to each other and to the instructors. Few said in so many words, but many implied, that the course had given them a new outlook on medicine. This was true especially at three interrelated points: their attitude toward patients, their attitude toward the causes of disease, and their treatment of chronic illness. These comments were made in the atmosphere of warmth and enthusiasm which characterized the course. More weight can be attached, perhaps, to what the same men had to say six months or more later, when seventeen answered new questionnaires about it, sixteen were seen in follow-up visits by one of the instructors and a member of the Commonwealth Fund staff, and fifteen attended a "reunion" or refresher course, a day and a half in length, held at the University of Minnesota in December 1946. All told, twenty-three of the twenty-five men were heard from in one or more of these ways.

They agreed that the principles they had been taught were of real and practical benefit in dealing with patients. Many of them had been through a period of hesitant experimentation to see if these principles would work in their own offices. Except for a few young veterans just establishing new practices, they found it hard to arrange time for the leisurely interviewing which the patient needs to ventilate his anxieties. But most of them had chosen a few patients on whom they thought it worth while to spend more time than usual, and had found the results rewarding. "I have been able to help a number of migraine patients,

* For samples of these comments see *Psychotherapy in General Medicine*, pages 29–32.

one asthma, a number of cases of vomiting and 'stomach trouble' in veterans who were in combat, etc.," wrote one man. Another: "I think I am distinctly less ill at ease in dealing with these countless 'headaches' and 'gas' and 'dizzy spells' and 'heart troubles.' " "While the results could hardly be described as brilliant, they do seem to be indicative of definite trends toward increasing adaptability and contentment on the part of most of the patients," wrote a young doctor who was fitting some psychotherapy around the schedule of a hospital residency. The oldest man in the group, noting that "the impact of the course was the biggest event in twenty-five years of professional life," gave this modest account of his experiences:

I take more time on my patients. Formerly I did most of the talking. Now I let them do it and it is so revealing—the stories that spout out that might bear on their illness. An eighty-nine-year-old woman told me yesterday, "You are the first doctor I've seen that isn't in a hurry to get me out of the office."

In my own "bull-in-the-china-shop" method I believe my results in general are very good. When a patient says, "Since I've talked with you my backache has disappeared," "My belly-ache is gone," I do not say they have been cured, but I say, "If you know why you have this 'headache' or 'belly-ache,' or what have you, then you are half-cured and the other half may clear up in time." I have learned not to promise too much. The patient usually understands and is satisfied.

Getting the patient half-well is comparatively easy. But getting the last half well is my difficulty, which denotes lack of training. I am trying to overcome this by more reading.

At the end of the course one thoughtful young physician, who had had striking success in one of his clinic cases, wrote thus:

This course has been most effective in enabling me to better handle my chronic cases. I have no illusions that I will be able to "cure" a large percentage of patients that come to me with emotional complaints simply by using the superficial psychotherapy we have been taught to handle in this course. A few I will help tremendously; many I will be able to help a little; but many more I will not be able to reach at all. But with all of them I will be more comfortable.

Six months later he had this to say:

While taking the course, I was discouraged by the thought that, since the level of psychotherapy we were being taught is really and necessarily only very superficial, our patients would show no real benefit. In practice, I am encouraged by the improvement even this superficial psychotherapy brings about.

"It has been a great satisfaction to see that 'it works,'" wrote a man who summed up his experience, in conversation, by saying that he was now getting a thrill from the very problems in medicine that he used to find most perplexing.

Obviously no one in the group had become, or could have been expected to become, a skillful psychotherapist. Some of them talked too much and listened too little; some tried to hurry their patients into insight; some felt at a loss in grappling with dimly seen difficulties. They all worked near the surface of the patient's problems. But this is where the general physician should work, and the patients they were helping at this level were precisely the patients whom they had previously been able to help very little or not at all. They were thinking straight, also, about patients they could not help. The doctor's own sense of frustration, and his irritation at the patients who frustrate him, have often tied his hands. These men had stopped blaming patients for neurotic behavior; they had accepted the fact that a neurosis is real, not imaginary, and that a patient in pain or distress can be just as sick in the absence of physical findings as in their presence. They had stopped blaming themselves for not being able, after due investigation, to pin the patient's troubles on an organic cause. Freedom from these two common sources of constraint had made them better doctors. They were happier in practice and therefore more helpful.

As one of the instructors said, there is a ladder of accomplishment, of which the first rung is interest; the second, understanding; the third, skill; and the fourth, judgment. These men all took the first and, in some measure, the second step. At the third level, some had a native skill in dealing with people which this experience reinforced. The fourth step, judgment, comes only through long experience. To take even the first and second steps was exciting and rewarding; it pointed the way toward better medicine.

General Orientation

THOMAS A. C. RENNIE, M.D.
AND WALTER BAUER, M.D.

MAY I say, in opening this course, that we are a group of doctors who have come here to share our experience with you? The majority of us are psychiatrists. We have come to share our experience in understanding and treating sick human beings. You will have a great deal to contribute to the understanding of patients, and we from our particular discipline shall have something to contribute to you, I hope, in the same task. We are not much interested in diagnostic terms or in classification of one or another kind of illness; we are profoundly interested in understanding what patients are like, what their emotional make-up and problems are, and how it all reflects upon the disease for which they come to a hospital or clinic or practicing doctor. We will try to maintain that focus as much as possible. At the outset, therefore, I would urge you not to be too concerned about whether a given disorder is a psychoneurosis or a depression or a psychosomatic situation. We hope the patients you will be seeing here are broadly representative of those who come to you in private practice. The aim of the course is to understand such people as human beings, with a view to a better and fuller knowledge of why they are sick.

We come to you as psychiatrists who are very much interested in the problems with which you as general practitioners are dealing. Remember that our specialty is relatively young. You perhaps do not know that as recently as 1900 there were only five psychiatric hospitals that provided treatment for specific psychiatric disorders. And as late as 1930 there were some medical schools that still taught no psychiatry at all. Now the picture has greatly changed. The psychiatrist has taken himself out of the isolated tower in which he so long worked, remote from general medicine, and brought himself back into the full activity of daily life. That represents, I believe, a very wise transition and development.

In the beginning a psychiatrist was sometimes called an alienist, a strange term meaning, I think, merely that he dealt with some kind of disorder that was considered alien or foreign to everyday human experience. Sometimes, indeed, he himself was considered a little alien and foreign to everyday living. Then he came to be called a psychiatrist. Two great figures in medicine, in psychiatry, helped to bring about that change—one in this country and one abroad. In this country Dr. Adolf Meyer was one of the first individuals to insist that the human being must be understood in his totality; that one must understand his somatic functions, his physiological functions, and all the organic processes that go into him if one is to understand what happens to him as a human being. Abroad, Freud, developing his theory at about the same time but in a vastly different fashion, had the courage and daring to explore certain areas of human personality that had not previously been understood or dealt with. Propelled largely by the genius of Freud and the practical common sense of Adolf Meyer, we psychiatrists have moved closer and closer to the everyday problems of the ordinary individual who goes to a doctor. That is really a very interesting and very heartening development.

When I did my internship in internal medicine, which was, to be sure, a number of years ago, we went on "grand rounds," and we wheeled about large cases of autopsy material—kidneys, lungs, or some pathological material illustrating what the poor patient was presumably suffering from. We wheeled these out before the patient, and we discussed in front of him all the details of his condition in a conversation which might go somewhat like one I heard a week ago in a large hospital in New York City. A seventeen-year-old boy lay in his bed, and about twenty doctors were grouped around him. They discussed the pros and cons of what the pathology in his abdomen might be. One doctor said, "I think he has a hypernephroma." Another offered his tentative diagnosis, and a third said, "Why he's exactly like that patient we had on the third floor a couple of months ago." Someone asked, "What happened to him?" "Oh, he died. He died last week." A fifth doctor said, "Have we any slides of this thing?" Whereupon another doctor said, "Of course we haven't any slides; the patient is still living." Then the doctor who had asked about the slides said,

"Well, we'll probably get them in a couple of months from now." And the seventeen-year-old patient lay in bed listening to this conversation. I find it very interesting that the man under whom I studied internal medicine, who used to permit the wheeling around of these various pathological specimens, subsequently became the editor of a textbook in psychiatry.

It was some fifteen to twenty years ago that psychiatrists began to come out of their special hospitals and evidence interest in the kinds of patients on whom they had received their initial training in medicine. They went back into the medical and surgical services from which they had originally come, taking with them some of the new point of view that they had acquired in their rather specialized science. Out of that has grown the large interest in the area now popularly known as psychosomatic medicine—that is, the study of sick human beings that utilizes the knowledge of both internal medicine and psychiatry. I hope, therefore, that we are finally out of our isolated areas and back once more where we belong and where many of us have always wanted to be.

War has contributed very largely to the development of this situation. Last week, for example, I had thirty-five young doctors apply for residencies in psychiatric training at a veterans' hospital; they've been coming in at the rate of ten, fifteen, or twenty a week. We haven't enough places in this country to train the people who want to learn psychiatry. That interests me, for fifteen years ago, when I was teaching in medical school, we felt very proud of our record if one or two men in any graduating class said that they were interested in or wanted to study psychiatry. Now we have an incredible phenomenon—literally hundreds of young doctors coming out of the service have decided that this is the area of medicine in which they wish to specialize. I think that could hardly be otherwise in view of what happened during the war. Remember that out of about fifteen million presumably able-bodied healthy young men who were called out by Selective Service for examination, approximately four and a quarter million were rejected. Of those, some thirty per cent, almost a million and a half, were rejected for neuropsychiatric reasons—that is, because of difficulties in their personality or emotional make-up which rendered them unfit to serve in the war. Remember, too, that once war got under way the largest single reason for discharging men from the service was this same kind of disability. Approximately half a million were so discharged, constituting about forty-five per cent of all the medical discharges from the armed services, the largest single reason for disability discharge. By a very conservative estimate at least another quarter of a million were discharged for physical, or somatic, diseases in which the emotional component was so large that they must be regarded as psychosomatic disorders. In brief, then, well over two million men found disabled by circumstances of war had disabilities of the kind we will be discussing in these next two weeks.

That finding created a tremendous interest and a tremendous stir in American medicine. Few doctors went through the service without having had acutely and poignantly brought home to them the importance of this area of medicine. They saw friends develop emotional difficulties; they saw large numbers of men sent into hospitals with such disorders. Out of this experience came a heightened appreciation not only of the disorders themselves but of what could be done about them by new and modern techniques of therapy. So the young doctors' interest in psychiatry is perfectly understandable. They saw this orientation of medicine effectively at work and producing results. Their interest was heightened, and now by the hundreds they are asking for more training in this specialty.

More than that, something happened to America in general. I, who had something to do with a rehabilitation clinic for the treatment of these men after they were back in civilian life, have watched an incredible phenomenon taking place. The first people to pick up the idea that psychiatry was interesting and fresh and unusual news were the newspaper man, the magazine writer, the radio script writer, the movie scenarist. For quite a while, some two years ago, we were deluged by people wanting to write about this interesting subject. Very shortly thereafter other groups became interested. One of the first was a group of industrialists who suddenly said, "But we have to reemploy these people, and we don't know anything about emotional difficulties. We don't know how to place them back in jobs. Can you give us any orientation?" Very closely behind them came the ministers and the priests, who suddenly said, "Yes, we, too, have a place in this, but we have not been prepared for it, and we need orientation." Then universities began realizing that they were going to be swamped by men who might have some emotional difficulties, and they did not know what to do about it. Lastly, the general public began manifesting a very keen interest in these things. Indeed, we have been accused of overselling our specialty. That may or may not be true. At any rate, to a very interesting degree, we have helped to alert many people to emotional disorders, and we hope that we have helped them to understand these disorders.

What can we do about it now that we have discovered these interesting facts? There is very little that we psychiatrists can do, for, as you know, there are not more than thirty-five hundred psychiatrists in this entire country, out of the total population of about a hundred and eighty-five thousand doctors. So we have come to realize with no equivocation that if these emotionally sick human beings are to receive help, it will not be from psychiatrists for the most part but from general practitioners and men in internal medicine and surgery and other specialties, who must now, somewhat belatedly, get some kind of orientation to the understanding and handling of these problems. So I say to you, the problem is essentially yours. You know that; you have it every day in your practice. The problem is the general practicing doctor's. Unless in some fashion he can come not only to recognize emotional problems but also to get enough courage to do something about them, obviously vast numbers of emotionally disabled people will go untreated. That, frankly, is the major reason why we are here for these two weeks.

About a year ago an interesting conference at Hershey, Pennsylvania, called by the Commonwealth Fund, discussed just these problems. Out of the conference came the realization that the only hope for relief of these people lay in the practicing doctors. To live up to this hope the practicing doctor has to get more orientation to psychiatry than he traditionally receives in medical school. I think of the many students who have gone through medical school in my days of teaching, and I think of the many objections they have raised to a psychiatric point of view. They say, "We won't understand psychiatry. It's nebulous; it's not scientific; it's not something that can be weighed and measured. You use such strange terms; you use such incomprehensible words." Well, we do have some specific terms, and in the course of these two weeks you will hear some of them. We will try to keep them to a minimum. If you don't understand them, demand an explanation or translation into everyday words. But in any scientific area a few new terms are inevitable. I usually reply to my students, "You don't complain when you enter gross anatomy and have to learn several thousands of terms with which you are not familiar. Why do you complain so about having to learn at most fifty to a hundred new words in this area of medicine?"

Since you are the people who are going to be treating these patients, I want to reemphasize the responsibility you have for acquiring a better understanding of the workings of some emotional factors. I need not tell you the kind of problems you will meet. You know them better than I do. You know the patient with a general organic illness who does not respond to ordinary medical manipulation or medication or surgical procedures, who indeed may become worse as a result of such treatment. His condition may be long drawn out, his convalescence may be delayed because the doctor lacks an appreciation of the emotional reactions accompanying his disorder. I'd like to use for example the situation that is represented by an amputation. I've known surgeons who have said, "That's the most beautiful job I've ever done. That man's leg is off, and he's had a fine recovery." They were not interested in knowing that the man's capacity for earning had been seriously reduced or ended, that he had a whole set of family problems related to this, that he had several children who would not be able to go to school because of economic privation. A whole new set of emotional factors had been set loose as a result of that surgical procedure. It is very interesting, indeed, how human beings respond to procedures of that kind. One person may lose a hand and may thereby have a sense of justification for failure, may feel curiously relieved; to another the amputation may be a crippling, disabling experience that breaks the entire pattern of his life.

You know, too, a second large group of disorders—the conditions in which certain common somatic aberrations or changes are related to fluctuations or changes in the emotional life of the individual—those common conditions, such as ulcers and hypertension and asthma and many others, in which the best understanding of the disorder comes from the combined curiosity and investigation of the internist and the psychiatrist. That is the group largely known now as the psychosomatic conditions.

You have learned to recognize also that emotions can produce physical complaints affecting any or all organs of the body, complaints not adequately accounted for by the findings of your physical examinations. Related to these are the conditions in which the patients complain primarily of disabling exhaustion and fatigue.

There are also conditions in which emotions operate in a somewhat different way, producing symptoms that we are apt to regard as more specifically mental or psychological—namely, the disorders of those individuals who have fears or phobias and recurrent disturbing thoughts that they cannot shake off, which we call obsessions, or the need to repeat endlessly certain activities, which we call compulsions. Then, too, there is the interesting group of individuals who suffer from repeated accidents, the ones we speak of as accident-prone people. They have an interesting and rather special kind of personality make-up. Industrial physicians are apt to recognize this type, for they know that the majority of accidents in a plant occur regularly among a relatively small group of individuals. These are the common, everyday problems that come to practitioners. It is with some of them that we shall be dealing during the two weeks you are here.

We have chosen to limit this course to the study of sick human beings who represent some of these more common categories—specifically, the psychosomatic or psychoneurotic varieties. We have little interest in taking any of the time of these two weeks to go beyond that rather common range of disorders. Now, at the very outset of our consideration of these conditions, let us recognize that we are to deal with human emotions primarily. Perhaps, the simplest analogy for you would be what happens under anxiety. You all know anxiety; you've all had it. There's no one who, under certain circumstances, hasn't experienced it. You know it because of the dryness of the throat and the tremors and the shaking of the knees and the tachycardia and the perspiration.

These are common expressions in every human being of a very prevalent kind of emotion. We have studied anxiety in much greater detail, and we have learned interesting facts about its effects. We've seen the general range of somatic responses to it. We know something about the blood pressure changes during it. We know that the white count may become elevated under anxiety. We know that blood-sugar changes commonly take place. We know that these and a variety of other manifestations are part and parcel of the anxiety experience.

Now let me go a little further. What happens in most emotionally sick human beings can best be understood on that simple basis of response to anxiety. Each of us handles the emotion of anxiety in a different way. There are many different ways in which we can manage it. Each patient is best understood on the rather simple basis that his illness represents his way of dealing with anxiety, his defense against the discomfort of anxiety, or his translation of anxiety into a different area. Thus some people experience anxiety directly, in acute, overwhelming form. They experience it with all the physiological, somatic discomfort that is implied in a sense of impending disaster or fear of death. Their anxiety is characteristically expressed through the cardiovascular apparatus, in terms of palpitation, irregularities of rhythm, precordial discomforts, dyspnea, a sense of choking in the throat. If the anxiety is felt in this manner—immediately and with all its attendant discomfort —we are likely to speak of it as an anxiety state or an anxiety disorder.

Not all individuals, however, handle anxieties in that way. The human being has many methods of attempting to ward off his discomforts. For example, he may blot the anxiety experience out of his conscious recognition and develop, as a substitute for it, certain rather characteristic symptoms that lie commonly in the realm of what we technically call hysteria or hysterical reactions. The substitutions may show a rather dramatic resemblance to known organic pictures; that is, they may clinically resemble organic neurological diseases but not be substantiated by adequate neurological findings.

Anxiety can be handled in still other ways. It is commonly mediated directly through organs and somatic functions. This is perhaps best illustrated in the area of psychosomatic disturbances. In these cases the anxiety is mediated through the autonomic nervous system and translated into functional disorders of various organs or parts. We now know that emotions, in a broad sense, can be etiological in these conditions; they can explain fluctuations in the degree of symptoms; they have a great deal to do with the course and outcome of organ dysfunctions; and they may spell the difference between acuteness and chronicity in these conditions. We also know that certain physiological processes, once set off on the wrong functioning path by overwhelming anxiety, sometimes become irreversible and can no longer be turned back into normal channels. Anxiety may sometimes be handled by focusing it on certain experiences, such as specific fear of high places, closed places, animals, dirt, insanity, cancer, etc. This kind of anxiety with a highly topical focus has a special content of thinking regarding it. Then, too, anxiety may be thinly disguised and lead to obsessive thinking or compulsive activities, or it may be disowned by the individual and projected onto others in terms of suspicion and distrust.

There are a variety of ways, then, in which a human being may manage his anxiety experience. In none of them is the condition deliberate or feigned; in all of them the fundamental situation is unrecognized by the individual. To be sure, the individual knows he is sick and to that degree may have partial insight that something is wrong, but he rarely, if ever, knows completely what is wrong. In other words, the real sources of his anxiety are unconscious. A great number of other emotions besides anxiety may produce these same effects; the same variety of manifestations can result from anger, fear, rage, and resentment. Throughout our course, then, we shall be dealing with anxiety or other emotional reactions in human beings; it is their nature which we have to understand before we can be effective as therapists with these individuals.

If one takes the time and interest to elicit the emotional factors, it is surprisingly common to find that with the onset of an illness certain experiences or events highly charged with emotion have occurred in the individual's life. It may be, however, that the fundamental emotional difficulty lies far back in the past. It is our task, then, to scrutinize the complaint or the illness in terms of the emotional factors operating at the time it began and in terms of the entire background of the personality of the individual and his particular emotional make-up. When we do, we find interesting facts. We commonly find that the illness coincides with, or begins at the time of, particular emotional stress or strain. The individual may have experienced death in his family, financial loss, or other events in the external environment, or it may be that the emotional problems and conflicts lie within himself and are not so much determined by external precipitating events. In our final understanding of the patient we have to realize that there are several aspects that have to be kept in balance as we consider them. First, his degree of constitutional toughness or capacity to withstand stress and strain. Second, the extent and degree of the noxious stimuli represented by the life experiences operating at the time his illness began. Third, the extent and degree of his present internal and emotional complexity or conflicts. We often find that an outward event is merely the trigger to set off within the person the vast range of emotional experiences that result in the illness as such. Let us recognize, then, that unhealthy states of emotion may protract an organic, physical disorder and may delay recovery and sometimes actually prevent recovery. Unhealthy states of emotion can also be productive of specific bodily or physical complaints, which will be described later as psychosomatic reactions. And finally, emotions, emotional imbalances, can be productive of certain symptoms more essentially mental in type, the obsessive, compulsive, phobic varieties of psychoneurosis.

Sometimes, indeed, the very nature of the patient's complaint gives you clues as to these kinds of reaction. You are all acquainted with the patient who has persistent bodily complaints that shift from one organ to another, somewhat inconsistent, often so entrenched as to assume almost the proportions of a delusion or a conviction that the organs are actually damaged. To that group we might attach a technical term— hypochondriasis. Other patients complain largely of exhaustion, of generalized irritability, of waking tired in the morning and staying tired all day, and of never being relieved of fatigue. To be sure, you have to be very certain you are not dealing with an Addison's disease or a hypoglycemic reaction. In the main, however, I think that in most of these cases you will find that you are dealing with emotional reactions to life—that special kind of complaining we designate as neurasthenia. Other complaints have to do with the irregularity of essentially normally functioning organs—the rapid heart rate in the presence of a presumably intact cardiac status; the entire battery of human complaints related to functional imbalances of specific organs, which takes you into the realm of all the specialties of medicine. All textbooks tell you about a fourth kind of specific complaint, the hysterical, but you will rarely come across it. This is a very dramatic condition in which the patient suddenly develops blindness or inability to talk or paralysis of an arm or leg or areas of anesthesia on the body which you cannot substantiate by ordinary neurological examination. Then you will find that some patients complain, not about their bodies, but about recurrent disturbing thoughts, about fears which they cannot throw off. They have to repeat acts over and over because not to do so results in too great anxiety. From these special kinds of complaints, then, you get certain leads as to the essentially emotional nature of the patient's disorders.

These conditions of psychoneurosis and psychosomatic disturbance are not diagnosed by merely excluding the relevant organic pathology. They are diagnosed far more importantly by the positive indication that something is wrong in the emotional life of the patient. It is not sufficient merely to have a completely negative physical examination to come to the conclusion that the disorder must be either emotional or psychoneurotic. It is equally important to spend time with the individual to ascertain the known emotional facts that give a positive clue to emotional imbalances in his life. In doing this, of course, your main tool is language. It is what the patient tells you that is important; it is what you can elicit by sensitive and understanding listening, sharing, giving the patient a chance to tell you what the major complaint really is. Do not be fooled by the first complaint the patient offers, for it so often does not give you the real picture of what is disturbing him. It is out of the process of history-taking that you get the positive indications that somewhere along the line of the emotional development of that human being things have gone sadly awry. Such material you will get in a highly characteristic fashion—through the medium of talking, through the medium of the patient's expressing to an understanding person some of these emotional perplexities that have troubled him, either in an immediate situation or in his past.

Let me emphasize very strongly that the method to be used is not one of digging for confessions or striving for a complete history, such as you might obtain by following an outline. The method is that of creating a special situation in which the patient feels that he is understood, that he has time to talk, that the doctor really hears what he is saying, that he can talk about many personal matters that he has had no previous opportunity to bring out, knowing that his story will be respected as valid material worthy of a doctor's time and interest. That objective, of course, is best attained by creating a sensitive, understanding atmosphere which permits such material to emerge spontaneously from the patient. Consequently, the patient will do most of the talking and the doctor will do very little of the talking, if he is a wise therapist. The patient, like everybody else, is seeking for a human being who understands him, a human being who stands behind him ready to support him and encourage him and give him insight and understanding. In the wise therapist he finds a human being to whom he may go with his problems, a person who understands and protects him and has a nonpunitive attitude toward him, and who gives him, primarily, the opportunity to talk and talk and to get out of his system many of these emotional matters that he has previously kept bottled up.

Now there are certain dangers in a process of this kind. One can do too much examining of the patient, particularly from the physical standpoint. With emotionally disturbed patients it is important to get the somatic status settled as soon as possible, to ask promptly for any additional physical examinations or laboratory studies that you need in order to feel confident and secure when you tell the patient that you are more interested in the emotional aspect than in the physical findings that you have elicited. This procedure is best for all patients, as a matter of fact. Physical, somatic issues should not be reopened unless for very specific indications, for to protract your examinations or to reopen them days or weeks afterwards is inevitably to raise a doubt in your patient's mind that you were thorough enough in the first place or that you had the right to tell him that he was organically sound.

That, I think, should suffice as a brief orientation for you. As the course goes on, you will learn a great deal more about intricate interrelations of emotional factors, some conscious, many on an unconscious level. You will learn more about the actual nature and structure of a psychoneurosis or psychosomatic condition. We are primarily concerned that you learn during the course the importance of an attitude toward the patient which permits him freedom and which keeps your own emotional reactions toward him as much in the background as is humanly possible. With these comments I'll retire and turn the session over to Dr. Walter Bauer, who will make some further comments and answer questions.

DISCUSSION

DR. BAUER. This recent emphasis on the psychiatric aspects of illness is vital to all of us. I'm sure that your very presence here indicates that you feel that this is a point of view which is essential to every phase of clinical practice, to all illness, which every physician, be he general practitioner, internist, psychiatrist, or surgeon, should possess. The fact, I think, that has disturbed all of us as practitioners of medicine is that soon after entering practice we found ourselves incapable of handling many problems that came to us. One doesn't have to practice medicine very long to get some idea of the frequency of the problems Dr. Rennie has discussed. Our first private patient may have been a neurotic. It was then that we fully appreciated for the first time our lack of understanding of the neuroses and their treatment. We may have said, "I feel reasonably certain that he's a neurotic but what can I do about it?" Many of us have found ourselves in this embarrassing position.

This, in part, is a deficiency in American medical education as we experienced it. As medical students we were exposed to a few lectures on the diseases of insanity and we saw a few patients who represented various disorders of conduct or thought, and that was about the end of it. Yet soon after entering practice we found a patient sitting in our office who had a variety of complaints which we felt reasonably sure were functional in nature but which we did not know how to handle. Most of our instructors had ignored them, exhibited very little interest in them, and at best prescribed either a sedative or a placebo. Many of us followed suit, only to find the patient back in our office with the same or other complaints. Then we tried a variety of prescriptions that didn't do

the trick, as witnessed by the fact that by the end of two years the patient had reappeared in the office probably twenty-four times, and we
wondered what we could do next. It was perfectly obvious that, if the
patient cared to, he had every right to say, "You're not much of a doctor, are you? I've been here twenty-four times, I've had twenty-four
prescriptions, I'm still sick." It's surprising more patients don't say
that. The reason they don't is that something has gone on between the
two of us. We've established a certain relationship with the patient
without understanding its full significance. That is the reason he continues to reappear in our office.

After going through this experience time and again, I finally came
to the conclusion that one of two decisions had to be made. If I was going to continue in the practice of medicine and be reasonably happy, I
had to learn something about human beings and had to do it with a
meager background and with no formal training. It was either that or
quitting, and I preferred to practice medicine. I'm sure that many of
you are here today for similar reasons. You know that from fifty to
seventy-five per cent of your practice involves problems of the sort that
Dr. Rennie has described. Some of them are relatively simple situational affairs which most of us can handle with relative ease; at least we
can bring the patient back to his previous baseline. Others are more
complex. We went through medical school, unfortunately, under the
influence of too many organic-minded physicians. Naturally one has to
learn how to take a medical history and acquaint himself with all the
details of doing a complete physical examination. Otherwise, we should
be lost; we should have no idea as to how to proceed. We were also
taught that there are certain laboratory procedures that should be employed to substantiate the impression gained from the history and
physical examination. Yet I'm sure that you all have seen far too much
reliance placed on laboratory studies. For example, a patient comes in
complaining of palpitation; he has been to see a number of doctors and
has been told by several of them that there is nothing wrong with his
heart. The last doctor he saw obtained an electrocardiogram, found the
T wave in lead I a little abnormal. Despite the fact that he knew that
the patient had no symptoms or physical findings of heart disease, he
just didn't have the courage to stick by his guns but said to himself,

"Well, maybe this means the patient does have a little myocardial involvement. Perhaps I'd better tell him to go easy or take him off the job for three months." If we're not careful, we as physicians can be responsible for such marked fixation of symptoms as to make it extremely difficult some fifteen or twenty years later to do much about them. I can cite other situations—such as the patient who comes in complaining of being tired and weak, no pep, and so a basal metabolism is done. The recorded result may or may not be correct. Say it is, say the reading is minus 20, using a method where the lower limit of normal is minus 15. Doctors sometimes tell such a patient that he has thyroid deficiency and will have to take thyroid the rest of his life. In many of these instances, however, the basal metabolic reading probably represents what we term a low-rate case, an individual who was born with a rate of minus 20, who will always have a rate of minus 20, and yet has a normally functioning thyroid.

Many physicians have said that they are not interested in psychiatry, they don't understand it, they are afraid of it, they don't know how to interview people, they don't know how to interpret the information they obtain. All of that may or may not be true. Those same physicians fail to appreciate that they practice psychiatry seven days a week whether they're aware of it or not. Each time they see a new patient they establish a certain doctor-patient relationship, which in most instances is good or at least reasonably favorable or the patient wouldn't keep coming back. Psychotherapy begins when we first see the patient. If we're wide awake, we make certain observations as the patient comes across the threshold of our office, as he sits in our office; during the physical examination we should take these findings into account in trying to decide the nature of the patient's illness. We see combinations of disorders. We see people who have somatic complaints that are psychic in origin; we see people with various diseases that have a psychic component. As practitioners of medicine we must weigh all factors in each and every case.

Clinical Problems

I*

HISTORY-TAKING

HISTORY-TAKING is a term which we use in medicine to cover the broader term "interviewing." As you know, interviewing runs a very wide gamut—from census-taking and interviews about schools, jobs, credit ratings, and so on, to the more subtle and complex forms which ministers, lawyers, social workers, and doctors employ. The essential difference between interviewing in census-taking and interviewing in medicine is that in the latter situation the person interviewed is sick and usually somewhat frightened about the threat that sickness involves. The object of the medical interview is to acquire information that will help the doctor understand what the problem is, who really has the problem, and what the doctor can do to help the person with the problem. Through the medium of the interview, and because of it, a relationship between doctor and patient is established. This relationship is different from the usual relationships with friends and associates, for the patient is in trouble and he comes to the doctor for help. Consequently, the patient will be in some degree dependent on the doctor. The doctor represents to him support and authority, a person on whom he is calling for help and guidance. Because of that, and because of his illness and his troubled feelings about it, the patient may have some difficulty in talking about his problems—he may resort to subterfuges and to circuitous speech, he may be long-winded in his descriptions.

Since the medical interview, the history-taking, leads to the establishment of a relationship through which certain data are to be acquired, we must consider what the doctor should feel and do about it.

* This chapter was compiled by the editor from recorded discussions that took place in various section meetings on April 1 and later.

I think everyone will agree that by far the most important thing in history-taking is the attitude of the doctor—that is, he must have an attitude which generates confidence and understanding. The attitude one has to stress all the time is "I am for you; I am for you in your trouble." This must be wholly an attitude. Never put it in words, for words are sure to sound patronizing. And don't put out a sheet of paper to write down, as they did in the Army, name, rank, and serial number. Putting a piece of paper out in front of a patient means the same thing as rank, name, and serial number. It says, "Here you're a number, you're just another who's going into the catalog." When you're facing the patient and you're giving of yourself to the patient, it is so much better. The patient feels he's got you; you are his spiritual support. We'll go into that in later lectures, where you will see that ill patients are like children; they regress to a childish dependence on the doctor. That is the basis of the patient-doctor relationship. We have to utilize that situation, without manipulation and management, for all the effectiveness there is in it. And we must create the situation intuitively and naturally.

To utilize this relationship the doctor must have the capacity to deal with other people's anxieties without becoming maudlin or sentimental, without identifying with the patient's problems blindly, without being punitive or moralistic. In teaching medical students we point out that each of us has some emotional scotomata—blind spots—and that one is fortunate if he has a reasonable understanding of his own blind spots, prejudices, and biases about other people, about minority groups, about certain personality types. If you are able to be objective about your own feelings, you are able to see more clearly than otherwise what is happening in the patient. The attitude of the doctor, then, should be one of confidence and understanding and of interest in the patient, and the doctor should convey the feeling that he has lots of time. A lots-of-time attitude may seem to be impossible in general practice and in the practice of internal medicine, but this attitude—whether you actually have lots of time or not—is a tremendous help in eliciting historical data from patients.

In addition to having the proper attitude, the doctor should allow the patient to talk as freely as possible and should do what may be called "active listening." This means having an attentive, understanding facial expression, occasionally nodding the head, occasionally asking, "Yes?" and "Just how do you interpret that?" or "Just what does that mean?" or "I'm not sure I understand that"—questions which are not leading but which may provoke the patient into fruitful channels of information.

Then, for successful history-taking, one should avoid premature optimism and premature reassurance about problems. Many patients, when reassured too early or with too much enthusiasm, lose confidence in the doctor because they feel that they have not had an opportunity to tell him their complaints. That being so, they are likely to doubt his assurance that everything will be all right. There is danger, then, in too early a pronouncement as to diagnostic status and the reversibility of a disease process. That doesn't mean, however, that you should be pessimistic or cold or aloof or indifferent. Rather, you should be realistic about the problem and should not make dogmatic or definite statements about reversibility until you have a fairly good idea of what is wrong.

Next, avoid too much humor. At times humor may help, but at other times jocularity or depreciating the significance of certain symptoms may annoy patients. They say to themselves, "I'm sick, and while I'm thankful for the doctor's interest and his helping me about some of these things, the problem isn't as funny as he seems to think it is."

Another point to be remembered is the importance of the doctor's facial expression. Once the patient has talked about his difficulties and has looked at your face while he has talked, he feels some security. The doctor's expression is a magnifying reflector and must be carefully guarded, for instance, when you are making a cardiac examination. Listen too long in a particular spot and the patient is sure you have found something, even though you deny it.

The physical examination, as you know, lends itself admirably to history-taking. The physical intimacy of the examination, and the dependence of the patient on the doctor while it is going on, entrench and implement a bond between them. We have found that asking the patient after the physical examination if he has anything else to say often leads to more positive or more direct data than were secured before. This is because the patient's anxiety has been allayed somewhat and his confidence has increased after the physical examination.

To sum up, then, allow the patient to talk; engage in "active listening"; guide the interview through nonleading interrogation, questioning only when the material that is emerging seems fruitless or when a vicious circle seems to be developing. Avoid judgmental values, avoid moral values, acquire a facial expression and a demeanor of dignity and of quietness and repose. All these things have tremendous significance to sick people and they generate the giving of confidences. The essence of successful history-taking is to give the patient dignity.

*

In general practice you may be accustomed to using history outlines. Such an outline was prepared for use in this course, and I shall give it to you now.* There are various comments to be made about it, however, and it may be that the outline will prove useful chiefly as a list of topics we consider of importance rather than as an actual device to be used in interviewing.

The principal point to be made about this or any outline for history-taking is that if a doctor is thoroughly aware of what he wants and why he wants it, he will get the necessary data regardless of the order in which the material is presented and without much recourse to direct questioning. If an outline is used, it should not be slavishly followed; rather, the history should be worked out by getting the patient to tell his own story and to feel comfortable with you. Obviously, you can't ask intimate questions when the patient is still a stranger to you. You have to establish a relationship; otherwise the patient won't understand why such intimate questions are asked. You spend most of the time listening until you see that your patient feels that he's in on your wave length, that you're in on that wave length together.

Although allowing the patient to speak freely, try to keep the discourse in relatively fruitful channels. Work back from the present ill-

* See page 58.

ness, and then use the outline as a check on whether the needed points have been covered. It often isn't necessary to have the outline in evidence at all. Sometimes you can look it over after seeing the patient and after writing your notes, to find out whether there are any broad topics that you have missed, so that you can cover them next time. A good case history can't be elicited immediately from the patient in *a, b, c* order. It has to be compiled more heterogeneously. After one has collected certain data and has seen their relative value and their position in the constellation of the problem, the history outline can be used to organize the material into a more meaningful whole.

There are a number of areas you need to explore in almost every case. They are here in this history outline. You know them, I'm sure, as well as I do. Formalized history-taking is of value only in the very early part of your career. The sooner you learn to collect the needed data in a casual way while you, as a good hound dog, are chasing the scent of the person's illness, the better your work will be. You somehow automatically judge the patient's intelligence. You get to be pretty good at that after a while. You ask him a little bit about his educational history and what went on in school and how he related himself to people in school. Before you know it, much of the so-called formal mental-status examination is something that is completely on the periphery of your line of endeavor. The same is true of the question of delusions or hallucinations. Whether or not the patient is leading a life of emotional frustration is something which very frequently you can discover by indirection. So, although you must have clearly in mind all the areas you want to know about, you don't have to sit down with a pencil and check off the various details. The sooner you are able to get away from formalized history-taking, the sooner the limited time you have at your disposal will be productive. I find that I automatically cover the points made in this history outline without any special endeavor, as I go sniffing along and trying to chase down the significant trends in the patient's life.

Now, a few comments on particular topics in the outline for history-taking. First, the patient's "chief complaint." By and large, one should start with this. The present illness is what the person comes to you for and what he wants to be helped with. It is usually possible to branch out and make avenues of progress from the present complaint and then work back to its history. In eliciting the chief complaint, don't insist on keeping strictly to the symptoms. If you allow the patient to talk freely, he is pretty likely to slide off into a discussion of other matters which may be very revealing and important. Giving the patient a chance to tell his story is particularly important in cases of episodic pain, convulsions, epilepsy, asthma, and the like. In such cases what you especially want to discover is the trigger mechanism that brings on the attack. For instance, one asthma patient related her attacks to fear of pregnancy. When this sort of thing comes up in an interview, don't interpret its meaning to the patient; just try to put things in such perspective that the data become self-revealing.

On the topic "past illnesses" the main point to be remembered is that neurosis tends to be a recurring pattern. Menopausal difficulties, for example, are often experienced by women who had difficulties at puberty. Childhood diseases may determine that a particular somatic system shall be the vulnerable spot around which later difficulties center. The age at which such illnesses occur is an important factor in suggesting what inferences to draw from this aspect of the history.

Under the topic "family history" it is usually very unwise to ask directly, "Have you ever had a person in your family who was insane?" You may be skeptical, of course, as to how you can get information on this point without asking such a question. You will find, however, that by tactful circumlocution even this fact can be secured. If you do ask the question directly, you are likely to get the answer, "What do you think, doc, I'm crazy?" Then, too, when you get a history of family difficulties, be sure not to take sides. The doctor's attitude on such a point should be one of neutral sympathy.

The purpose of getting a "history of neurotic tendencies in childhood" is to find out whether there has been a neurotic trend throughout the patient's life. Repetition is personality, you will learn in this course. Accordingly, in judging the nature of a patient's complaint, you feel more certain if the case has an inner consistency. When something doesn't fit the pattern, you begin to suspect an organic difficulty.

The purpose of the whole history-taking procedure is to reexamine and utilize material that is readily available, not to get a lot of new material. Throughout, the important point to keep in mind is what the data mean to the patient. It is this that really matters. For example, "marital history, children or lack of them." These facts are not very important in themselves. We ask about them primarily to discover how the patient feels about these important areas of his life.

Often the presenting complaint gives you the lead. For instance, a boy comes into my clinic office, where I don't have much leisure. His chief complaint is lack of concentration. "Tell me about it," I say. "Well, I'm having great difficulty. I'd been working in the radiation lab, and when I was working there everything was swell. But now that I'm back at school, this thing has come back on me again." "Oh, you had it before?" "Yeah." "When was that?" "When I was an undergraduate at Yale." "Well, tell me how it was when you were an undergraduate at Yale." So I go into that. You see he's a second-generation Italian, a poor kid from New Haven. "How many in your family?" I ask. "I don't know—nine or ten," he replies. And he's the last along the line. So now I begin to see a number of important leads in this history. Second-generation Italian; insecurity, family who lived according to the old-country pattern; going to Yale, de luxe, tremendous. He was the baby of the family; you know what Italian families are like and how much they shower on their young children. I begin to see why he is an insecure lad and why he's likely to be especially sensitive to rivalry situations. Next I begin going into what his reaction to rivalry situations is. So I'm off on my history-taking.

As you're talking about matters like these, you are automatically covering the ground. Little by little, starting from the chief complaint, you get into the history of the present illness, then into the background areas, then perhaps you come to the religious history. There you try to find out what religion means to the individual. You know, perhaps, that he's a Catholic; you know he goes to church. But you want to find out what religion *means* to him. In the case I've been talking about, religion had much meaning to the boy. In part it meant an identification with his father and in part, on account of his obsessive, compulsive character, it provided an area in which he could indulge in theological tugs-of-war. So go back and find out what religion means to your patient, what an authoritarian figure, such as the church, means to him. It's of no value to say, "Religious history, Catholic, check," and let it go at that. What you really work for all the time is to find the dynamic meaning of feelings and events in the individual's life.

Now, a word about note-taking. It's up to you. Personally, I think the fewer notes you take the better. If you need to make a minor notation, O.K. But don't sit there and say, "Yeah, now let me see. Age? How many cigarettes do you smoke a day?" If you do, you destroy the relationship. Don't let note-taking be in the foreground. Personally, I never even sit behind a desk. I always get my chair out from behind the desk. I never put a desk between me and the patient. I don't want that authoritarian point of view; I don't want the protection of that desk. I want this out in the open. The patient's got a chair just as I have, and we're sitting there talking. So if I were to take notes, this is the way I should do it. Talking to the patient (even when I write I'm facing the patient), I should just make a little heading with perhaps just enough of a notation to start me off on my later dictation. Of course, as busy practitioners you have many things to think of, but you will find you have an amazing capacity for remembering these things once you really relate yourself to the patient emotionally and learn to like being in on the inner areas of the emotional life. Your memory becomes very good then.

I must admit, however, that note-taking is a subject on which opinions vary. Certainly each doctor should be guided by what he wants to do. I do think there is danger in becoming too slavish about writing notes. It probably all harks back to our medical school days, when in the latter part of the sophomore or junior year we were introduced to history-taking and each was given a little red or black or blue book with its system of questions. In our anxiety over this new experience of interviewing sick people, we were so anxious to get the data that our attention and vision were directed almost entirely toward the little book. Our questions, preferably monosyllabic, came out of the book. Sometimes we didn't even look at the patient, we were so anxious to get the questions answered. These are experiences that all of us have gone through. The experienced physician knows that such behavior has two results. First, it provokes the patient into not giving the needed information, and second, it provides a tremendous amount of information of little or no value.

These, then, are some of the main points to be made about history-taking. I'll leave it to you now to ask questions.

DISCUSSION

STUDENT.   It has often seemed to me that the first thing you say to a patient is of importance. I've often wondered what the first sentence should be when the patient doesn't voluntarily say something immediately. I've used such expressions as "What can I do for you?" or "What is your problem today?"

DR. ROMANO.   It depends a great deal on who the person is and what your experiences have been with him in the past. I think it is safe to say that most people who come to see a doctor are anxious in one way or another, and that the magnitude of their anxiety or anxiousness has two variables: one is the acuteness or the severity of their illness; the other is their own preparation for anxiety—how well compensated they have been in taking care of the inner and outer stresses of their lives.

The present illness, therefore, seems to be the point at which one should start out, after an overture of pleasantries designed to put the patient at ease. If the patient wants to smoke or walk around while talking—that is perfectly all right. Some patients may want to open a window or do this or that to allay some of their anxiety. One should be quite flexible in this matter. Then one could ask, "Why do you come here to see me?" or "Do you have some trouble?" or "Do you feel all right?" or "How long has it been that you have not been feeling well?" and then go on to some of the details. I feel—and I probably am prejudiced—that one should avoid question-and-answer techniques as much as possible, for they usually don't give you very important information. Allow the patient to speak as freely as possible and in your own mind note a number of things. In this connection I think it's important to remember that speech is not only a means of communication but also a means of disguising and camouflaging emotions; hence the doctor should note not only what the person says but how he says it. In other words, not only the content but also the form and organization of the patient's presentation are important.

There may be certain things which the patient refers to recurrently. There may be striking omissions in a chronological account of an illness. There may be physiologic concomitants of what the patient says. He may speak about his mother's death with tears in his eyes; that's as valid a datum as whether the liver margin is or is not palpable. Similarly, if a patient blushes or sweats profusely or if in the middle of an interview, at a point which may be critical in the story, he asks to take off his coat or to go to the toilet or shows an increased motor discharge by a great deal of fumbling with clothing or twisting and turning or thumbing his hair—all these are valid and significant data that indicate an overdischarge of emotional tension which may or may not be provoked by the material the patient is presenting.

To come back to opening remarks, one that is usually not good is "What's wrong with you?" "What's wrong with you" is a moral indictment, for the patient doesn't know what's wrong with him, and, in addition, he may be ashamed of the fact that he's acting this way. He doesn't know why he's acting this way, and a question like that may provoke even more anxiety. There are cases, however, in which it is a very good question to ask, for right off the bat you may get an idea about the patient's attitude. But when you ask that question, you have to be on the alert to see whether the patient has an indifferent attitude or whether he is trying to pull something on you or feels he is being persecuted or something like that. Valuable information may be gained by using the question, but there is risk of losing your relationship with the patient. In general I think it is wiser to use indirection.

DR. BAUER. Don't you think that at the end of your history a somewhat similar question is very much to the point? After you have done a certain amount of interrogating you may ask, "What do you think causes this trouble? What do you think is wrong?" Such a question has to come very late, however; it has to be one of the last questions.

DR. ROMANO. Yes, I have found that a very valuable question. The patient may reply, "Well, I'm not a doctor." Then you say, "I know you're not a doctor, but, after all, you're the person who has had this trouble for a long time and you may have some ideas about it. I'd like to hear your ideas because many times patients' ideas are more helpful than anything else." Then the patient may say, "Well, as a matter of fact, doctor, sometimes I get these headaches when I feel angry at my wife or mother but can't say so." Such an answer may be of great significance, for the patient may be afraid to be angry at a person he likes so much. So sometimes this question is fruitful, and sometimes it isn't.

STUDENT.   Suppose you haven't been able to crystallize your own ideas. Suppose you need more data. How do you allay the patient's anxiety and not leave him feeling up in the air at the end of the interview?

DR. BAUER.   Suppose you have taken an ulcer history with too many inconsistencies in it. You then say to the patient, "You may have an ulcer, but there are many other things you and I will have to discuss even if you do. I don't believe you have one. We're going to find out about that, we're going to get an x-ray. I am going to be very surprised if you do have an ulcer, but even if you do, we still have other things to talk about." That's about the way I handle a situation of this sort, even if I only have fifteen minutes. You have to give the patient some idea what you're thinking about, in so far as the case permits.

DR. ROMANO.   Another point to be considered is the length of time you spend with a patient. Personally, I don't see how some general practitioners do as much as they do. For example, I know some doctors who see from seventy to a hundred patients a day. Now, granted that any of you, particularly small-town general practitioners, are very much harassed because there are too few doctors, it still seems to me that you can actually save time by having longer interviews. There are many instances in which another fifteen minutes may avoid second, third, fourth, and sixty-fourth visits.

STUDENT.   I have noticed that in small towns people are very reticent about bringing their troubles to you because they have contact with you socially. I have found that awfully difficult. I am wondering whether it is going to limit us in doing the kind of work we've been discussing here.

DR. MURRAY. I think that in many cases a skillful approach will break through this barrier you speak of, particularly if you wait for the right time. Timing is everything. Timing in psychotherapy is as important as it is in blacksmithing—the metal has to be just right before you start to hit it. If you are called, for instance, to see a woman in an anxiety attack, this barrier is quite ready to rupture because of the terrific pressure of the patient's internal emotions. Your awareness of that throughout the weeks you were waiting for this to happen makes you yourself ready to come in.

DR. RENNIE. You sometimes have to stop and say to a patient, "I have to ask you some things that you may or may not answer. No matter what you say it will not go out of this office." Unless you are consistent about keeping your patients' confidences, you will not get anywhere in a small community. This means you cannot share confidences with your wife, or with anybody else.

As to treating your friends, that is another situation. Some friends will come to you, some will not. If they are chiefly concerned with maintaining your friendship and respect they are apt not to come; they will go to somebody completely outside the social circle. On the other hand, plenty come quite frankly. Again, it is a matter of convincingly reassuring them that whatever is said in the office is absolutely sacred. If they bring up the question of your secretary and whether you dictate your notes, you might say, "If the idea of my dictating notes makes you uncomfortable, I won't do it. I will take only a few pencil notes."

DR. JENSEN. I wonder if there isn't another factor here—that a good many patients haven't learned that physicians are interested in these things we have been talking about. Once you give them a chance to talk, they will pick right up and go on because they know you are interested in some of these matters that other physicians apparently pay no attention to.

DR. RENNIE. A young internist friend of mind came out of medical school with a strong opposition to the psychological aspects of medicine. In the course of ten years of practice he began waking up. In getting medical histories he now finds it just as simple to ask about problems in the home, finances, or the job as to ask about alcohol, etc. You don't have to apologize because you are going to ask certain questions; you ask them casually. If you can create an attitude of casualness, you can do a lot.

STUDENT.   Do you feel you have to have several visits with your patient before making a psychiatric evaluation?

DR. RENNIE.   That will have infinite individual variation. Certainly a psychiatrist in his first interview begins just as you do. I should never dream of saying to a patient, "You are here to talk about your emotional troubles." I start just as you do, "Why did you come to see a doctor?" I may spend twenty minutes out of the hour on the somatic aspects of his difficulties. Only after I think I have given the patient ample opportunity to tell me about the somatic complaint do I start on anything else. I usually begin with some innocuous question such as, "Your story of headache interests me a great deal. Does it change any from day to day? Are there days when it is better or worse?" Then I lead into, "Have you any idea why it should be better sometimes and worse at others? Might it be that you are more worried or more upset at one time than another and that makes it worse?"

STUDENT.   The average patient who comes in to see a general practitioner has some physical complaint, such as palpitation, which he thinks is organic. You check him over and find this isn't so. Then you have to get over to the patient that it isn't organic. That's where we have our big problem. Should you tell him that? Or how should you go after it?

DR. MURRAY.   Wait until you've worked the case up and got the data. At that time you can say, "No, we will have to seek some other place for an explanation of your symptoms. Now, we know that psychological factors can be as important noxious agents as chemical poisons or bacterial invasions. So let's go into your life situation." You don't necessarily mention emotional conflict, but you yourself know that where there's anxiety there's conflict. You don't tell the patient that in so many words, but you let the patient feel that this is the next area in which you are going to work.

STUDENT.   The thing that amazes me with patients I have referred to psychiatrists is the terrific amount of information that the psychiatrists get from them.

DR. RENNIE. The psychiatrist gets a lot in his first interview partly by creating an atmosphere in which the patient realizes that the doctor is interested in these things. It is partly that; it is partly that after considerable experience in history-taking you know that every human being has certain areas in which there may be difficulties and you do a fairly systematic review of that. You start with the least sensitive questions: "Where were you born? Are your mother and father living? Brothers and sisters? Your childhood, do you remember much about it?" When the patient has had a chance to tell you what comes up spontaneously, you ask about other aspects. "Were you particularly nervous, high-strung? Did you ever walk in your sleep, have nightmares, or temper?" From there most patients will go on to tell you about schooling and attitudes toward school. Then you can go into jobs, marriage, the sexual part of marriage. If at that point the patient is very much upset, drop the problem and come back later on. If the patient shows no indication of being upset you can get further facts about sex at that point. The psychiatrist gets so many facts because he pursues a fairly orderly process.

STUDENT. Do you find that patients respond differently according to the type of conflict they present or the type of somatic condition? In another course I took they talked about a patient with an ulcer having a feeling of insecurity for which he was trying to compensate.

DR. RENNIE. I feel very strongly that the important thing is not to jump to conclusions about personality structure in certain somatic diseases but, rather, to approach every patient with openmindedness.

DR. ROMANO. In that connection I'd like to point out the danger of becoming selectively deaf—that is, of only hearing what we want to hear. We hear about a pain and the first thing we say to ourselves is, "Peptic ulcer—unless proven otherwise." You can do the same thing in the psychological sphere. A person may have a certain symptom— let's say hypertension. You think, "Aha! Hypertension is related to repressed rage. I have to find out what this man's resentments are and show them to him." Well, that may or may not be right. One has to be intellectually honest and emotionally objective enough to get the data as they come and then aggregate them and not make premature judgments or be biased by what may prove to be an unsound hypothesis.

STUDENT.   How do you steer a patient who just opens the flood-gates and tells you everything? This seems to be the unfortunate result sometimes of following the injunction "Just let the patient talk."

DR. KAUFMAN.   In such situations you have to decide which of two things you are trying to do. If you are trying to give the patient relief by catharsis of long-suppressed stuff, the flood may be all right. If, on the other hand, your object is to get a picture of the situation as a basis for treatment, it's a good technique—without rebuffing or definitely in-terrupting the patient—to repeat once in a while a key phrase that is along your line of interest. For instance, if a patient mentions his sister in a way that suggests there is something important there and then rat-tles on to something else, the doctor might just say, "Your sister?" By this technique it is usually easy to bring the conversation back time after time to pertinent material. Whitehorn once said that nothing a patient tells you is irrelevant, but this is true only when long-time treat-ment is in question. You are sometimes equally interested in what the patient doesn't say. When the natural sequence of his story requires him to go in another direction and he forks off, you will often find that by going back to the fork you will pick up something important. Never-theless, never confront a patient with something he can't tolerate. And don't push for information too strongly; the patient may be ready to give it two minutes later.

STUDENT.   One of my chief difficulties, too, is learning when and how to cut off a patient when he starts off on a long, irrelevant talk.

DR. ROMANO.   Well, there are some pointers as to what to do. You may ask a question. The patient may be starting to talk about what he thinks his problem is. For instance, I remember one patient who talked about his bowels and gave many details about his stool—the qualities of it, the color, how difficult it was for him to evacuate his colon, when the movement happened, what he thought about it, and so on. You might listen to that sort of talk for a while and then you might say, "Is there anything else that troubles you?" "No, it's just that," says the patient. Well, then you can jump—no, not jump but lead from there. You might ask about length of time. "How long have you been trou-bled this way?" Then you can ask, "Are there times when you have more difficulty or less difficulty?" And so on. Then you can ask about other things.

Now, the fact that a patient will not talk about other things is an important diagnostic point in and of itself. You have the feeling that this man is tenaciously holding on to this symptom. His whole life seems to revolve around whether his stool is normal or not. Then the question comes up, Why this tenacity? What factors are at play here to keep this man reacting in this way? Here you say to him, "You're a man, you have to live, you have a family, and you need a house—you have to be sheltered, and you have to work—what about those things?" But he'll come right back to this colon business again. Then if the discussion is too fruitless and too trifling and you get into a vicious circle, you perhaps can be aggressive and positive and simply say, "Look, I would like to hear something about some other things." This depends, of course, on your relationship with the patient and on just what you sense is going on in him.

There are many other tricks. One is to note, as we've said before, what he talks about. Second, what he holds on to. Next, the recurrent theme—what he comes back to all the time. Then, what he doesn't tell you, what omissions, what breaks, what gaps or inconsistencies there may be in his talk. His facial expression or body movements during talking are also important. All those things, taken together, may help you get some idea of the relative importance of various matters to him.

DR. COTTRELL. I think a patient usually tries to please his physician. So if you are interested in a subject, he will tend to bring more of that to you. That's a general rule. If we as physicians seem extremely interested in one part of him he will tend to tell us more about that. If we lose interest in it, he will tend to lose interest, too. We don't need to become preoccupied about the patient's stool just because he is. If you show less interest in it and more interest in other parts of his personality, I think he will gradually get the idea.

DR. ROMANO. That's a very good point. At times the doctor may infect the patient with his own anxiety about the stool, for instance. The doctor asks detailed questions about it. Even in a routine examination we do those things, you know. The patient begins to think, "This is really important." One must sense the relative values of these things. You realize that the stool business is probably very unimportant from a medical, biological point of view. But psychologically, what this man's great interest in his stool means is that a great number of other problems are being displaced upon it. So your trick is to try to help him get off that topic and get on to other, more pertinent matters. But you can't do that by repeated questions about the stool.

STUDENT.   How about the use of personality evaluation tests?

DR. RENNIE.   There are a number of those tests available, and at times they have a certain value. They may give you the feeling that you are short-cutting a lot of investigation, that you are getting more immediately to the evaluation of the personality, but they don't help the patient. There are times when such tests are indicated, of course. There may be specific situations in which you would like very much to know the intelligence rating as accurately as possible. That would be particularly true for school children or adolescents.

STUDENT.   There are no short cuts, then? You have to develop the personality background?

DR. RENNIE.   No short cuts. Start with the first step of establishing trust and respect and go on from there.

SUGGESTED HISTORY OUTLINE

The physician confronted by a patient with psychoneurotic problems often finds it difficult to obtain a systematic history. The complaints are frequently vague or multiple, or both. The patient is apt to wander in his recital and to ask as many questions as he answers. However disturbing this behavior might seem in the ordinary office or clinic interview, it must not be forgotten that the essence of psychotherapy is giving the patient an opportunity to unburden himself, and what he volunteers may be fully as important as his answers to specific questions.

Up to a point it is better to let the patient talk as he will, while the physician keeps the necessary questions in reserve until the way is clear for them. Many of these questions touch on subjects which many people are reluctant to discuss. Nothing is gained by pursuing them when the patient is unwilling to cooperate, because either false or evasive answers are furnished or the patient seeks another physician. It is far better to temporize until the patient is ready to confide. In so far as possible the patient should be allowed to tell the story of his illness in his own words. When he digresses or becomes excessively circumstantial, pertinent questions may be asked to clarify the development of the symptomatology.

The history should bring into focus the facts of the present illness, the setting in which it occurs, and, what is more important, the patient's attitude toward the facts, in respect to his social and family situation; his personality, including his occasional and prevailing moods, his ups and downs, irregular or rhythmic; his aspirations; his work, ambitions, and achievement; his economic situation; his social activity, standards, and needs; his sexual activity; and special immediate personal problems or conflicts not touched on elsewhere. These may be ascertained by covering the topics listed below. It should be remembered always that the facts about the patient should be associated with his own attitude toward his own behavior. Only by this means can his standards, aims, and frustrations be brought into clear relief.

I. CHRONOLOGICAL HISTORY OF PRESENT COMPLAINT

A. Symptoms. Do the principal symptoms concern the heart, gastrointestinal tract, or other organ systems? When did they begin? How do the symptoms affect the patient? Do they fluctuate from day to day, from morning to evening, from hour to hour? Are they affected by eating, exercise, work, social or other special situations? What brings relief, temporary or otherwise?

B. Setting—Life Situation. Often a detailed play-by-play review of the patient's daily pattern from waking time to waking time gives a better conception of attitudes and values than a systematic survey of symptoms and evidence of life stress. Patients may not recognize the tensions or moods associated with daily living. Were there any known precipitating factors, such as worry, accidents, disappointment, bereavement, fright, financial or other strain? Any previous period of similar difficulties? Describe onset, duration, symptoms, special situations. Did anyone frighten him about his condition? What have other doctors said? Was the patient depressed, elated, anxious, apprehensive? Does worry affect the symptoms? If he becomes upset about anything do the symptoms get worse?

II. HISTORY OF PAST ILLNESSES

Review of past illnesses with particular attention to the following disturbances: nervous breakdown; headache; fainting, dizzy spells; convulsions; visual and hearing disturbances; changes in taste sensation; cardiovascular symptoms; respiratory symptoms, including sighing respiration; gastrointestinal symptoms, particularly appetite, food intake, food fads, periods of nausea, heartburn, diarrhea or constipation, and migratory abdominal pain; genitourinary symptoms; locomotor symptoms. What are his habits, including sleep and exercise?

III. FAMILY HISTORY

What is his attitude toward home life? How many are there in the family and what is the patient's relationship to them? Describe individual personality types. What is the economic and social status of the family? Place in the community? Security? Have there been serious illnesses or deaths in the family? If so, what was the patient's age at the time? Current health of members of family? Family atmosphere pleasant or unpleasant? What kind of home— ample, meager, crowded? Did parents get along together harmoniously or otherwise? Attitude of parents to the patient and to other children? Disposition of parents: placid, calm; cheerful or morose; active, talkative; tolerant, indulgent; dominating; strict or lax, changeable; silent, distant; irascible, display of temper; habits as to alcohol; able or poor managers? Did parents separate and remarry? If so, what was patient's reaction to this? Reaction of patient to step-relative? Any nervous or mental trouble in the family? Any condition like the patient's in the family? Much illness in the family?

IV. PERSONAL HISTORY

A. Childhood and Early Development. Breast fed? Delay in learning to walk or talk? Nail-biting, nose-picking, enuresis, temper tantrums, easy weeping, eating problems, nightmares, sleep walking, "allergies"? Relation to brothers and sisters? Was there anything unusual about childhood? Was patient considered nervous or high-strung?

B. Schooling. When did schooling begin? End? Did patient like school? Were his grades high or low? Did he have any failures? How did he get along in school with teachers and other pupils? Why did he leave school?

C. Work History. First job, kind and duration? Why did he leave? What kinds of jobs has he had? How long did they last? Why did he leave? Work satisfactory? Salary? Is he satisfied with his present job and getting along well at it? Is he well treated? Relation to his boss and other workers? Is the work a strain? Hours? Ambition? Future? Does he like the kind of work he is doing? What is his concept of "success"?

The aim here is, of course, to determine whether the present job constitutes a strain, a source of tension, or a source of frustration.

D. Sexual and Marital History. When did menarche occur, and what was patient's attitude? What is the interval of menstruation? Duration? Amount? Dysmenorrhea: cramps, backache, fainting, days in bed, prostration? LMP? Symptoms associated with menopause: headaches, depression, hot flushes, asthenia, palpitation, fainting?

Is patient married? Happily? Difficulties with wife (husband)? Any children? Are they well? Does he worry about them? How is the sexual part of marriage? Satisfactory to both? Does wife (or husband) enjoy it? How frequent is intercourse? Is that often enough, too often, or just right? Any contraceptives? Fear of pregnancy? Does he want more children? (If patient is a Catholic, the contraceptive issue must be handled with caution.) Does the patient feel relaxed and satisfied after intercourse? Any interest in anyone else? Any sex relations with anyone else since marriage? Does he worry about it? If over twenty-five and not married, why not? Any special reason? Is he in love? Does he worry about it? Anything in past sex life that worries him? Worry about masturbation?

Has he had advances by individuals of his own sex? Any homosexual experience?

Any increase or decrease in sexual desire during this illness? Worry about it? Are symptoms connected with sex activity? Are they worse after intercourse?

E. Financial Status. What are his economic resources and reaction to them? Enough to live on? Any worries? Debts? Own own home? Provision for future? How important is money to his feeling of security?

F. Social Adjustment. Ethics, religion, politics? Standards of social behavior, games, parties, dances? Attitude toward need for social contact and the esteem of others? Does he get along with his family? With people in general? Number of friends? Does he avoid people? Do people treat him right? Talk about him? Make fun of him? Laugh at him? Try to harm him? Any enemies?

V. PERSONALITY FEATURES

Note abnormalities when indicated in general appearance and attitude, stream of talk, mood, content, orientation, general information, calculation, remote and recent memory, retention and recall, insight, judgment, speech, and handwriting. Estimate intellectual level.

Is he energetic, aggressive, outgoing, self-confident, sociable, affectionate, or is he withdrawn, passive, submissive? Is he easily offended, shy, shut-in, a daydreamer, hard to approach? Is he eager for sympathy? Is he retiring, bashful? Does he depreciate himself, feel inadequate? Is he frank or evasive? Is he suspicious, envious, or jealous? Is he rigid, stubborn, obstinate, or plastic? Is he suggestible and easily flattered? Is he impulsive? Is he anxious, worrisome, fearful, or timid? Is he perfectionistic, neat, orderly, meticulous? Is he responsible or irresponsible? Does he have temper outbursts or is he phlegmatic and placid? Does he bear resentments or forgive easily? Is he generous or cautious? Does he greatly respect authority or is he rebellious? Is he critical, quarrelsome, or easygoing? Is he stoical or complaining? Is he overdependent or assertively independent? Does he mix easily with people, or is he "standoffish" and aloof? How does he take criticism? Is he preoccupied with fair play? Is he cynical? Does he need to be thought well of and is he "politic"?

Where possible compare adult personality features with those of childhood and adolescence.

In such personality investigations it is well to remember that outstanding personality features often have counterparts in strong contrast, such as docility and rebelliousness, or amiability and resentment. By thus realizing that the opposite qualities are likely to occur, one will not be confused by these apparent contradictions. Yet such contradictions need to be understood and resolved by the patient before personal harmony is possible.

What is the patient's attitude toward his assets and deficits?

Insight—is the patient aware of being tense, anxious, ill at ease, emotionally disturbed? What is the usual visceral response to fear? Any evidence of diarrhea, constipation, polyuria, dry throat, trembling, sweating? (Use such questions as "How would you respond if you suddenly had to give a speech? If you witnessed a serious accident?") What are his usual methods of showing fear? What kind of dreams? Frightening or pleasant? Fantasies? Does he recognize that life situations have any bearing on the way he feels, that his temperament is related to this illness? Does he consider himself an emotional or nervous person?

The Patient-Physician Relationship

M. RALPH KAUFMAN, M.D.

AS doctors we have two kinds of relationship with our patients. One is what we might call a reality relationship. We are physicians. We are people to whom other people come because they are ill and we have knowledge and skill in helping them. That's one relationship and a very important one. The other is a symbolic relationship. We have a kind of symbolic value to a sick individual. In psychotherapy both these relationships are important.

Let me give you an example of the symbolic relationship. Some patients come to us with much fear and trembling. Others don't come to us at all, because they have anxiety about illness and they fear that once a doctor has examined them they will really have an illness. Those of you who have worked with t.b. patients know that an individual may suspect that he has tuberculosis, he may have a cough, he may have symptoms which he knows are tubercular. Usually somebody in his family has had tuberculosis. But he doesn't come to a doctor, for as long as a doctor hasn't made that diagnosis he feels, in some magical way, that he doesn't have tuberculosis. You're familiar with that type of problem. It's part of our difficulty in tuberculosis prevention, and it's also part of our difficulty in dealing with psychoneurosis.

One of you raised the question this morning as to what to say first to a patient who comes to see you. I think one has to realize that from the very first interview the fact that the patient has chosen you rather than some other doctor is significant. Similarly, the first words that you have with a patient may determine just what kind of relationship is going to develop between you and him. Certain individuals will respond to an authoritative approach. Others come to a doctor because they want sympathy. Others come because they want to get certain things that they can't get at home. They come to a doctor because they have problems that they want to discuss with somebody. They can't talk about them at home, they can't go to the minister, and so they come to a doctor. Consequently, part of the patient-physician relationship may develop before the patient actually comes to the doctor's office.

Once the individual consults a physician a symbolic kind of relationship is established—a relationship to authority, a relationship to a person who knows about medical matters, who has certain therapeutic powers and also certain magical powers. For some patients just coming into a doctor's office is enough to allay a certain amount of anxiety, while for others this step increases tension and anxiety. In the development of the first part of the doctor-patient relationship, one has to be aware of these possibilities, so that one doesn't increase an individual's anxiety by a too abrupt approach to his problem. You are going to learn a good deal about taking a history. Suppose the first question a doctor asks is, "How often do you masturbate?" This approach to the patient is not beyond the realm of possibility. I've frequently heard that question or its equivalent asked because the doctor felt he had to plunge right into the heart of the problem and expected the patient to tell him the most intimate details just because he was a doctor. In such cases, however, the patient will either look askance at the doctor or get out of his office as soon as he can, or he will say this, that, or the other thing in answer to the question. Your first approach may determine the kind of relationship the patient is going to have with you.

The same principle applies to taking a history. With the taking of the patient's history there is the beginning of the patient-physician relationship and the beginning of the therapeutic relationship. How the doctor takes a history may determine what the initial relationship is going to be. If he is sympathetic and interested in the patient, the patient will gain what we call rapport with him and will be willing to tell him about certain aspects of his problem which heretofore he has either been unwilling to discuss or hasn't had an opportunity to discuss with any doctor. Very frequently we psychiatrists have had a patient come to us after trying half a dozen doctors and have had him say, after we have put him at ease and let him tell his story, "You know, doctor, you're the first one who ever let me tell those things." That in itself is the initial situation for the establishment of a psychotherapeutic relationship.

There are other aspects of the patient-physician relationship which go beyond this initial one of establishing confidence or rapport. When we describe the development of personality and the significance of a neurosis, you will hear that an individual tends to repeat throughout his life the patterns of behavior he has laid down in childhood. An individual's relationship to his mother, father, teacher—whether it is a relationship of authority or the relationship of love—determines what kind of relationship he will later have in situations that carry similar implications. The tendency is, by and large, to repeat his early relationships. In working intensively with patients over a long period of time, the doctor finds some for whom he takes the place of a good father, and he may therefore have projected upon him certain aspects of the patients' experience and personality needs. On the other hand, individuals who resent authority and resent an older person may become what we call our "bad" patients. A patient who doesn't take our recommendations seriously, a patient who won't stick to a diet even though it has been very carefully explained to him why he should—we find in such cases that it isn't so much a question of the diet as of the attitude of the patient toward the physician.

There are always two aspects to a patient-physician relationship. Most of the time we see only one aspect—the positive. That we do not see the negative aspect is not because it isn't there but because everyone of us likes to be liked. We like to be told, either directly or in very subtle ways, that we're great guys, we're good doctors, we know what it's all about, we hit it right on the button. We take a subtle, near-conscious delight in being told how bad another doctor is, how he misunderstood completely what the problem was. Frequently all this may be true, but whether it is or not, we always have a slight tendency to overvalue ourselves. On the basis of a positive relationship a tremendous amount can be accomplished, for the patient is likely to take advice and to accept suggestions. When the patient develops negative attitudes toward us, we tend to take them even more personally than the positive attitudes. In other words, when a patient tends to overvalue us we are likely to believe we're not quite so good as that, but pretty nearly as good. But the minute a patient is hostile toward us we are sure he doesn't know what he's talking about. In such cases there's something wrong with the patient, he's not a good patient, and we can't do anything for him, for we can't tolerate hostility. If, however, we search for the basis of hostile reactions, we usually find that patients are merely repeating with the physician their previous patterns of behavior. This explanation must not be used to cover all cases, of course. Let's not go so far as to say that whenever a patient becomes angry with us or hostile to us or thinks we're lousy doctors it is only transference. Sometimes the patient's right. Sometimes there are reality situations we have missed and so have created this reaction, but even in reality situations there is a certain amount of projection to us of hostile attitudes.

The psychiatrist is accustomed not to judge himself by the patient's overvaluation or underestimation. When overpositive or negative reactions are evinced, the psychiatrist tries to discover just what the patient's earlier relationships were. That acts as a kind of buffer, a kind of safety valve for the doctor's own self-respect and ego. If you can remember that not all your hostile patients are hostile because you're Joe Doakes and that's the kind of fellow you are, then I think you can accept a certain amount of hostility. By and large, we can all handle a patient's positive feelings, and we utilize them consciously or unconsciously. But when it comes to the negative aspects, most of us become a little bit hot under the collar, whether we recognize it or not, and we try to get rid of that particular patient. If, however, you understand that when hostility is shown to you, when certain negative feelings appear (a patient may break an appointment or not be cooperative in relation to medicine or a prescription; there are many subtle ways of showing hostility), when you understand that at least part of this hostility is not directed against you personally, then it becomes easier to handle that kind of situation. If there is hostility, it is best not to go into a deep analysis of it but to give the patient an opportunity to discuss his feelings toward you.

If we hold ourselves sacrosanct and inviolate, so that nobody can tell us anything that we don't like to hear, then we're going to lose a lot of patients or a lot of our patients are not going to get well. Patients sometimes lose their symptoms not because we're good therapists or because we've hit on the right kind of prescription, or because the detail man has left us something which is really modern and up-to-date and we've given it to the patient; a lot of our patients get well because they have secured in their relationship with us something that they have unconsciously wanted. They may have wanted sympathy and understanding, so that when they developed a positive relationship to us their symptoms disappeared. This is due to the fact, which we'll discuss at greater length in the future, that a neurotic difficulty is a kind of compromise situation where the patient is trying the half-a-loaf principle—where half a loaf is better than none. For various reasons he can't get what he wants, and the neurotic difficulty is a compromise. If he develops a positive relationship to the doctor and gets the protection or sympathy or whatever it is that he wants, then he doesn't need his symptoms and so he gives them up. If, on the other hand, he develops a hostile attitude toward us, then he's got us by a very simple maneuver. All he has to do is not give up the symptoms and then we're lousy doctors. Consequently, the positive and negative attitudes of the patient become important immediately in relation to the patient's holding on or not holding on to his symptoms.

As I said before, the positive relationship is much easier for us to accept than the negative relationship. It may, however, create inner tension and difficulties in ourselves, for a lot depends on what kind of demands a patient makes. You start with a patient who has an ordinary positive relationship toward a doctor. He has confidence in him, feels he is sympathetic, and so on. He may begin to come to your office at odd hours, may begin to insist that you practically give up your practice and confine yourself to taking care of him. You've had patients like that, I'm sure, who make tremendous demands on you. Then we do one of two things. Either we say, "This is impossible, I just can't do it; you had better go to see somebody else," or we become angry with the patient because the demands he makes are so great. On the other hand, if the patient shows some hostility toward us, we can't take that either. Either we try to slough the patient off or, as I said before, we regard him as a bad patient—somebody who doesn't follow our advice or somebody who doesn't like us. It's easier for us to take love and affection and adoration (I deliberately use those terms) than it is to take hostility.

Now there are two sides to this patient-physician relationship. One is the patient. I've roughly indicated the sources of some of his attitudes: namely, his life patterns and relationships. The other is the physician himself—certain of his own personality traits and characteristics —and that's awfully important for a physician to know. I don't mean that every one of you here, every doctor, has to sit down and analyze himself to find out just what makes him tick. But he does have to know just what kind of relationships he generally builds up with his patients.

Some of us have only "good" patients, only patients who like us, who send us Christmas cards and presents. We rather deliberately, though unconsciously, build up that kind of relationship. It has value up to a certain point. It is important to realize, however, that not only the positive relationship but also the negative relationship is important, for only when the negative comes to the forefront can you have a patient talk about his hostility, bring it out, and face it. The fact that the hostility may be directed against you at first provides a leverage for bringing to the patient the fact that he has both negative and positive feelings toward key figures in his environment, such as his father.

If a patient can admit to only conventional attitudes (that one must have only love for one's wife, only honor for one's parents), and if we expect only that kind of relationship between him and the doctor, we never can get down to what the patient finds it difficult to face. The individual's problem may not be his love for his parents; it may be his hostility, his anger toward them. If, however, he were only angry, there wouldn't be any problem, for if one is only angry one can talk about it. But there are two sides to every relationship—both love and hostility. The patient is afraid that if he brings out hostility something may happen to the other side of the relationship; this makes it necessary for him to bury or repress the hostile feeling. Say you have a patient with hypertension or diarrhea or peptic ulcer whose problems center around emotions of anger and resentment and the inability to tolerate such feelings. Sometimes the only way you get a hint of what there is underneath is by a change in the patient's attitude toward you. The minute you take that change personally, you're licked. If, however, you understand that a doctor has a significance for the patient over and beyond his being Doctor A or Doctor B, then you can utilize that feeling to bring out the patient's emotional attitudes.

Later on in these lectures we shall talk about therapy. You will see that some therapeutic procedures are based on working along with a positive rapport; by and large that is the relationship between the patient and the physician. On a more or less superficial level one can maintain a good therapeutic relationship and achieve certain results. In contacts with patients that are of necessity rather short and not carried out over a long period of time, one has to work with the more superficial aspects. But one must not allow oneself to fall into the trap of thinking that a patient must only overvalue a doctor. One must always be aware of the other possibility. In any long-continued relationship between patient and physician, both sides are of significance and importance. The positive side has been called rapport, it has been called a feeling of confidence in the physician, it's been called by analysts transference, and so on. The name isn't as important as the awareness of that kind of relationship.

In an intensive kind of psychotherapy, the more complicated aspects of the relationship that I have been talking about become an actual part of the therapy. That, however, doesn't concern us at the moment. What I want to bring to focus here is the fact that a relationship between a patient and a physician, which is a bilateral sort of thing, does exist in every case and that it extends beyond the reality situation. This relationship is contingent, for the most part, on two factors: first, what kind of doctor you are and whether you have or haven't given the patient reality reasons for feeling one way or the other; second, what the patient's attitudes toward the key figures in his life have been.

I think that on the whole what I've talked about today is something that all of you are aware of. What I really want to do is just to put it in a somewhat different perspective. Any doctor who practices medicine is actually aware of these problems, and if he allows his awareness to become part of his automatic thinking, then he doesn't get into trouble. But don't say to yourself when you sit down with your next patient, "What does this patient think of me? Yes? No?" That's like riding a bicycle and thinking each time whether you put your foot down here or there. That's not much fun, and it doesn't get you anywhere.

Now are there any questions so far before we go on? Is the thesis clear to you or isn't it? Is it something you recognize from your own experience?

DISCUSSION

STUDENT.   What is the technique of finding out where hostility originated?

DR. KAUFMAN.   Well, you can do it in a number of ways. If the patient has shown some overt hostility to you, instead of just passing it by, you can draw his attention to it. You can just say to him, "You're angry with me for something. Why are you angry?" Now if you say to him, "You're angry at me. What the hell do you mean?" he'll say, "Who? Me? No, I'm not." But if you just say to him in a matter-of-fact way, "It seems to me that you've got something against me," or "Have I done anything?" or "Has anything happened?" the patient usually will hem and haw a little bit and then start to tell you why. Then you listen to him tell you why he's angry with you, and pretty soon you will find, even in the most superficial kind of therapeutic relationship, that what he's telling you has really little to do with what *you* have actually done. If you know something about this patient's background, you will find that he has apparently been talking to you about something similar that has happened to him before.

At this point you have to be careful (that's why I've been a little hesitant in bringing this formulation out) how deeply you go. For instance, you don't want to bring out a patient's hostility to his father if it is very deep. It would be almost impossible for the patient to face that without cracking up, for after all he can't just talk about hating his father's guts, wanting to kill him, and so on. He can, however, talk about the fact that he sometimes resents what his father did to him, in the way of discipline, for instance. In other words, as long as you keep your discussion to matters that the patient knows about it's likely to be all right. By and large, in the kind of work that I do in the outpatient clinic, I *recognize* unconscious sources but I don't *deal with* unconscious sources. In other words, I don't do a laparotomy if an examination will suffice to show me what's going on. In the kind of situation you're in, you don't go into what we analysts call purely primitive, regressive, oral sadistic fantasies about hating the father.

You will find that there are many patients—such as those with hypertension—who will not take the opportunity to talk about their resentments. If you ask them why they won't talk about it, they will tell you that they've never been able to talk about being angry. If you ask them, "What do you do about your anger?" some of them will say, "You know, doctor, I swallow it." That is a very frequent way of putting it. They swallow it; they just allow it to tear them up inside. In such a situation it isn't the thing to say to the patient, "Now, look, you're angry." But you can draw his attention to it, using yourself and the relationship to you as the primary lever for pushing back and allowing some of this material to come out.

This is not a very difficult technique, provided you do not act in an accusatory way. The minute you accuse a patient, he will withdraw, because that's a bit too much for him. After all, the patient also has a certain attitude toward the doctor. We used to grow beards and wear striped pants and wing collars to build up this symbolic part of the relationship. We don't do that now. We wear sport jackets, we smoke cigars when we talk with our patients, and we talk to them about golf. We do all kinds of things. But still the fundamental relationship is there.

Another thing that I think is important in knowing about the patient-physician relationship is that once you recognize the type of patient you are dealing with you can expect that he will develop certain characteristic attitudes toward you. For instance, the compulsive, obsessive type of individual. I'll describe in just a few words the kind of person he is and you'll recognize him. This kind of individual is very meticulous, very careful; he pays your bill on the first of the month without having to be dunned for it; he is always very, very polite and gracious to you, but he never gets well. You know that patient, don't you? This obsessive kind of person never expresses any kind of anger or resentment, always accepts everything you have to say. One of his main problems is this handling of aggression and hostility, which he has buried under this pseudo graciousness and quiet, peace-loving manner. If you work with that kind of patient, you find that some of his inner thoughts and ideas, some of the ideas that come to him that he may complain to you about, deal with aggression and murder and things of that sort.

Another kind of patient is the woman who is rather coy, who always wants just five more minutes of your time than you are prepared to give, who prefers that you make your visits sometime in the middle of the night, who, in general, wants a great deal of evidence that she has a very special place in your set-up. Very roughly, that's the kind we call an hysterical personality. In short, then, the patient's personality structure and his needs determine to a greater or lesser degree what kind of relationship there is going to be between him and the physician.

The doctor's personality also determines how much hostility is allowed to come out and how long he is able to tolerate the patient who shows hostility. I know psychiatrists who work only with a positive transference. They try to keep only a positive relationship, on the theory that with such a relationship the patient's needs are minimized and he won't have to keep his symptoms.

Very frequently you find that a patient with whom you've worked for a long time and cleared up quite a number of problems either will not get well or suddenly gets up and leaves you. Then she goes to a new doctor who has just moved to town and after one visit loses all her symptoms. You are familiar with that type of patient. You've really worked with her; you've read all the textbooks and you've listened to all the lectures, put in a lot of time with that patient, and she just hasn't quite got well. Then old Joe Doakes comes out of the Army; she goes to him once and then she says, "Dr. Doakes is a grand doctor. He really knows. I spent two years with Dr. Smith and he just couldn't do a thing about it." If one is aware of the fact that there are various attitudes within the patient-physician relationship, it makes for a much freer kind of relationship than if one constantly wonders why this patient to whom you've done nothing or for whom you've done so much is behaving in this way. "There must be something in me," you say, "something I did or something I didn't do that caused that reaction." Actually, it may be that in the relationship with you the patient is trying to work out something which has nothing to do with you as such, and it's a comforting thought to know that, after all, this reaction gives you a lead as to what you're going to be able to do with your patient.

There are all kinds of patients. There is the patient who develops an overwhelmingly positive relationship to you after one visit. The ordinary, well-adjusted patient develops a feeling of confidence in relation to his doctor, but he just doesn't go around talking about what a wonderful doctor you are. Beware of that. If you have a patient who thinks you're the most marvelous doctor in the whole wide world, look for the other side to appear, too. Some day that patient will turn right around. Unless you're aware of both sides of such an attitude, you're going to miss its essential significance.

When we come to explaining why patients lose their symptoms (that is, "get well"), I think you'll find that, by and large, it's the doctor-patient relationship that is the significant factor and not necessarily the kind of medicine that we use. Or it may be *how* we use the medicine that's important. This is not only true for the patient who is psychoneurotic or otherwise a psychiatric case; it's just as true of the cardiac patient or the one with a fractured femur, or anybody else. This patient-physician relationship is not something that concerns only neurotic patients. It concerns every patient, regardless of what the illness is. One can see it most clearly if the relationship continues over a length of time. And it's particularly important in relation to convalescence; whether the patient is going to get well or not may be determined by the relationship.

There are lots of factors that enter into convalescence. For instance, if a patient gains something out of having the doctor come to see her every day, then she will stay in bed so that the doctor will come every day. Of course that isn't the only factor that keeps a patient from getting well, but we must be aware of it. She may have a positive attachment to the doctor, and this is the only way she can see him; or she may hate his guts so much that this is the only way she can pay him back. Remember that possibility when you're dealing with human beings.

One of the things we psychiatrists have been accused of so frequently is that we think we can eat our cake and have it too; for now I tell you a patient may stay sick because she has a very positive relationship to you, and then I turn right around and say that she may stay sick because she hates your guts. You say, "Which one of these things is true?" They may both be true. Staying sick may achieve a different objective for each particular patient. You have to understand that completely opposite emotions or attitudes may achieve gratification by exactly the same actions. We see that constantly. A patient may do one thing for positive reasons and then, when his attitude changes, do exactly the same thing with a completely different motivation. You have to be aware of all these possibilities.

By and large, I think that when one is working with the kinds of problems we're discussing here, the ability to talk quite freely to the patient about these matters has the great therapeutic value of catharsis; in addition, it indicates to the patient that he doesn't have to keep his emotions under cover. Consequently, some of us work very consciously with the patient-physician attitudes. Others understand what is going on and try to use that in their therapeutic effort.

STUDENT.   Would you say a little more about the fact that aggressive and hostile feelings are normal?

DR. KAUFMAN.   I'm glad you brought that up because, being an aggressive fellow, I am apt to take for granted that aggressive and hostile feelings are normal. When we talk about aggression and resentment and hostility and so on, it sounds a little bit as if people don't have these feelings unless they're neurotic. Actually, these feelings are part and parcel of the ordinary, normal developmental picture. If a mother loves a child and pays all the attention in the world to him, the more attention she pays him and the more she gives him the easier it's going to be for that child to develop hostility and aggression; for to such a child a mere "no" means that "mother doesn't love me any more." Now, whether the hostile or aggressive feeling can be expressed or not is something else; the feelings in themselves are normal.

There is no relationship between people that doesn't have as a normal part of it some hostility and aggression. Just visualize for yourself any relationship between two people that you know of, and you'll immediately see that at some time or other, no matter how positive that relationship is, there has been some hostility or aggression. Consequently, if it becomes necessary to understand the relationship, we miss the most important thing if we concentrate only on the positive side. The child who is good, particularly in our culture, has to *deny* these aggressive and hostile feelings, but they are still present. Therefore it becomes very important, in working with individuals, to give them an opportunity to bring these feelings out. But when the patient brings them out, when you see them, that doesn't always mean that you're dealing with a *neurotic* aggression or a *neurotic* hostility. Aggression and hostility may be part and parcel of a normal reaction. The way they are handled may be neurotic. The inability to express any kind of aggression or hostility is neurotic, not the hostility and aggression themselves. A type of person I have already described, the one who is so sweet and innocent that you want to kick him in the pants, because he just doesn't appear to be normal—that kind of person is neurotic.

I think the more a doctor regards aggression and hostility as normal, the easier it is for him to handle such feelings and allow the patient to bring them out. There are certain kinds of aggression and hostility that definitely are pathological, of course, but that's another problem. I think that one can go further than hostility, aggression, and so on, and point out that all emotions are part and parcel of normal development. Their intensity, their quantity, the kinds of events that trigger them off, which of them are pushed aside, those are the factors that determine pathogenesis, not the emotions themselves.

In understanding a patient one not only has to get the information but also has to put it together in perspective. One has to understand what the relationships between factors are. Just to understand that there is a positive relationship to the doctor, or a negative relationship, is not sufficient. One has to put the facts together so that one understands them. I'll tell you a story. I don't know that it's apropos, but it's a good story in relation to this business of putting things together in a proper perspective and drawing the proper conclusions.

Two men graduated from medical school in the same class. One was Jones and the other was Smith. Jones graduated at the top of his class and Smith graduated somewhere down in the lower third. About ten years later they happened to run into each other. Smith was sitting in a large car, chauffeur-driven, and Jones was kind of bobbing along, rather shabby, and they stopped and started to talk to each other. Jones said, "You know, Smith, I can't understand what's wrong with me. I was a pretty good student. I graduated top of my class, but since I've been out somehow I just can't make this practice of medicine click. And here you are, you're apparently very successful."

Smith said, "Yes, I'm doing pretty well. I know what's the matter with you, Jones. I knew it when you were in medical school. Come on, I'll show you something. I'll show you how you have to handle patients. I'm just on my way to see a patient. Come on."

So they went up to a rather shabby third floor, and there was an Italian writhing on the bed with a terrific belly pain. Smith talked to him, took a very good history, told him that he'd be all right, and gave him some medicine, saying, "Now be absolutely certain you take this three times a day, and you'll be all right within twenty-four hours." Just as he was about to walk out, he turned back and said, "And another thing, don't eat so many peanuts." At that the patient got right out of bed and said, "Yes, doctor, that's it. I think you're right on that."

Well, the two doctors walked downstairs and Jones, very complimentary, said, "You know that was a very good examination. I see something as to what I've missed in this about my patients. How did you know that he ate so many peanuts?" Smith said, "Well, that's the one thing about observation. If you'd looked around, you would have seen that underneath his bed the floor was covered with peanut shells." Jones thought that was absolutely marvelous. That was something he was going to remember.

About three weeks later Smith was driving by a doorway and somebody sped out as if he'd been thrown out, and there was Jones. Smith stopped his car and asked, "What's the matter?" "I don't know, I don't know. It's very funny. I had a patient just like the one you had. Identical symptoms. He was also an Italian. Identical symptoms. I gave him the same medicine, but when I said to him, 'Don't eat so much horsemeat,' he threw me out."

And Smith said, "Horsemeat? Why did you say that?"

"Well, this fellow had a harness under the bed."

So just hearing about these matters isn't the important thing in itself. You've got to put the proper interpretations on them.

STUDENT.   Do you have any advice about patients who shop around, who go from doctor to doctor to compare notes?

DR. KAUFMAN.   Well, the patients haven't been satisfied. Sometimes we can't satisfy them. Some patients shop from doctor to cultist, to Christian Science, to magnetic healing, to all kinds of things. Why do they do that? It's not only because they're superstitious or psychotic or this, that, and the other thing. It's because somewhere along the line medicine can't give them what they want. If a patient becomes a Christian Scientist it isn't necessarily because a doctor doesn't know how to handle him; it may be because the patient is so afraid of illness that he believes there is no such thing as illness. What better way is there for the solution of that particular problem than Christian Science? It's a complete denial. There is no such thing as matter, reality, or illness, and so there isn't any need to be anxious.

The fact that patients can't get from a doctor what they need—not in terms of medicine but in terms of inner security, sympathy, understanding—is another reason why they go from doctor to doctor. One of the things that sometimes keeps a patient from shopping around is the ability of the doctor to listen. In New York there used to be people who advertised as "listeners," and they charged five dollars per half hour. They were flooded with clients. They never gave any advice or said anything; they just listened. Not all the people who went to them had psychosomatic illnesses, but a large number of them, I'm quite sure, had the kinds of problems that a good many of us hear about in general practice. People have a great need to unburden themselves. If they go from doctor to doctor and nobody gives them an opportunity, then they keep on shopping around.

Now that isn't the only reason why patients shop around. Some patients may want to get a diagnosis which suits them, a diagnosis which they like. A diagnosis of heart disease or tuberculosis may not suit them, and they'll go around until they find a doctor who doesn't make that diagnosis, and then they don't need to have anxiety. Others are trying to find a doctor who will actually give them some help. Not all shop for the same reason. But a good many of them do it because they cannot get from the doctor what they feel they are entitled, and actually are entitled, to get. If you start out as a new doctor in a new town, you get on this shoppers' list. Sometimes some of them will stay with you if you sit down and give them enough time to tell their story, if they can develop a relationship to you.

I must add a word about this relationship. We were talking about positive and negative attitudes. Some patients can tolerate positive feelings for anybody only up to a certain point; beyond that it becomes too dangerous for them in one way or another. Hence allowing a positive feeling to build up in certain individuals is not of any value, for if it reaches a certain point then the individual has to run away. One of the most effective ways of handling these attitudes is to allow the patient to talk about his feelings when an opportunity presents itself in relation to the problem. We mustn't be afraid. You see, some of us are so afraid of becoming implicated or involved. We have a fantasy of ourselves as a sort of automaton. Actually, this is a pseudo-professional attitude which most of us can develop pretty easily. Almost every doctor can stand by and pat a dying patient on the tummy and talk rather casually, if the dying patient doesn't happen to be his child. So we try not to get involved in any kind of relationship. Now we can't allow ourselves to be involved from our side, of course. We mustn't take sides with the patient, we mustn't begin to play back with the patient into his own attitudes, but we still need to understand.

STUDENT. What should you do when a patient comes into your office and you feel there's a real clash of personality?

DR. KAUFMAN. If this happens often, then there's something that the doctor ought to attend to in relation to himself. But after all we, too, are human and sometimes, for one reason or another, there are patients that we just cannot handle. Dr. Bauer says that when he gets into that situation he tells the patient, after talking with him, that perhaps it would be better that he go to another doctor. I think we ought not to try to encompass everything and feel that we can handle every problem. But if it happens too often, then that's a completely different problem. I think we should try to see what it is that's wrong with us. Put it another way—if all our patients love us, I think it's time we stopped and asked why. If all our patients hate us, we also ought to ask why. If we hate all our patients the same thing is true. In other words, we can't have everything going in one direction without something being wrong.

Normal Personality Development

JOHN M. MURRAY, M.D.

I

TODAY we begin a formal consideration of the psychology of people. We start with the child, the infant. Roughly speaking, the way to learn psychology is to watch the infant and the child and gain some idea of what the behavior of these little people is. So today we start with the infant. To understand his psychology and that of the child there is one point always to remember—that is dependency. Underline that three times. The way the child expresses his dependency needs—if you understand that, you have indeed made a proper beginning to your understanding of all human behavior.

At birth the human being is completely dependent for his life upon the support and supplements of others. That goes for everything, of course: for food, for protection, for shelter, for everything that the child needs to carry on his life. Without such support the child cannot live. But there is another set of factors, factors whose influence is much more difficult to see, and these are the emotional aspects of his situation. To see and to understand the interrelationship of these two sets of factors—the practical things the child needs for survival and the emotional constellations centered around his biological needs—is to make the right beginning to understanding the psychology of the child and the adult human being. In fact, it is when these emotional needs—this second type of need that I've been speaking of—are not gratified that you find a child going into certain types of behavior upon which later neurotic symptomatology is based.

What is a child's first relationship to another human being? A child is not like an adult. He is not born loaded with love and loaded with an intellectual organization of ideas and an orientation toward other people. A child can express his dependency needs in one way alone, and that is in a somatic way, in some type of bodily function. Right after birth, that somatic way is through the use of his mouth. The child forms his first relationship with an object in the world with his mouth. That statement, too, you can underline. In this way the child finds sustenance close to the mother's body; he finds warmth and security; and he finds also a relief from unpleasant somatic tensions, particularly those associated with the gastrointestinal tract. It is safe to assume that at this time the child does not differentiate the world outside his own body from himself. To make such a differentiation is a capacity that develops later.

So we see, in this first stage of development, the child fulfills his practical dependency needs by a relationship with another human being. Later on, certain other elements of this relationship, which are not essential for the carrying on of life itself, prove to be very important in the emotional life of the child. Even at this early stage the child experiences gratification in his relationship with his mother, a somatic gratification. The pleasure which he derives from the tactile impulses he receives around the lips and the mouth from the warmth and softness of the breast is an important element in his life. Sometimes a child's stomach may be filled, but his need for this somatic gratification is not filled. If the nursing period is over before this particular need is fulfilled, what you get, as all of you doctors know, is thumb-sucking. Thumb-sucking gives the child a feeling of security. Later on, when the child is a year or two old, thumb-sucking usually indicates that the child is a bit unhappy and is seeking a feeling of security by this extension of the normal way of getting emotional gratification.

The child, then, has a practical need for the use of his mouth in relation to his mother, and also has an emotional need for that relationship. To use a technical word, the child erotizes the feeding situation, from which he is able to derive intense somatic gratification. This latter capacity meets a very important and vital need in the child's emotional life. As the child develops in his relationship with human beings, we shall see what an important part deviation from the capacity to express these emotional needs normally plays in his life.

The child goes through this early phase of oral relationship with his mother unable at first to appreciate the fact that the breast is not part of himself. Later he realizes that the breast comes and goes, that it isn't there all the time. Later still, he finds that it belongs to somebody else, that there is another body in the world. Then the conception of mother develops and, later, the conception of father and other children in the family. All the time the child is elaborating these conceptions of other people in the world around him and is relating himself emotionally to these people.

The child may fulfill his dependency needs in this manner with a feeling of security or with a feeling of insecurity—that is, with a feeling of gratification or of lack of gratification. He may fail to adjust well to this transient and recurring loss of his mother. Now, why is it that a child so early in his life can, somehow or other, strangely formulate within himself the fact that he is in an insecure position? The work which has been done with infants by Margaretha Ribble and others provides some understanding of this phenomenon. Dr. Ribble studied a series of infants in nurseries who had serious gastrointestinal disturbances. This type of child seems to lose his sucking reflex and to regress to an intrauterine pattern; sometimes the blood goes back into the portal circulation again, dams back into the liver, and it is necessary to use intravenous feeding if the child is to live. Ribble found out that in practically all the cases in her series the mother did not want the child —was so cold and unreceptive that even in the first days of life the child was aware (certainly not conscious but nevertheless aware) of the situation and expressed his emotion about it in a somatic way.

The child grows and develops, gets up to the age of a year, let us say. By this time he is aware of objects and is developing the capacity to relate himself to his mother as the demands of the world dictate. He may accept these demands in a normal way for his age, or, if he doesn't find adequate security, he may need such additional devices as thumb-sucking, or tantrumlike reactions when his mother is absent. In subsequent months the early oral relationships begin to become less intense, while the other areas in which the child meets the world are becoming more pronounced. The child's awareness of other objects is the beginning of his intellectual, or thought, capacity, which is the basis of his later ability to slough off the intensity of his somatic relationship with the world and develop a more realistic—a budding ideational—relationship with it. The mouth begins to diminish in importance as the predominant zone of somatic relationship and the child begins to take an intense interest in the other end of his gastrointestinal tract. I want you to conceive of the child at this age as essentially a gastrointestinal individual; it is the gastrointestinal tract that is the all-important thing to him at this time of life. So now the opposite end of the gastrointestinal tract becomes important; it is as important as the oral zone for a brief period in the emotional development of the child.

Let's now take a child who is beginning to show some signs of insecurity in life, and let's follow what oftentimes is the history of such a child in his somatic relationships with people around him. Let's say the mother is somewhat neurotic. She's not happy in her relationship with the father. She is overprotective of the child because of her lack of adequate emotional relationship with her husband. The child senses this. He is not adequately weaned from his early and powerful emotional dependencies on his mother, and so, finding an inadequate gratification in the relationship situation, he begins to suck his thumb. Let's say, now, that when the kid gets to be about eighteen or twenty months old the father doesn't like this and wants something done about it. And something is done about it. The child's hands are tied down, the father slaps the child, or the parents paint his thumb with some vile paste in order to break him. Perhaps the dentist has threatened that the child's teeth will be deformed. You all know what is apt to be said and done in a situation like that. Somehow or other the child is intimidated to a point where he gives up the habit.

Now what happens? Well, the commonest thing that happens is that the child develops constipation at about two years of age. Somehow or other it seems as if the child derives a sort of devilish gratification in saying, "Well, even though you can do this to me and pull my thumb, I've got you fooled at the other end because there's no handle on that that you can take and pull down!" It is a fact that the child can play that same game at the other end of the intestinal tract and, by the tactile sensation of the body with the stools, can find a sensory gratification that supplants the old somatic gratification experienced in thumbsucking. And not only that. The process of intellectual growth and development has begun, and the child now is keenly aware of some of the emotional relationships in the family. Oftentimes he is clever enough to manipulate his relationship with his mother and to secure certain other emotional gratifications. For instance, the mother's anxiety over his not having a bowel movement every morning is something which the child becomes readily aware of, and something which he cleverly utilizes in order to manipulate his relationship with her. If he cannot get adequate gratification for his emotional needs in a normal relationship with his mother, then the child, even at this stage of life, finds a surreptitious gratification in utilizing the symptom of constipation to obtain interest from her.

These, then, are the first two important elements in the child's emotional relationship with life. I want to repeat them. I apologize for the reiteration, but I want you to see again the two components involved in the situation: first, the practical aspects, the things that are perfectly apparent to the child, and second, the hidden, inner emotional meaning to the child.

As the child becomes older, the zones of intense interest shift. The gastrointestinal tract, with its two orifices, passes into the background and the genital and urinary zones begin to take a forward place in the scheme of things. If, by the age of three and a half, our hypothetical child has been successfully weaned from his thumb-sucking and his constipation, he will now turn to touching the genital zones for the same type of gratification that he has experienced in the two earlier stages. As the genital zone has become the most sensitive area of the body, the gratification which was experienced earlier in the mouth and in the anus is now related to the genital area. Indeed, frequently the family or the doctor is successful in curing constipation merely because the child has found a new zone of interest.

I want to say here, as Dr. Kaufman said yesterday afternoon, that these stages should not be regarded as manifestations of psychopathology. They are not. These are normal stages in the development of a child, stages which go on step by step. If the child makes them step by step, he makes a correct journey on the road to normalcy. If for one or another reason—either through an excessive need for the particular type of gratification or through intense fear aroused by too abrupt or overly zealous frustrations of it—the child becomes attached to these earlier types of pleasure, we know that this will be at the expense of later normal development. If the child is held back to these zones of the gastrointestinal tract and expresses his need of them in later life, this expression will be at the expense of his capacity to express normally his emotional needs in terms of the genital zone.

To continue, our child now passes over to his interest in the genital zone and not only becomes interested in his own body but also in the activities of other people in terms of this special body area. He becomes interested in what the parents do in their intimate life. He asks the eternal question "Where do babies come from?" One day you may tell him. I did so with my own children. Tell him the truth about where babies come from. Babies come from inside mother. The child knows this and accepts it intuitively, but on the other hand he denies it and says, "It isn't true; the stork brings them."

My older boy went through a tremendously intense time of asking questions about this, that, or the other thing, coming back ten minutes later time and time again to ask the same question. So finally one day I said, "Johnny, you keep asking me these questions over and over again. You know what I think is going on? I think there is something you want to know about but don't dare ask me, and so you just ask me all these other questions and you're never satisfied." And he said, "You think so, Daddy?" I said, "Yeah." And he said, "Well, what do you think I want to know about?" And I said, "I think you want to know where babies come from." "Oh, no, I don't want to know where babies come from, Daddy." "O.K., Johnny." But in about ten minutes he came back again and said, "Well, I don't know, Daddy. Maybe I would like to know." So I told him and for the rest of that day he asked no further questions. The next day I overheard him say to his nursemaid, "Emmie, do you know where babies come from?" And Emmie said, "Why, where do they come from?" He said, "The stork brings them." You see, at this time this idea of mother and father and babies was too over-whelming, too exciting, too interesting, for him to digest adequately, and so he retreated again to the childish conception which was a safe idea for him. However, I know that the other idea was there at the same time and that the two conflicting ideas were going along hand in hand without mutual interference. The capacity for that kind of reaction is characteristic of children's psychology.

At about four or five years of age, then, the child becomes interested in the activities of other people in regard to the genital zone. And the other people who are closest to the child, of course, are the other members of his family. It very naturally follows that this powerful and intense interest turns to these people for whom the child has a powerful emotional concern. The child goes through an intensely active period, therefore, of wondering what mother and daddy do together at times when he is excluded. Somehow, too, the child becomes desirous at times of taking the place of the parent of his sex and has ideas of intimate interest toward the parent of the opposite sex.

You can picture, then, this child, caught in the rip tide of a situation which has no solution but one of retreat. He is still dominated by powerful dependency needs. Even though his actual dependency for food and shelter is not so strong at this time, nevertheless the emotional needs persist with tremendous intensity, and so he cannot be happy unless he is normally and securely related emotionally to his parents. On the other hand, he is developing a tremendously powerful fantasy life, which is going on contrary to his need for a secure dependency relationship with his parents. It is, as I say, the rip tide of the emotions that the child is caught in at this time of life. This is the time when, as all you doctors know, the child is constantly getting himself into trouble. He may be overly aggressive and overactive; he probably is having nightmares; he may be going through eras of minor phobias —dog phobias, fear of going out of the yard, or something of that kind. Those phobias and other symptoms and that emotional intensity are expressions of the inner turmoil that is going on within him—on the one hand, his search for the intense, exciting, and interesting expression of the inner emotional needs which he senses to be taboo and, on the other, his need to behave so that, first, he will not be punished and, second, he will receive expressions of love from his parents.

These are the vitally important moments in the development of the character of the human being. At this time, in order to show how that works, I shall go back again to my experience with my own children. Remember, now, that the child needs, first, to feel secure in being loved and, second, to be free from the fear of punishment. Remember, also, that there is within him this seething, inner world of fantasy about forbidden impulses. Consequently, an eternal tug-of-war goes on in the mind of the child at this age. Throughout this period he is continually experiencing denials or frustrations at the hands of his parents. As he grows and develops and normally learns to give up his socially unacceptable impulses, he does so at the behest of numerous thou-shalt-nots from his parents. In this connection a very important development occurs. The child begins to identify himself with the person who is advancing the thou-shalt-nots.

I want to show you through an experience of my own what I mean by this word "identification." Jimmy got pneumonia, and he went to the hospital. He wasn't very sick. When he came home he wouldn't stay in bed. In the evening he'd be a little excited and not want to settle down and go to sleep. I was downstairs reading in the quiet house and heard those little feet going on the floor above, and so I went upstairs and said, "Come on now, Jimmy, and get into bed. You know you'll get cold again and you'll get sick again and will probably have to go back to the hospital." He looked at me as though he wasn't used to this big bum telling him what to do. As he had apparently got his own way pretty well in the hospital, he didn't like this very well and I could see it in the look I got. I went downstairs again, and five minutes later I was back upstairs. "Come on now, Jim. Go on back to bed and stay there." Well, that happened five or six times, and the old man being what he is got a little bit sore. I said, "Come on now, Jimmy. If you do that again I'll smack you; I don't want you to get sick again." I went downstairs and pretty soon feet were going along the floor in just the same way. So I went out and cut a little switch from a bush in the yard. As I went upstairs, Jimmy heard me coming and he headed for the bed. Just as he got to the bed, I gave him one little quick clip with the switch across his bare feet. Then he hopped into bed and began crying. He cried for a while, and I went downstairs. He cried some more, and then about ten minutes later his mother, who was upstairs, heard him talking to himself, and this is what he said, "Now, you be a good boy and stay in bed. If you don't, I'll sock you."

What I want you to get out of that story is this: that lad was a different lad from the one he had been before he got hit. He had taken an infinitesimal part of me inside himself. This experience of being frustrated and of being hurt a little caused a reaction, and his response was to take a part of me inside himself. If he would follow that part of me, he would be spared further conflict along this line. I want you to remember that little story because it is out of thousands or tens of thousands or hundreds of thousands of such experiences that the conscience is born. The conscience is a very, very important thing in the life of the adult person, particularly when you are dealing with psychoneurosis and neurotic manifestations. It is from literally thousands, tens of thousands of such thou-shalt-nots that the structure of the child's conscience is made up. At this time of life, in the hectic activity of his need for somatic pleasure, the child is very sensitive to the demands of the thou-shalt-nots, for he is afraid, as I said before, of punishment and of loss of love.

To substantiate that I ask you to think for a moment of the subjects of the children's stories that have come down through the generations. By and large you will find that their themes are the themes of these two important things in the life of the child. One, fear of loss of love. Remember the little match girl who died when the last match went out, alone and cold outside the warm house at Christmas time. Or remember the babes in the woods who were lost when the birds ate up the crumbs. Two, fear of punishment or mutilation. Jack the Giant Killer, Little Red Ridinghood, and so on. Those are the themes with which the child is eternally concerned at this phase of his life. Those are the thoughts which the child cannot resist. Those are the stories the child asks for again and again. The reason is quite simple. They are the themes with which the child is most occupied in his inner life at this period of his existence.

At this time a very important step in the development of the child takes place. If the child has adequately passed through the early phases, he is now ready for an intense growth in the development of his capacity to meet the world in terms of ideas instead of somatically. He is now ready to be taught. His interest is now not so much in what he can do to get pleasure as in what makes the wheels go round. If I handed a child a watch at age two he would stick it in his mouth; he would relate himself to the watch in a somatic way. But at age six the child listens to the watch tick. He is ready to replace a somatic relationship by ideas associated with the purpose of things. So at this time we send the child to school.

We've come to the point where we begin to see a decline in the intensity of the child's emotional activity. There's been a gradual developmental process which seems to come to a head at the point where the child translates his need for intense somatic gratification into a capacity for intellectual activity. You all know that at this period many a child becomes a much more placid, a much more serene, a much less active and driving person. Sometimes it seems to happen almost overnight. The little girl who has been a tomboy, struggling like the devil to keep up with the lads and to be one of them, suddenly takes up with a doll. In her capacity to love this doll she finds security, and now she can let all this other hectic activity and identification with boys go down the river. Now one of the important things that have happened is the organization, the formulation, or the structuralization of the conscience. The tens or hundreds of thousands of thou-shalt-nots activated by the fear of punishment or the fear of loss of love have been built into a social core within the child that makes him want to live within the framework of what the world—chiefly the family, the school, and so forth—says he should do and to be happy within that framework. The thin, still voice within now tells the child to do this, to do that, that he will be happier if he does. For illustration, the child comes in hungry at five o'clock. The child knows it's half an hour before supper. He's tired; maybe he has a little hypoglycemia at this time. It's been an active day of play, and here on the table is some candy. The old instinctual life inside says, "Go get it. It's good, it tastes good, you'll feel better." But the conscience speaks up, "If I take that mother won't love me, or daddy will slap me." On the one hand, the gratification. On the other hand, the loss of love or the punishment. They are weighed in the balance. In a sense, conscience is the activating force of that balance, and what the child does depends upon the whole series of its yesterdays. And whether the child takes the candy, and is punished by his parent, or is mature enough to say, "I can have a piece of candy after supper; I'll wait until then," is a vitally important thing in terms of the development of that child's personality and his capacity to meet the world as he should be able to at this level of age and development.

To summarize, then, the important problem in the development of the child—this bundle of energy that expresses itself in the need to live —is to form a personality whose specific function is to relate the child and his inner needs to the environment which either grants, denies, or postpones the fulfillment of these needs. The secure and peaceful child is one who can form such a personality.

Notice here that the most important elements in the child's outside world are people, other personalities, and that the child has his own characteristic attitudes toward these personalities. Now we can go back for a moment to yesterday's lectures. Dr. Rennie, Dr. Bauer, and Dr. Kaufman spoke of the importance of interpersonal relationships in the lives of people. They elaborated upon the relationship of chief importance professionally to a doctor—what happens to the patient when he comes into the doctor's office. In the light of what we have discussed this morning, we can see that these early, infantile dependency relationships are reactivated when a sick, troubled, suffering person enters into a relationship with a person from whom he expects help. Here lies the basis of the doctor-patient relationship. If you stop to think about it, you can see why or how that is true. Patients do, in a sense, attribute godlike qualities to the doctor in much the same way as the child endows his parents with omnipotence. They do expect great things from you—things which their mature intelligence would tell them they could not reasonably expect. In this relationship, however, it is not the logic of the intelligence that is working but rather the logic of the emotions of the small child, of that primitive, inner part which remains with us as long as we live and which the neurotic unfortunately carries less comfortably than his more happy, more maturely developed brother or sister.

To help you formulate these ideas specifically, I shall do what Dr. Rennie yesterday said would be dangerous—apply a few technical terms to these concepts I have been talking about. We have seen the need of the child for experiencing emotional gratification in his personal relationships, at first somatically and later with an ideational quality. This driving need psychiatrists have formulated as instinct. It is the basis of what is known as instinct psychology—that the child instinctually seeks these gratifications, that the child has emotions or energies

within him that continually well up and seek expression in relationships
with people. A part of the personality—a primitive, unorganized part
—is conceived as a wellspring from which these emotions continually
arise, sometimes giving gratification and sometimes giving pain because
society says "no." When I come to this point I am always reminded of
Show Boat and Old Man River. Why can't I be like the river, starting
up there, flowing down to the sea in a gradual, complacent, and easy
manner, never disturbed, never ruffled, never suffering, just flowing
along in a casual way? "He don't plant 'taters, he don't plant cotton, and
them that plants 'em is soon forgotten. Get a little drunk and you land
in jail." Get your emotion tensed up inside of you, go out and get drunk
to relieve it, and you land in jail, but Old Man River just goes rolling
along. I think that became a great song because, by and large, it expressed the thing that all human beings strive for—the capacity to keep
these inner surging emotions, these instinctual drives, continuously
moving into the outside world in such a manner that we find gratification or at least a minimum of suffering.

This powerful source of the inner instinctual life seeking gratification is sometimes called the *id*. *Id*, as you know, is the Latin for "it";
it simply signifies that undifferentiated source or wellspring of energy,
that element that Old Man River represented for the singer. Second,
we have seen the development of the personality, of the *ego*, the
"I," that part of me which makes me different from everybody else.
This is developed in order to act as a buffer between the inner instinctual being and the outside world which man organizes. Third, we have
seen that a highly specialized part of the personality, the conscience,
develops. This is sometimes called the *super-ego*. This part of the individual has as its executive force tremendous quantities of anxiety in order to make us behave. In a sense, that unhappiness and depression
which children experience when they are not lined up well with their
parents we likewise experience as adults when we live estranged from
our conscience. Super-ego, conscience, is especially important to us as
doctors, for by and large we always find in neurotic patients gross mal-
formations of the conscience, with the result that the individual cannot
fulfill his need for normal gratification.

I'll turn the meeting over to Dr. Rennie now, who is chairman for the questions.

DISCUSSION

DR. RENNIE.   I am tempted to take just a few minutes before you launch into your questions to make some remarks about the course and the relation of various sections to it. You may wonder why on the second day of a course on the psychoneuroses and psychosomatic disturbances we choose to tell you about the early developmental period of every human being. I think the answer is pretty obvious. You are not going to be able to treat human beings unless you understand human beings. There are a number of ways of attempting to understand adult human beings. For instance, there are a variety of tests or questionnaires that aim to give you some picture of what a personality structure is like. They have some limited value in giving you an immediate, rather brief picture of what a personality consists of, but they do not give you all of the picture. Indeed, there is only one way to get all of the picture and that is the biographic way—going back to the beginning and getting step by step, as accurately as possible, the various stages in the evolution or development of the human being. Now that is pre-eminently the method used by the biographer, sometimes by the novelist. Biographers and novelists know, without scientific training, that the full picture of what goes into the making of a human being is only completely understood when you start at the beginning and follow it through step by step. So we want you to have the biographic story of all human beings—yourselves, your patients, your friends, everyone. The essential biography of all of us is what Dr. Murray has been telling you this morning. He was talking not only of the neurotic individual. This is not the life story of neurotic people only; it is the life story of all people, yourselves included.

While we would like you to have that framework, I might warn you that you are not likely in the next two weeks to get such understanding from the interviews that you are going to have with patients. To amass material of this kind about a human being is a long, time-consuming process.

You might ask what right Dr. Murray has to say what is going on inside the infant. Why does science say this and that occur at such and such a stage? Well, there are two main reasons why we are sure that what we are saying is true. First, there have been people who have devoted years of study to the infant and the small child and have watched their behavior and have come to pretty much these conclusions. Dr. Murray has told you about Dr. Ribble's work, that fascinating work on newborn and very young infants in which she found that if they don't get enough feeding or sucking activity they may go into actual surgical shock and even die. We also know from the work of men like Gesell at Yale that these things do occur—if you open your eyes and put aside your prejudices and observe what is actually going on. Second, the other main body of evidence comes from the study of adults over a long period of time; it is from Freud and his pupils that a great deal of this information has derived. If any one of you were to devote one hour a day five days a week for a period of one year, or two, or more, to thorough-going psychoanalytic investigation and treatment, you'd be amazed to find how soon you'd stop talking about contemporary matters and begin bringing up memories of experiences that are very much like those you have heard about this morning. These two large bodies of evidence lead us to believe that what we have been saying is valid and can be counted upon.

Essentially, then, what we're aiming at in these lectures is to show you the development of the adult personality structure. These structures and processes that you have heard about are inevitably interwoven into the ultimate character that marks us as grown-up persons. Indeed, you may be surprised many times to see, if you are honest, how many remnants of these things exist in you at the present time. All the need for oral activity does not drop out in infancy. Strange remnants of it persist into adulthood, and the same is true for the lower end of the gastrointestinal tract. Consider, for example, how many of your friends enjoy sitting on the toilet fifteen minutes for a function that legitimately requires only one or two minutes. Consider the prevalence of cigarettes and chewing gum, and other objects that can be put into the mouth, as a manifestation of how much oral needs persist openly in the adult human being.

In the clinic you're going to be dealing with patients who have had real difficulties in personality development. As time goes on (I'm anticipating a little of what you will hear later, but I think it's wise to do so for your over-all orientation), you will realize that when these psychoneurotic individuals are beset by difficulties in contemporary life they sometimes, indeed frequently, revert to modes of satisfaction that really belong to these earlier periods of life. Hence, you may actually be dealing with some of the material discussed this morning in a treatment situation with an adult psychoneurotic individual.

From what Dr. Murray told you this morning, I think you can appreciate that all adults, and particularly psychoneurotic adults, have a very great need for the satisfaction of those primitive cravings for affection and acceptance and security. I bring that point up because it ties us back into what Dr. Kaufman said yesterday about the patient-physician relationship. Individuals who have an inordinate need for security and acceptance and affection are inevitably going to project something of that need upon you as doctors, and they are going to invest you with the qualities that they are looking for in order to satisfy those needs. That's all I want to say at the present time. I have gone forward and back a little in the course because I want you to see this biographic, historical material in the perspective of the entire course and what we are doing with the patients.

STUDENT. I would like to ask a question about the conscience and discipline. It seems that, from what has been said here, a properly balanced individual needs that conscience. The thing, I think, that worries young parents is how much discipline they can carry on without danger. It seems that for the proper balance a certain degree of fear is necessary. Fear is an instinct that has a good purpose, but I would like a little discussion of the dangers of discipline.

DR. MURRAY. I give one rule that you can apply to this—when you frustrate a child, do it only to a degree to which the child can accept and master the frustration. In other words, don't frustrate a child to such an intensity that the child feels overwhelmed and washed under by his inability to relate himself to what you want him to do. Somewhere between the outside limits of spoiling the child by granting him too much and excessively inhibiting the child by overintense restrictions and taboos is the mid-line which the child can normally accept. If you don't restrict the child enough, the child becomes afraid of his own powerful instinctual needs, which seem different from those of people around him. If you repress too much, then the intensity of the child's conscience induces fear or anxiety. The ideal is the mid-line of holding the child just enough, so that he can absorb and understand and can live with his emotions.

STUDENT.   If you stop a child who has done something, or you punish him, is it necessary that you leave him with what you might call a substitute for his gratification? Is that part of punishment?

DR. MURRAY.   A child can have an equal amount of gratification in identification. That is one of the most important ways to handle a child. If you want to stop a child from sucking his thumb in a way that will not be traumatic to the child, do it in this manner—by identification. "Daddy doesn't suck his thumb; mother doesn't suck her thumb." Say that day after day, and finally the child will get greater gratification from doing things the way the parent does them than from thumb-sucking. In that way you are doing what you said—substituting one gratification for another, but in a manner which aids the child to master his instinct. Consequently he does not develop anxiety. The child then grows in relation to himself and to the world around him in a way that's mutually agreeable.

DR. RENNIE.   Dr. Jensen, you're a child psychiatrist. Do you want to add anything to that?

DR. JENSEN.   Well, I think I'd like to say a word about the use of terms. I think many times we get confused. The two I am referring to that have been used here are discipline and punishment. I think there is a good deal of difference between them. Learning to live comfortably with one another is a discipline. We are having our limits defined for us from the very beginning. Some of us learn it more, some less. Now, if we exceed those limits, punishment comes in to get us back to those limits, which we might call discipline. If we can think of the two terms in that way we won't get mixed up so much. We're all being disciplined all along the line, but not necessarily punished.

I think there is another thing that enters into this matter of punishment, and that is the degree of comfort with which the adult does it. If the parents can move directly, easily, and confidently in administering punishment, they can minimize some of the fear and some of the other overwhelming reactions of the child and bring about this identification that Dr. Murray rightfully referred to. In going back over the experience we've had with children who have been punished, I can't recall a single incident where the child resented being punished when he felt he had it coming. He certainly was filled with resentment, however, when he didn't feel he had it coming.

DR. RENNIE. I would like to add that all this can be done by a parent either punitively (that is, as a counteraggressive reaction from the parent which the child immediately senses) or it can be done with sustained affection.

STUDENT. But do you feel that you can accomplish all purposes by the sense of security and love and example? Don't we sometimes actually need punitive measures?

DR. KAUFMAN. It seems to me that the question the doctor raised is a very important one, not only in relation to this particular problem but in relation to therapy, for we mustn't forget that what we do to a patient may also be regarded as punishment and discipline. It seems to me that one good rule is to punish with discipline but still allow the child to maintain his self-respect. As Dr. Murray said, if we overwhelm a child and, as Dr. Jensen said, if we punish him, not to fit the crime but to satisfy our hatred for him, then we have done something which is almost irreparable to the formation of his conscience.

A certain amount of discipline is necessary. We learned that, incidentally, to our cost. If I may digress a little here, when analysis consisted mostly of reading a book, there arose a very curious phenomenon in relation to the bringing up of children. We found that neurotic difficulties were caused by repression. So we said, ergo, let us bring up our children without repressing them at all. And we had the damnedest brats you ever saw. I had a case the other day at the hospital which brought this out clearly. The patient was a very neurotic woman who had been raised as a foster child, who lived with her aunt and uncle and little cousin. When the cousin did wrong, the aunt and uncle punished her (smacked her or something); but when it came to our patient, they had a conference about her and didn't punish her. What she wanted was to be smacked, just like the other child. So punishment in itself isn't always an evidence of lack of love. Besides, it is something which a child unconsciously needs. So I think, to epitomize in a rather general way, punishment and discipline which allow the individual to maintain his self-respect will create a normal kind of a conscience and personality rather than the overwhelming thing that we sometimes see.

II

WE left the lad yesterday about six years old, having quieted down somewhat in the intensity of his emotional pressures, having found a new capacity for meeting life with his intellect and letting down on his need for somatic expression. This is commonly called the latency period. During this period the child's interest in tabooed items continues, but at a reduced pace. The latency period in the ordinary child extends to what we might call pre-puberty—around eleven, twelve, thirteen years of age. Twelve is a good average. At that time a number of physiological changes begin taking place in the lad's growth, evidenced, of course, by change in voice, appearance of hair, secondary sex characteristics, etc. You know those as well as I do. There are a number of very important emotional changes which also begin to take place in his life at this time. The first is an intense drive toward activity.

In the latency period the lad's character is marked by strong identifications. In a sense you might say that he has borrowed his character from the important people in his milieu; he has not built the strong substance of his character by this time, and it is one of the functions of the puberty period to accomplish this. Now, one of the important psychological changes we note at this time is the solution of a number of these identifications. I know that you men are aware of this process in boys. (By the way, I shall speak mostly about boys. Later on, I may say a word about girls if we have time.) As I say, you have all seen examples of this beginning change. A good father walks into your office. He's been a kindly and understanding parent to his boy. And he says, "I can't understand Johnny now. Everything I tell him to do, he does the opposite. He's irritable. He's grouchy. He never wants to do anything that I tell him, and I just don't know what to make of him."

Well, psychologically what has taken place is very simple. Johnny has given up his identification with his father. Up to this time he may have been as exemplary a son as the father could ask for—quite passive in his relationship with his father, accepting his father's leadership and domination even though the father has not insisted on such an attitude. But at this time, under the impact and intensity of the puberty emotions, dominance by the father becomes unwelcome to the lad. There are strange stirrings within him that cannot let him accept this condition any longer. He must break through the cocoon of this emotional situation, and he does, at times rather dramatically. Sometimes there is a terrific intensity to deny and reject everything there is about the father.

I have spoken of the good father, the kind father, the very acceptable father. Of course, if the father is not of this variety and the lad has a strong character, the storm may be even of a greater intensity. But in either case the lad is breaking up these old dominances, is unwilling to be passive any longer; the old identifications are unsatisfactory. He may shift entirely away from identification with his father and now want to be like the kids, perhaps like some tough guys he's picked up playing on the ball team. I think you all hear accounts of situations like that.

To make matters worse, there is a hard something within the boy that seems to give him the feeling he has a right to do all this, something that makes it very difficult at times for him to try to stand in the way of these new urges. In other words, his conscience, that directive influence which he has borrowed from numerous identifications, now becomes weakened (at the same time that inner drives are so strong), for his relationship with those people who were models for his conscience has become loose.

I'll have to go into a little detail in explaining this phenomenon to you so that you can understand just why this change takes place. I shall use Aichhorn's way of putting it. In his lectures in Vienna, Aichhorn used to picture the boy as having a certain number of pounds of libido or emotional feeling, most of which he needed to deposit on objects in the outside world. He'd give his mother, say, fifteen pounds and his father fifteen pounds, and he'd give his brother eight, his younger brother seven, and his little sister maybe three or four, the dog maybe three—his toys and all his possessions, they too would be given so many pounds of libido. What Aichhorn was really saying was that there is an emotional something within us which we deposit on the outside world and by means of which we relate ourselves to the world. That "something" is the cement that binds human relationships.

In this giving out of libido, however, the child keeps some for himself. Now what happens in puberty is that as identifications become less strong with parents, teachers, and others who have been ideal figures to the individual, the pounds of libido return to their original reservoir and increase its size. The individual now has a tremendous amount of libido in relation to himself or, if you will, a greatly increased self-concern. This continues during the years in which he tries to reorient himself, to find new figures with which he can relate himself and fulfill his emotional needs. To do so may take some time, and during this period you may see bizarre behavior on the lad's part. You may see, on the one hand, tremendous capacity for idealistic behavior; with this heightened interest in the self he is able to rise to great heights of supersocial interests. Likewise, he's very capable of intense attachments to his friends. At the same time, he is able to do things of exactly opposite nature—to throw all this aside, to abandon restraint and do things strongly against the direction of his own conscience and, consequently, to suffer bitterly in the mildly depressed states that occur during adolescence. We see this particularly in his marked ambivalence toward sex activity. At one time, a strong idealist, the next time, masturbating but with tremendous guilt.

So much for the general psychological background of the individual in adolescence. Let us go now more specifically to his sexuality, which is a very important part of his problem at this time. Sexuality takes up at puberty in more or less the same vein that it left off around six. The boy's interest is at first still on older people. Hence the tremendous tendency for the lad to develop a crush on his school teacher, for we know that the object of his most intense concern back in childhood was usually his mother, or perhaps his older sisters, and when his sex interest picks up again it is on the same basis as earlier. The teacher, a substitute for the mother, is oftentimes its first object. Following this, there may be an intense rebound, an intense denial of all of this interest in the opposite sex and a turning back to the gang again.

This phase has to be gone through. There have been powerful taboos and inhibitions of sexuality put on the lad during the early phases of childhood—a necessity, mind you, an absolute need if culture is to persist. These taboos are very strong, and so at adolescence the lad experiences anxiety as powerful impulses arise again and meet the taboos. That is why it is so common for lads to gang up and have a tremendous amount of emotion in their relationships with other lads. We see that all during the period of adolescence, sublimated satisfactorily perhaps in the way they follow the activities of their sports team. You know how intense that is—how loyal is the attachment to the home team and how completely "no good" are the rivals.

The hostilities in the lad are also very strong at this time and, unless kept well in hand, are apt to express themselves in outbursts of delinquent behavior, antisocial activities, particularly if the lad has failed to make identifications during his latency period. Such failure occurs usually in families in which the father is overstrong, as well as in those in which he is weak or is brutal to the mother. In none of these situations can the lad easily identify himself with his father; as a result he has a defective conscience, which is not able to hold within bounds the aggressive emotion he feels at puberty.

Now we go back to our main theme again, the boy's sexuality. This sexuality seeks sublimation, as we call it (a satisfactory social expression), in the tendency to form gangs. It takes more direct outlets also, usually in masturbation. This behavior is often accompanied by great guilt. Repeated masturbation characterized by a great sense of guilt is something to be expected at puberty and is of no clinical significance in the ordinary case. If the lad engages in what we speak of as compulsive masturbation, however, it is of some concern. In other words, if an intense state has been induced by anxiety over the struggles of adolescence and the lad tries to relieve his feeling of tension by repeated masturbation, consequently developing minor depressive swings as he feels more and more unable to find an adequate adjustment to life, we do have a problem. It is not that the masturbation is hurting the lad; the difficulty lies in the fact that his guilt and depression and the associated symptoms are taking away from him the ability to progress in normal growth and development. In such cases all that is usually required is to step in and break up the guilt reaction and nature will restore itself, with masturbation taking its normal course during this era of the lad's life.

As the years of puberty go on, the boy begins to dissolve the intensity of his gang attachments and his isolation from the opposite sex and becomes interested in girls. Usually there is a definite splitting in his sexual feelings at this time. His attitudes toward girls are of a completely asexual nature, for the taboos of the earlier years are still existent and his sexual activities continue to be confined to masturbation. There are, of course, many variations from this pattern, and lads often pick up heterosexuality very early in puberty—for instance in lonely farmhouses where there isn't quite enough to do. This is rather unusual, however, and the pattern ordinarily followed in our culture is the one I have described.

During adolescence a series of neurotic symptoms may appear which we must regard as normal. These symptoms may be of a depth and intensity which ten years later would indeed be evidence of a malignant psychological process. They usually begin with difficulties in concentration. Sometimes there are sleep disturbances, restlessness on going to bed, appetite disturbances. Perhaps most characteristic of all are the minor depressive swings that I spoke of. Sometimes even schizoid reactions are evident, strong tendencies toward introversion, a turning away from the world and toward the self and its luxurious fantasy life. Even such symptoms, although they show strong regressive tendencies, are not of very great significance and in many cases are only fleeting.

There is one other area of the lad's activities during the puberty period I should speak of now, and that is rivalry. If you would understand the boy and his emotional problems, you must have a pretty clear-cut picture of the nature of his rivalries, the inferiority he is experiencing, and the anxiety he has because he feels he cannot rise to meet those he wants to be like. Such feelings may be traceable back to childhood and may reflect the traumatic influence of the arrival of additional children in the family. At two or three the child, deeply attached to his parents, is oftentimes very loath to share with them the emotion they now must give to the newborn baby. Even if he did not have such experiences in childhood, the boy's feeling during adolescence that he cannot rise above his own group is indeed very intense. When he finds that his ability to compete is not adequate, he may begin to use various devices to evade normal competition. Many times this rivalry and the inability to meet it adequately force important symptoms to appear. Among these symptoms are the following: one, withdrawal into the self; isolation and aloofness; two, rejection of members of the opposite sex at the time such interest should appear; three, inability to study, growing out of the feeling that there is no sense in even trying because the rivals (an older brother, for instance) do so much better. Perhaps if the brother is not an athlete, the lad takes an intense interest in athletics and tries to become superior in order to prove that he's better than the brother in this area even if not in others. Over and over again we saw that in the Army Air Forces—neurotic younger brothers who, by getting wings and a bar, wanted to achieve a feeling of superiority over a brother they'd been struggling with all their lives. We found out that this was usually a pretty poor substitute for the wish really to fly and to serve, and ultimately the showdown would have to come. These are important things to be aware of as you evaluate what is going on in a lad during puberty.

There is one other angle which might have been taken up yesterday, but I have waited for this background to introduce it, and that is the concept of the unconscious. Some people, particularly psychologists, object to using the word "unconscious" as a noun, because you cannot bring it out in your hand and demonstrate it. They will accept the term as an adjective and say that there are certain things going on within the individual of which he is not consciously aware. Be that as it may, it is a fact that most of these conflicts around which neurotic difficulty is focused go on without the conscious awareness of the individual. It is usually also true that if we can succeed in making these conflicts conscious, the individual of normal intelligence and of normal adaptive capacity is on his way to making a more realistic adjustment.

Most of the impulses which produce serious conflicts—those which are chiefly associated with our sexual and our aggressive drives—take their origin deep within us in the unconscious areas, and the manifestations which show on the surface of consciousness have undergone very strong alterations before they appear there. Our social self, backed up by our conscience and our ideals, will not allow us to do many things we desire in the deep unconscious to do. Nevertheless, the pressure of the inner emotions for expression is as continuous, as definite, and as demanding of a solution as the pressure of the Mississippi moving on its way to the sea. That we attempt to deny the existence of these things and push them out of consciousness in no way alters the fact that they are there and will be heard. The conscience (the super-ego which we spoke of yesterday) is itself partly unconscious; in fact, most of the conscience functions in an unconscious capacity and only a small segment of it is at the service of our conscious activity.

There is a continuous conflict between powerful forces in the individual, perhaps never so powerful as during puberty. The game played inside each individual makes that of international politics a piker's game in its grabbing and its giving and taking of concessions, for the pleasure-seeking self is eternal and relentless. If you don't believe that you can ask Bergen. That's what he capitalizes on every Sunday night when he shows you how the clever little Charlie McCarthy that resides inside each of us is continually seeking to cut this corner, to cut that corner, to get this concession, to get that concession, in order to gratify our need for pleasure. That's the struggle that's going on in the individual all the time, and it is usually a struggle of which we are unaware. It is when this struggle becomes too great, when the forces of repression master the innate tendencies so strongly that a damming-back of activity ensues, that symptoms appear.

We have spoken of the struggles that go on in maintaining a normal balance during puberty. Let us speak for a moment now about the positive factors that lead the lad into normal development during this era. As we have seen, the lad's identifications with early figures, particularly with authoritarian figures, are very apt to be weakened. New figures as substitutes are avidly sought after by the young fellow. This is a very important step in the direction of maintaining a normal balance. The lad seeks an older person who combines some of the positive attributes of the rejected parent with something the lad is now reaching for that the parent doesn't have. Very frequently he finds this person in the coach of the sport he is interested in. If his repressions are very active, he may turn strongly toward the religious side and may find the substitute in a priest or minister or YMCA leader or other group worker. This new-found identification serves for the time being to bolster up the normal activities of the conscience and to help the lad through this stormy period of puberty.

The youth is also capable of great aesthetic and idealistic striving at this time. The conscience is still a powerful force even though some of its earlier moorings may have been loosed, and it may drive the lad in the direction of the aesthetic and idealistic. It is a strange phenomenon, too, that the powerful force which the conscience has at its disposal to stimulate such interests comes from the lad's primitive instinctual energy, originally directed toward sexual or aggressive aims. That may be hard for you to understand. It's rather like the old situation in Russia, where a few people were at the top, with the mass of the peasantry subject to their purposes. The Czar selected a number of powerful and strong younger men out of the mass, gave them rifles, trained them as soldiers, and redirected them against the peasantry in order to make them serve his purpose. Just so the conscience borrows its energy from the instinctual source of energy within the individual, remakes that energy for its own use, and directs it back against certain desires of the individual. Hence we find one individual approaching aesthetic endeavor with the same intensity as other individuals are approaching excessive sexual activity during puberty. This great capacity for turning toward the aesthetic and idealistic in puberty is one important means of development toward healthy maturity. These ideals drive the lad in the direction of achievement, and here again rivalry reinforces the other drives. As doctors all of us have been through that phase. In puberty all of us went through that phase of ambition which made us want to struggle through college and through medical school in the achievement of maturity. These, then, are the positive values which move the lad in the direction of health and normalcy through this stormy period of adolescence.

You may raise the question now, "When does adolescence end? When does the lad come out of this state?" The answer is that everyone is different. Some men become reserved and inflexible individuals early in life, other people never give up some of their adolescent attitudes and activities, even though in other respects they may be intensely mature. Perhaps old George Bernard Shaw is the outstanding example of that—a man of great maturity along one line but certainly a perennial adolescent along others, which increases the old duffer's capacity for enjoying life. I imagine that you doctors here in Minnesota see people mature rather early. Farmers with the grimness of the realities of the earth constantly before them are not likely to hold on to the joys of adolescence as long as others who are living in a more flexible situation. This seems particularly true of the wives of farmers we've seen here in the clinic; they come to middle age with deep regrets because they have not found something in life to replace what they've lost.

Here in brief, then, are a number of the important forces and counterforces which exercise influence during adolescence. We can see they are powerful crosscurrents and rip tides which push and twist and pull at the lad during this struggle of growing into maturity. The lad who comes successfully through that period settles down, for he feels he is reasonably sure to be the master of his ship. That is the thing which is of the utmost importance to the lad during puberty—to feel that he is capable of growing and developing to the point of being the master of his own destiny. He wants to leave behind his dependency on others for decisions; he wants to slough off the authoritarian figures who dominate him. Sometimes it isn't necessary that he should leave the family in order to assume an independent role, but in very few cases is he happy if he cannot feel that he is on his way toward achieving this independence. To help a lad achieve this, to effect an alteration in his identifications, so that he can feel he is on the road to attaining the independence of maturity, is a far more important task for the therapist than any immediate solution of the problem of sexuality.

DISCUSSION

STUDENT. What are the positive factors that induce the child to outgrow abnormal sibling rivalry and the negative factors that tend to exaggerate and prolong it?

DR. KAUFMAN. I think it's rather difficult to answer that question because we've first got to take into consideration everything that Dr. Murray has said about the development of the individual. What kind of sibling rivalry are you talking about? Rivalry between a younger brother and an older brother? What is the interval between the children? For instance, a child who comes when his older brother is five is in a different position from one who comes when his older brother is only a year old. The amount of aggression that was shown by the older brother to the younger brother, by the father to the younger brother or to the older brother—these are only some of the factors that enter into this question. So I think it's very difficult to make any general statements about how to handle the problem of sibling rivalry. The question can be answered only in relation to specific instances. One thing we must remember in dealing with our problem is this—a broad understanding is of great value provided we season it with a specific understanding of the situation. That's just as true here as it is of any problem in medicine. Every case has got to be studied and understood in terms of the specific situation, and you can do something about it only in relation to that specific situation.

I would like to reinforce, however, what Dr. Murray has pointed out—that sibling rivalry is not an abnormal, pathological kind of thing. It's part of the ordinary, human growing-up within a family. If you find a family where there isn't any sibling rivalry, you find a pathological situation. I think that's awfully important to remember.

STUDENT.   If a parent is aware of the emotional drives at the age of puberty, how should he attempt to guide the lad?

DR. MURRAY.   If a lad is showing symptoms and the parents come to you as a doctor to discuss the problem, first talk the matter over with them. Then see the lad, go into the thing from his standpoint. Then formulate the problem for yourself—the intensity of the lad's bewilderment symptomatology, the relationship of the parents to it. Having formulated your problem, come to a decision as to what you can do to help this boy. I think you, the doctor, must be the impelling force in the treatment situation. It is usually unwise to turn the problem over to the parents, for there is already too much emotional intensity for them to be effective. A neutral third party is needed as the pilot. As I look back over my cases of this sort, there are indeed very few of them in which I would want to turn the specific treatment over to the parent. The nonspecific treatment—perhaps, yes. You might say to a busy father,

"Your son loves you but you never have anything to do with him. Take some week-ends off and go hunting with him or to a football game, or go out and play golf with him. Do the things he wants to do." That's another thing, mind you. This general getting together for the purpose of letting the lad know that his father loves him, of giving the lad more access to his father for identification, that is all right. But I should be very loath to explain the specific handling of the inner situation to the parent and then let the parent take over.

STUDENT. How about a normal lad? Can the parent attempt any explanation?

DR. MURRAY. That would be all right, but on this basis—that the parent tell the child he's perfectly free to ask about these sexual matters if he ever wants to. It would be a mistake for the parent to walk into the lad's sexual life with any kind of descriptive talk. For this reason a parent can make the mistake of excessively inhibiting a lad by being critical of his masturbatory tendencies. He can hurt him even more by telling him not to worry about it at all, that sex is all right. For the lad not only needs to express his erotic feelings, he also needs to express his ideals and to hold on to the assets he is using every day in inhibiting these tendencies. His problem is to keep his sexual tendencies well under control from within. So you can hurt the lad even more deeply, if in some way you violate that, than if you inhibit him too much. If the father goes to the boy and says, "Any time you want to talk to me about sex, it's O.K. You're as free to talk with me about that as about anything else," that's all right. But to force it on him is a mistake, for it may make the boy retreat within himself. Generally, I'd say it is better that some neutral person bring these facts to the boy's attention, someone for whom the lad has a lot of respect, whom he likes very much.

STUDENT. Dr. Murray, the lecture this morning was on boy psychology. Is girl psychology very different from that?

DR. MURRAY. Yes, yes, it's quite different. If you're interested in that, I'd refer to the chapters on preadolescence and adolescence in Helene Deutsch's book, *Psychology of Women*.*

* Helene Deutsch. Psychology of Women: A Psychoanalytic Interpretation. Volume 1, Girlhood, 1944; Volume 2, Motherhood, 1945. New York, Grune and Stratton, Inc.

Clinical Problems*

II

1. A PATIENT WITH BACKACHE

Complaint. This patient is a housewife, aged fifty-five, whose complaint is pain in the back. The pain began at the time of an illness, probably an acute arthritic episode, sixteen years ago. At that time she had a series of intravenous vaccine shots. She obtained almost complete relief, except for this residual pain in her back. Her present back pain started about nine years ago. She began noticing pain over the right sacroiliac region, occasionally transmitted to the leg. The pain is not affected by coughing or sneezing or by any particular activity except hanging up clothes or doing housework. She has no relief from it in bed; in fact, sometimes she has as much difficulty in bed as when she is up. The pain is no better and no worse in the morning than in the evening. She describes the pain as a shooting pain—like needles going through her back. Some days, she says, she feels fine; other days not so good, in fact, simply terrible. She now receives vaccine treatment once a month, and for two days after that her pain is completely gone. In addition to this difficulty with her back, the woman has diabetes but this is under good control and does not cause her much concern.

Personal History. This woman was born in Poland and came to the United States when she was nineteen. Her religion is Jewish. Little was learned about her education. She married shortly after she came to this country and had three children. Her husband died in an accident, about the time that her present pain started. Shortly after this one daughter had a nervous breakdown and was put in a rest home. Two years later, because of criticism, she brought her daughter home, although she had not recovered. Subsequently, as the result of an accident, the daughter became partly para-

---

* Excerpts from discussion in section meetings when patients had been seen but once. In the cases reported under the heading "Clinical Problems," histories have been condensed and organized under formal headings for the reader's convenience. In these cases, and also in the dry clinic cases reported later, personal data have been altered freely and many details elicited by the physician have been omitted in order to mask the patient's identity.

lyzed. The daughter can now walk with crutches but the mother says she is really not much improved.

As to finances, this woman is dependent on the earnings of another daughter and a married son. Her chief concern about home matters is that she has sole responsibility for the care of this invalid daughter and for the housework. She spoke matter-of-factly about her daughter, however. Her one show of resentment came out when, in connection with finances, she was asked whether she was receiving an old age pension. She flared up and said, "I'm not as old as I look. I'm only fifty-five. After all, remember what I've been through. I've worked so hard, my daughter is an invalid, and my husband was killed."

DR. ROMANO. Backache, then, is this patient's principal complaint?

DR. S. (STUDENT). Yes, aside from all the hard work she has to do, which she seems to think is the cause of her backache.

DR. ROMANO. How disabled is she because of the backache?

DR. S. Not very much disabled. She does all her housework—baking, cleaning, washing, all those things.

DR. ROMANO. And yet she has been coming to this hospital for sixteen years? Did you get any data regarding the onset of the complaint?

DR. S. She dates some of it to the acute arthritic episode sixteen years ago. At that time she had an acute attack—pain, fever, and so on—which was apparently very much benefited by therapy but not completely cured. She continued to have some episodes of backache. The onset of the present exacerbation dated partly from her husband's death and very definitely from her daughter's illness.

DR. ROMANO. What determines the fluctuations in the pain?

DR. S. Nothing that I could learn of. She says there are days when she feels wonderful and then, without cause or reason, come days when she has to go to bed.

DR. ROMANO. Did you examine her physically? What did you find?

DR. S. There was nothing particular that we noted, although we did not have all the necessary instruments. Her back movement was very good. Standing with toes and heels together, she could bend forwards, backwards, sidewards, and twist. There was no tenderness on percussion of the spine. She had had x-rays. They showed a hypertrophic type of arthritis of the entire spine, more marked in the dorsal region than in the lumbar. Her pain is all in the lumbar region.

DR. ROMANO. Were you able to get any information about her early life?

DR. S. She came here at nineteen. Her parents died many years ago.

DR. ROMANO. So you have no idea what experiences she had as a child or what her relations with her parents were?

DR. S. No, all we know is her family life since marriage. Her husband was a second-hand-clothes dealer.

DR. ROMANO. As I understand it, you are now faced with the problem of determining how far the patient's symptoms are related to or caused by psychological factors and also of determining whether her symptoms are neurotic. Unfortunately, the practice of reaching a diagnosis of neurosis through exclusion of demonstrable physical or laboratory signs continues. The diagnosis of neurosis, like the diagnosis of any illness, must be determined by positive data. We know, too, that the presence of physical signs does not necessarily exclude neurosis. Positive data are usually obtained by getting information about (1) the onset of the illness, its acuteness, social setting; (2) the emotional climate of the patient at that time; (3) the precipitating factor; (4) the presence or absence of a pertinent area of conflicting emotions; (5) the gains or purposes of the illness; (6) the determinants of the "choice" of the symptom.

Other factors include the nature of her family, her early life experiences as they relate to feeding, weaning, toilet-training, discipline and siblings; to her performance in school, work, and play; to her sexual maturity; to the cultural pattern in which she lives; to changes she's had to adapt to; to illness and to responsibility. In this latter regard you want to get an idea of which adaptive devices the patient has used, how effectively they have been used, and when failure occurred.

From what you tell me, this woman may have had one or more precipitating factors; the death of her husband, the disability of her daughter, the responsibility of caring for this dependent daughter, may certainly be focal points which could generate a number of these reactions. She may be thinking, "Here I am working my fingers to the bone taking care of her. Who's taking care of me?" That would be one thing. "I've lost my husband. Not only have I lost him but now I have to continue to take care of a child." This may provoke many other feelings.

Some women, some mothers, may utilize such an experience to control or smother a child. I think it would be necessary to get more information before one could go further.

DR. COTTRELL. It would be interesting to know more about the daughter. Certainly we wonder what kind of relationship there is between mother and daughter, and what was the cause for the onset of the daughter's original illness. I think Dr. S. did mention that the patient felt she had to bring her daughter home. Jewish people, as you know, don't tolerate the thought of having their children in institutions, so with the pressure of the community and of her friends, who apparently felt she should bring her daughter home, she did so.

DR. ROMANO. I think that's a very important point, which may have a number of interpretations. However, it's difficult for me to know exactly what's going on, because I don't know the nature of the daughter's illness. Mrs. Wickman, what would be your thoughts about this as a case worker?

MRS. WICKMAN. I was thinking in terms of the possible ambivalent feeling between mother and daughter.

DR. ROMANO. This whole matter of the care by family members of a sick person, whether it be parent or child, brings up what Mrs. Wickman calls ambivalence. Ambivalence is a technical term to describe the harboring of love and hate at the same time. When one finds a situation such as this, where a patient may have had a traumatic experience (in this case, the death of her husband), it may generate a great number of emotional reactions. Later we will discuss grief. When grief is prolonged, it becomes abnormal, what we call a depression, clinically. Many times it has to do with ambivalent feelings toward the lost loved person. This ambivalence is often seen in the emotional attitudes of members of the family toward the sick or disabled members of the family. The mother or son or daughter who has the responsibility of caring for a sick and dependent child or parent often feels guilt over his occasional annoyance, anger, resentment in being shouldered with this responsibility. With chronic illness, disability, deformity, or mutilation, this may be exaggerated.

I think it may be possible, on a superficial level, to explain to this woman that it is natural at times to feel oppressed by the burden of taking care of a sick person and that it's all right to have occasional hostile thoughts.

I should think that a case worker could be of considerable help in respect to lightening this woman's burden. Perhaps a housekeeper could be utilized or perhaps the daughter should be hospitalized. That decision should be shared with this woman so that her own guilt in making arrangements would be lightened. But through environmental help and through the use of social case work, I believe she could be helped and we would learn more about her.

If I were to have this woman as a patient in my clinic, I'd talk with her and try to find out whether she is ready to have a case worker visit her in her home. If so, the case worker would attempt to see how sick and incapacitated the daughter is and to determine the nature of the relationship between mother and daughter. What is the financial situation? How much gratification does the woman get out of coming to the hospital? Those of us who work in urban areas know that for some chronically ill or disabled patients the chief pleasure in life is taking the trolley car to the hospital once a week. If that's the situation with this woman, it would be wrong to take that pleasure away from her at this time. So I think that the first step would be to find out whether she is ready to have somebody help her.

I would go about it that way, because in an instance like this, at the level at which we are operating, what you want to do is to get a picture of the social situation and see how healthy or how neurotic this woman's attitudes are to the life which she lives and to the situation which this life presents to her. From that you may see that the backache may be utilized in a great number of ways. The backache may be her need to say, "I am sick, too," or "I am a martyr, for even with my backache I have to be the good mother and the kind mother to the disabled child."

You have to remember, too, the religious factor and the minority group's code in respect to protection of the group and keeping everything within the family. What has to be done for the girl? There are so many questions to be answered. Of chief importance is the question, What pressure is there for the mother in assuming that whole responsibility?

When you have a disabled person on whom the family spends all their time (as in the case of some feeble-minded children), there is likely to be very great ambivalence about it. Doctors will say, "Well, Mrs. Jones, I think the wisest thing to do and the kindest thing to do for yourself and the family and the other children and for the child would be for you to place the child in an institution." "I'll never do that," says the mother. "While there's life in my body I'll take care of this child." When that leads to the detriment of the family structure, it is harmful. You cannot by edict say, "You should do this," but you can perhaps help the mother and father to find out why they are so tenacious in their insistence, for some of that insistence is based on feeling guilty.

STUDENT. When we were students in medical school and had a Jewish patient, the first thing that entered our minds was that, whether or not he had something physically wrong with him, this person was neurotic. In this case you have a patient who has some hypertrophic arthritis. How are you going to judge how much physical pain she is having when you know that basically she is emotionally unstable? Where do you draw the line?

DR. ROMANO. You have two points there. First, about the incidence of neurosis among people of the Jewish religion. (They are a religious group; not a nationality or a race.) Personally I think the incidence of neurosis among them has been greatly exaggerated. When you deal with large groups of people of all religions and cultures and intelligence levels, as we do in large city clinics, you find there is no marked propensity for any one group to have any specific kind of symptoms.

Your second question is, "How much of this pain is real (that is, structural) and how much is due to emotional forces?" That brings us back to the point we started from and that is, "How does one make a diagnosis of a neurosis? Does one make it by excluding physical disease?" The answer is no. One doesn't make the diagnosis by excluding physical disease alone, one has to have *positive* data.

My hunch in this instance would be, with the insufficient data, that the patient is unconsciously utilizing the experience which she had sixteen years ago, the acute febrile arthritic episode. At that time she probably was cared for and so that has special meaning for her. It has meaning not only because it was a period in which she was sick but also because it was a period in which she was dependent. She was cared for and she was loved. It was also a period before her husband's death, which may have been a period of normal gratification for her. So now, when she is facing frustrations and difficulties, she may have some pain from this arthritis. She does have pain, but whether the pain is due to these actual spicules of the bone or whether the pain is due to the psychological utilization of this whole experience is something that we don't know.

My thought in this case would be that this woman may be utilizing to a certain degree, in a neurotic fashion, a pain which she formerly experienced, probably to help her solve her present conflict as to what she should do. She is a widow; she is dependent upon her children for sustenance. She, in turn, has another daughter dependent on her for her day-to-day living. Can that generate a conflict? Yes, it can—namely, this, "I have been deprived of certain things; I'm not getting very much out of life. Why should I have to spend all my time and energy in order to take care of my daughter? But I can't think of a thing like that—that's awful." That's what her unconscious may be saying to her. "I can't let a thought like that even exist. I can't even talk about such a thing, much less think about it. I just can't let it come out. It's too bad—too wrong." Further information and study will confirm or correct our initial impressions. Are you going to see this patient again?

DR. COTTRELL.   We're going to see her again, and then we are going to ask some of these questions that have been brought up and ascertain whether or not she wants further help and, if so, of what nature. If we find that, although she's a relatively unstable person, this burden is some sort of gratification to her, we'll have to consider whether it is not best to let sleeping dogs lie.

DR. ROMANO.   That's quite right. Your job really is to find out whether the dogs are sleeping. It is very important for a doctor to know when not to do something. A great surgeon knows when not to operate. We should learn when not to interfere. If this woman is reasonably well compensated, leave her alone, especially if you do not have the facilities to carry through with psychological treatment.

I think that this is a point that young doctors and case workers find hard to accept. Experience and maturity help one to keep one's therapeutic intent in spite of limitations, but to direct it wisely and to avoid becoming quixotic. We have to be able to handle our own anxieties when dealing with the anxieties of other people. When you have a reasonable degree of understanding of your own emotional problems and are able to be reasonably objective in studying other people's problems and don't get too disturbed about them, then you are a good doctor.

STUDENT. Would you say that if a patient comes to a doctor with the symptoms this woman has he is not compensated?

DR. ROMANO. No, it depends on the degree of disability. If, for instance, this woman's backache led her to stay in bed, so that the active daughter had to give up her work to take care of her mother and sister, then I would say she was decompensated. But since this woman is able to do the laundry and other housework, I'd say she is getting along fairly well. But we don't know yet why she comes back to the hospital repetitively—whether it's just on the doctor's request or whether she gets some gratification out of coming. If the latter is the case, I'd say let her come back. There are many people we have to see on a supportive basis in an outpatient clinic.

DR. COTTRELL. This woman has a friendly feeling toward the hospital. The hospital has done a lot for her, and I think she enjoys coming here once in a while. By coming here she gets away from home and becomes a person with definite rights and privileges. We must remember that she isn't urging that something be done. After all, she has a right to have some help once in a while in doing the washing and all that, and since she can't get that help, at least she has a right to say she has a backache. Coming to the hospital confirms that right.

DR. ROMANO. That's a very good point. In fact, I think that if there's going to be a second interview with this woman, the doctor should make her understand that he is aware of some of her difficulties. There is danger in going too far in that direction: you don't want to make an invalid out of her, you want to keep her going. However, the doctor's attitude of understanding and acceptance will probably help her to share with him some of her more important emotional attitudes to her family and to her backache.

2. A PATIENT WITH HEADACHE

Complaint. This girl, aged twenty, has as her chief complaint blurring of vision, blacking-out, and headaches. The onset was very specific; a year ago, when she was sitting at home with guests, she suddenly was able to see only part of the people around her. The blurring vision lasted about fifteen minutes, followed by a severe headache. There was no vomiting; she never has had any vomiting with her headaches. The headaches have gradually increased until now they occur several times a week. Sometimes there is no blurring of vision; at other times there is blurring of vision and no headache. The headaches have never been so severe that they have interfered with her scholastic work, but she has had to miss school at times. She has been coming to this clinic for about a year but has had no relief. Now she is to have a spinal puncture. She's been told her condition may be due to nerves.

As to past physical history, this girl had polio at the age of sixteen. There was involvement of the muscles of the legs from polio and some atrophy, especially of the calf group. However, she had Kenny treatment for eight months, almost from the onset, and is able to get along quite well—dances, goes out, and apparently she does not pay too much attention to this defect. At least, she said she doesn't. She did state, however, that she has crying spells and gets depressed for no reason that she can see. She made this statement only at the very end of the interview.

Personal History. The girl's parents are living and well; her mother, however, is nervous. The patient was rather indefinite as to her father's occupation. She has one brother and one sister, both well. Nobody in the family has had sick headaches. The sister is a senior in a denominational college, where this girl is a freshman. The patient is probably not very happy about her school, for she prefers another one. She apparently has a good scholastic record, but her sister is brilliant and at the top of everything. The patient, however, says, very lightly, that she is perfectly satisfied; she hasn't flunked and school doesn't bother her much.

This girl has had a rather odd and confusing history of living arrangements. At the age of ten she went to live with an aunt and stayed there a year and a half. Then she returned home—for no special reason, she said; she just wanted to go home. Then after getting polio she was brought back here for treatment and again stayed with her aunt for a year or more. However, after returning home this last time she has visited her aunt only a few times. I understand from other sources that the aunt is a rather domineering person. The mother, too, the girl said, is the one who makes the decisions in the family.

DR. ROMANO. Will you describe this girl's behavior during the interview? What did she do, and what did she look like?

DR. F. (STUDENT). Well, it struck me that she certainly was unperturbed about her general condition. She seemed to try to make light of it. She was always smiling—I'd ask her a question and she would answer it and then smile. She had quite a few facial movements—arching her eyebrows and wrinkling up her face. There was no resentment of any kind that I could make out. This was a fine world—take it as it comes— happy-go-lucky type of appearance.

DR. ROMANO. She was somewhat coy, too, wasn't she? Here was a girl who was having very frequent headaches and yet wasn't especially disturbed about them. That was my feeling as I talked to her. The second thing was that in obtaining the history from her it was difficult to get an accurate chronological sequence. Both of those points are interesting and important. The one is her indifference, the disparity between the behavior of the patient and the nature of the presenting complaint. The second point is that whenever a patient has considerable difficulty in recounting details of past illnesses, particularly if they are recent, and is vague, circumstantial, or circuitous, or leaves gaps or omissions in the history, it usually means that some of these experiences are invested with special emotional charge or the patient is experiencing a disturbance of cerebral metabolism.

What are some of the significant points about which you would like further information for a better understanding of this girl's problem?

DR. F. Well, certainly we'll have to learn more about her attitude and relationship to her sister, who is apparently the shining light in the family. I also want to find out why she has had this peculiar mode of living, that is, living with her aunt when normally she would be at home. Third, I would like to know just why there was the onset of the original headache at this particular time. It looks like a migraine headache, but she was very specific about the onset. She was sitting at her aunt's home with guests—friends of the family—and for no reason that she knows of she had a sudden onset of scotomata—scintillating —something like looking up at the sun.

DR. ROMANO. In migraine headaches we're dealing *probably* with a mechanism which produces some change in the caliber of blood vessels, in the brain and outside the brain. Lately there has been evidence accumulated that migraine often occurs not in specific types of personality but in people who are experiencing some type of rage, anger, or hostility, which they do not express outwardly, which is not discharged in the normal channel of motor activity or speech but seems to be put away. The emotion, then, may have as a physiologic concomitant certain changes in the caliber of blood vessels. You can show that very clearly in the hand. With plethysmographic methods you can demonstrate vasoconstriction. The point is, does this also take place in the brain? There is some indirect evidence that it probably does. And also that the headache is probably due to vasodilatation which may follow vasoconstriction of the extracerebral vessels.

STUDENT. Should you be able to get a migraine, then, on a hypertension?

DR. ROMANO. There's supposed to be a distinction between headaches—hypertensive headaches and migrainous headaches—but I've seen a great number of patients who have migraine with hypertension.

There is another point in this case, another critical issue, I think— the girl's sexual adjustment. She's just twenty. We don't know much about her dating and parties. I think probably the polio has an emotional significance there. I'm sure she is what we call technically a somewhat narcissistic person, a person who has very little love going out, who keeps most of it inside. I think one would guess from her behavior that she is such a person. When you consider the significance of a physical disability, particularly of the leg and calf and thigh, to a young attractive girl with her need to be loved and to love herself, I think it would be quite a blow to be disfigured as this girl is.

DR. COTTRELL.   And that illness would have focused a lot of attention upon herself, too, with the continuous treatment in an important period of her developmental life.

DR. ROMANO.   Considering this case as an internist—for a decision and in outlining a program—I would want to see her a number of times. I very much question whether a lumbar puncture should be done on her. Her previous neurological examinations, I understand, were negative. I made another brief neurological examination yesterday, and there seemed to be no pertinent findings. What one would gain from a lumbar puncture I don't know. I think the harm that might come from it would outweigh any possible good.

Speaking of neurological examinations, I think you should make one every time you do a physical examination. Gross neurological screening can be done in three or four minutes and provides valuable clues. You can make three or four simple tests, and then if you do find something significant, you can be more detailed in your examination.

First, you can have the patient read a newspaper—one eye and then the other eye—and so get fairly good Snellen acuity in respect to vision; and you can test pupils very readily—much better with sunlight than with a flashlight. You can test extraocular movements, and of course you should use an ophthalmoscope. If the patient is able to hear the rubbing of your fingers at three inches, he usually has normal hearing, unless there are some particular subjective complaints. Movements of the head and grimacing, squeezing the eyes, and showing the teeth will show you facial innervations—upper and lower face. Have the patient stick out his tongue, bite, and then put out his hands, so that you can watch for a tremor; then the finger-to-nose test and the reflexes—knee and ankle jerks. (As to the pin test, a pin is a dangerous instrument; you get so many subjective interpretations of appreciation of pain, touch, and other things that if there is no specific disturbance you'd better not use it.) Then have the patient stand up, toes and heels together, look up at the ceiling, and close his eyes; and watch for sway. After stroking the sole of the foot for a plantar flexion or extension of the big toe, you have essentially completed a brief neurological examination. A good doctor would be able to do that in a very short time. If there are positive data of significance, you can go further.

I think everybody who has had headaches for a period of time should have that examination, but I don't think that a lumbar puncture is indicated as a matter of routine. Nor is there routine need for serial films of the skull or for an electroencephalogram, a brain wave. I think those examinations should be made only when there are indications for them. There are dangers, you know, in doing too many things and in protracting laboratory tests over a period of time. You keep a sword of Damocles over the patient's head, because you don't let him know what you think his trouble is due to. You have to have the courage of your convictions about what you think is wrong and get on to it and to the tests you think are indicated.

So I wouldn't do a lumbar puncture in this twenty-year-old girl who has symptoms which appear to indicate an hysterical utilization of migraine. Her appearance in the clinic was that of an hysterical girl. Her whole behavior indicated that, and I should think one would wish to know more about her. Why was she allowed to leave home? What was the significance of going to her aunt's? Did she find herself there the only child, a loved person, a fairy princess, away from the home where she had the rivalry of an older sister who was smart and got all the kudos? Now that she's going to the same school as the sister, and the sister gets all the honors and is outstanding in the senior class, while she is a lowly freshman, perhaps that rivalry and her feelings of hostility toward her sister play some part in this disorder of hers. I don't know, but one should consider such possibilities.

Now what should an internist do about a problem like this? Should he work with it himself or should he refer a girl like this to a psychiatrist? I can't answer these questions because we don't have enough information as yet about this girl. I feel that a girl like this could be helped to a certain degree by an internist who has some understanding of personality functions and of emotional relationships. I think that after two or more interviews it may be possible to find out just what issues the girl is facing and to help her see more clearly and more consciously some of her feelings toward her older sister. You could tell her, in a very superficial way, it's all right to want these things and to envy her sister. Tell her she may have assets of her own and may be able to achieve independence and maturity herself. Then, too, it might be possible in a case like this to make some environmental changes. I think perhaps going to a different school, which she is planning to do next year, may give her a chance for individual expression.

STUDENT. I'd like to know more about the contraindications for lumbar puncture in this case.

DR. ROMANO. A lumbar puncture should be done only when there are pertinent indications for it. This groping in the dark, looking for occasional data, looking for an answer to a puzzle without evidence that you may find it through a lumbar puncture is specious reasoning. The incidence of post-lumbar-puncture headache is high. It is a headache which physiologically is probably due to a decrease in the pressure of fluid in the subarachnoid space as a result of loss of fluid volume. There probably is a considerable amount of leakage from the area, even when one uses a small needle. And you can't use too small a bore, for then you don't get normal pressure readings. What happens is that the patient, twelve to eighteen hours after the lumbar puncture, has a headache, and it may be quite severe. With this there may be nausea, vomiting, a stiff neck, even fever, all of which may frighten the patient. Then the doctor may do another lumbar puncture because he is frightened, too. The headache is then prolonged for another few days.

Now the danger of doing a lumbar puncture on a girl like this, on any neurotic person, is, first, that there may be unconscious or conscious exploitation of it. "Something really must be wrong with me if the doctors do this!" Second, she may get sick from it, she may have a headache from it. If she does, that may be utilized unconsciously in a neurotic sense to prolong the disability. This girl may be striving for a return to the period of regression which she must have had during the polio attack, when she probably felt herself a loved child again. So those are the dangers—promoting invalidism, provoking pain, which in turn may be utilized. That's why any such procedure should be looked at very clearly and honestly. You must say, "Well, this is the information I'll get. Does it outweigh the disadvantages that the procedure may obtain?"

STUDENT. Is it usual for an individual who has had a period of regression to retrench or retreat to the same point when another problem arises? It seems to me that in this case the patient would be a little more apt to retrench in her rivalry with her sister by utilizing the polio.

DR. ROMANO. That is possible. You raise the question, Why this choice of symptom? I don't know. Let's assume it's a competitive rivalry situation that is the basic problem. Why doesn't she develop pain in her right leg or weakness there?

Theoretically this could happen and does happen many times. Theoretically, also, other things may happen. It may be that to a certain degree she is denying her polio; I think we both felt she was. She was minimizing her disability and to some extent whistling in the dark about it. It may be that her disability is compensated for by that mechanism. She has to use another one, then. But the question is pertinent. That's one of the fundamental points in diagnosis of a neurosis—what are the determinants that lead to the specific symptom? Why does unexpressed rage in one person lead to migraine, in another to hypertension, in a third to vasodepressor syncope, and in still another to a depression? I don't know. Modern psychology can't answer that as yet.

STUDENT. What would a normal reaction to her sister have been?

DR. ROMANO. A healthy reaction would have been to feel somewhat envious about her and somewhat competitive about her but to have been able to reach out for certain goals independently and to achieve some satisfactions, so that she didn't have to be so envious. We don't know which part rivalry may play in this instance. Both of us felt she was denying in an overdetermined way any degree of rivalry.

Psychotherapy

JOHN ROMANO, M.D.

THE concept of psychotherapy has been somewhat mysterious and confusing to many doctors. For a very simple and realistic definition, one could say that psychotherapy is the utilization of psychological measures in the treatment of sick people. In a very broad sense the variations of psychotherapy fall into two great types. The purpose of one type is to allay anxiety, to reassure, to bring about certain changes in the environment which may help to minimize the intensity of the noxious factors presented to the patient. The other type of therapy is sometimes called the uncovering type; it uses methods and techniques which aim at finding out some of the motivations for the behavior as they relate to inner forces which may come into conflict with other parts of the personality.

Now I think it is generally accepted that the type of psychotherapy which is practical and utilizable by general practitioners is the first type —namely, the type of psychotherapy that uses education, reassurance, and support, the management of patients' problems either directly or through the intermediary of other people or agencies. I shall speak in more detail about those methods later today.

I think, however, that the fundamental basis of psychotherapy consists of the patient-physician relationship, which Dr. Kaufman and Dr. Murray have been talking about in the past few days. As you remember, Dr. Kaufman told you that the traditional and conventional doctor-patient relationship is a blend of certain realistic factors and certain symbolic factors. Realistically, the doctor is a skilled person, the doctor is a person with special knowledge, the doctor is a person to whom one goes for help because of his experience and skill, and because of his special knowledge. Symbolically, the doctor represents something besides this realistic figure of a man with special skills and knowledge. The symbolic aspect of the relationship, we pointed out to you, is based essentially on the fact that a sick person, because of his anxiety and because of the threats to his integrity, is more dependent and more anxious than he would be if he were well, and therefore he has a corresponding need for the authoritative and protective figure he finds in the doctor. Now it seems to me that knowledge and understanding of the basic factors of the patient-physician relationship are the crux of all psychotherapy, that the limitations we are to speak of in a moment depend primarily on the nature and the integrity and substance of this doctor-patient relationship.

But first let's speak of aims. What are the aims of psychotherapy? I'm sure that many of the aims we speak of are complementary and overlapping. The aim may be to relieve symptoms or to promote a cure. The aim may be to increase the efficiency of a person in his daily life. It may be to increase his happiness. It may be to help him accept more maturely and more efficiently certain irreversible disabilities. The aim may be to enable the person to see more clearly some forces which he has not been aware of before, to help him bring them more closely to consciousness, to his awareness, so that he may deal less blindly, less impulsively, and more consciously and more maturely with the issues before him.

Now, which people, which types of patients, should receive psychotherapy? All sick people should receive and do receive, to a greater or lesser degree, some kind of psychotherapy. Psychotherapy is not exclusively directed to the treatment of flagrantly or obviously neurotic or psychotic patients. Psychotherapy should be and is directed to a great number of people who are experiencing only normal degrees of anxiety and distress in the course of acute illnesses, in the normal problems of convalescence, in chronic disease and chronic disability, after mutilation or after surgical intervention of one kind or another. The area of psychotherapy is very wide. It has to do, essentially, with utilizing psychological measures to help sick people. With those people who are sick primarily as a result of certain emotional forces, however, certain types of psychotherapy are used more or less specifically and of this we shall speak in more detail later.

As has been intimated in Dr. Murray's two morning lectures, we find that the neurotic symptom, neurotic behavior, represents a compromise. It is an attempt at a solution, at times partially successful, never completely successful, sometimes very little successful. The neurotic symptom must be understood logically as it relates to cause-and-effect relationships. And as has been said in the lectures, we have to deal at times with conflicts between the wellspring of instinctual needs, which Dr. Murray called technically the id, and other parts of the personality which are also unconscious, which he called the super-ego, the conscience. The id represents the primal needs, those relating to being loved, to expressing anger or rage of one kind or the other, to sexual excitation, while the conscience part of our personality is the incorporation of the do's and don't's of our parents. The conflict between these two parts of the personality is regulated by and modified by and controlled by the conscious part of our personality, the I, or ego. The ego has this constant problem of trying to satisfy one side of our needs as they arise from these primitive and instinctual drives, of holding them in check in order to satisfy the conscience part of our personality, which has been determined in great part by cultural acquisition, at the same time that it has to meet adequately the problems that come to it constantly from the outside world.

What are the limitations of psychotherapy? In the practice of medicine we all know that our therapeutic goals at times are quite modest and have to be realistic. With some patients you can help to bring about a cure that not only completely relieves the symptoms but leaves no residual disturbance of any kind. With others you are able to modify the symptoms or decrease their intensity to a certain degree, so as to make life more endurable. It may be possible to minimize certain external or provoking factors so that the course of the disease will be more mild or less intense. Then there are patients for whom the only thing that one can do is to give security and confidence, to allay anxiety and pain, for other matters seem to be irreversible. And there are some whom we cannot help at all. Similarly in psychotherapy, limitations are set by various determinants. One limiting determinant is the acuteness or the chronicity of the present illness. Another is the nature of the precipitating factor, its intensity, how realistic is the problem the patient faces. For instance, grief which is naturally experienced after the death of a loved person is a realistic, understandable, more or less normal, psychological experience of man. However, a depression simu-

lating grief may occur with no demonstrable or realistic factor to provoke it; it may have symptoms with a few exceptions similar to those of
grief, but the structure and the meaningfulness and the prognostic factors in the depression are quite different from those of a normal grief
reaction. In other words, the reality of the precipitating factor, its intensity, and its acuteness, are determining factors. They are in all illnesses.

The second determinant limiting psychotherapy is the nature of the
person who is sick. How flexible is he? How emotionally healthy is he?
How adequate has he been in accepting the normal day-by-day deprivations and frustrations that all of us have to face in this world? How
satisfactory has his adjustment been? What type of psychological defenses has he had to use in his life? Has he exaggerated these defenses? Has he inhibited himself too much? Has he become too passive,
too submissive, too quiet, too restrained? Is he unable to express even
the normal degree of aggression or normal degrees of hostile feeling
toward his friends and acquaintances and his family? On the other
hand, is he a person who seems to have too little control? Is he a person who is quite impulsive and acts everything out, let's say, without any
check or any inhibition, as if he were without conscience, as do some of
the patients that have been mentioned—the so-called psychopaths? So
the nature of the person is another limiting factor.

The third determinant is the setting in which the precipitating event
takes place. The setting, the actual timing, the patient's preparation
for the precipitating event are all important. The fourth limiting factor
lies in the skill and the knowledge and the abilities of the doctor—
what range, let's say, he has in understanding and in being able to follow through his understanding of the patient's problems. Finally, and
probably most important, is the nature of the doctor-patient relationship. What capacity has the patient, what capacity has the doctor, to
engage in this relationship, so that it can become a meaningful and productive one, a relationship in which the doctor may share the experience with the patient and help him either to discharge certain emotions
that can be discharged or to utilize other means of defense that may
prove more effective and more efficient than those he has been using?

So much for the aims, so much for the limitations—now let us consider some of the techniques available to the general practitioner. These, for the most part, have as their *Leitmotiv* the use of reassurance, the allaying of anxiety, the utilization of the doctor-patient relationship to give support and security, the manipulation of certain environmental factors to minimize noxious stimuli, and so on. I've jotted down some of the means that the doctor, the general practitioner, may use. In connection with these I would like to recommend to you three papers which deal specifically with some of these points—Dr. Kaufman's paper concerning psychotherapy in general practice* and two papers by Dr. John Whitehorn.† In a book written by Dr. Maurice Levine, *Psychotherapy in Medical Practice*,‡ you'll find in the second and third chapters detailed accounts of some specific means that the general practitioner may use.

One of the methods we spoke of could be called environmental management, the arranging of environmental factors, the altering of certain aspects of the patient's environment. The goal is to minimize certain of the noxious factors in the environment, to make the environment as pleasant as possible, although we know that in adult life and in the adult neurosis most of the problems come from within a person, not from without. For example, in problems relating to a person's behavior in industry, it may be possible to confer with the employer or to utilize intermediary persons such as a social case worker, in rural communities a visiting nurse or the county health officials or some of the social workers from county welfare organizations. In other words, get them to act as intermediaries in explaining rather simply to the employer or the teacher or at times the family members, if the latter are not accessible to the doctor, that some amelioration of the difficulty could be achieved if certain environmental modifications were made. Sometimes in urban

* M. Ralph Kaufman, M.D. Psychotherapy in general medical practice. *Journal of the Maine Medical Association*, 31:235–239, September 1940.

† J. C. Whitehorn, M.D. Psychotherapy. *In* David P. Barr, Editor, Modern Medical Therapy in General Practice, volume 1. Baltimore, William Wood & Co., 1940.

J. C. Whitehorn, M.D. Guide to interviewing and clinical personality study. *Archives of Neurology and Psychiatry*, 52:197–216, September 1944.

‡ Maurice Levine, M.D. Psychotherapy in Medical Practice. New York, The Macmillan Company, 1942.

communities a social case worker may be used not only to gather information, but also to work in association with the doctor to help the patient in his life relationships. At times material aid, such as supplementing the patient's income, may be utilized. At times a homemaker or housekeeper or the like may be put into the home by family agencies and children's agencies, which are being used more and more by general practitioners and internists in some urban areas. The essential principle is to try to alter certain aspects of the environment through explanations, through guidance, through suggestions, through various key people, whether they be schoolteachers, employers, members of the family. This manipulative method may at times involve helping a patient to plan a daily regimen, a daily set of activities—but not too rigidly, not too pedantically. At times planning may give the patient a feeling of security, a feeling of being buttressed by knowing what he should do in the next hour, or that afternoon, and so on. Together with this, there may be some encouragement for socialized living, for the use of groups such as the YMCA and clubs of one kind or the other.

There's a second method which may be called educational. This makes use of explanation—explaining matters to the patient, giving advice. Many times, most times, explanations and advice should be restricted to the current situation. We all know there is danger in giving advice too early or too dogmatically, but it is possible for the doctor to clear up certain misconceptions by explanation. There is a tremendous amount of information concerning health and disease being disseminated to the public today. I think that relations between medicine and the public should be improved and should be expanded, and some of this information is sound and good. But with it there is being spread a tremendous amount of misinformation, and also information which is not incorrect but which mobilizes the anxieties of patients about nutrition, disease, and emotional factors. So the physician has the right and the duty to explain certain superficial misconceptions and misconstructions.

A third type of therapy usable by general practitioners is what may be called supportive therapy. The physical examination may play a part in this. The physical examination has tremendous importance as a means of acquiring data concerning the emotional structure and the emotional problems of the patient; the degree of anxiety, the amount of sweating, blushing, blanching, exaggerated modesty, muscle tension, tremor, a hundred other facts may be noted during the examination. The physical examination may also be utilized as a means of reassurance. Explain procedures clearly and simply to the patient, avoid prolonging examinations and prolonging ancillary laboratory tests and keeping a sword of Damocles hanging over the patient's head for a long time. Avoid telling the patient about insignificant data which have no relevance to the problem at hand—the minimal cardiac murmur, the hemorrhoidal tag, the occasional bruise, the this or that, or the minor laboratory datum which seems to have no significance. This requires courageous conviction in coming to a definite diagnostic conclusion and in not resorting to unnecessary tests that allay the doctor's anxiety but not the patient's.

For the physical examination to be of considerable value, the doctor needs to have some understanding of the normal range of modesty, the normal range of anxiety of a woman, for instance, who is having a pelvic examination. He must be aware of the sensitivity of the adolescent boy who is afraid that his masturbation may be expressed in circles under his eyes or in the way he walks or acts. One needs to have awareness of the significance of the physical examination in order to utilize it constructively and directly as a means of reassurance.

There are also certain suggestive means of therapy. Hydrotherapy, for example, has been used since time immemorial. It is probably a combination of means of relaxing certain tensions: the patient meets with a host of very pleasant stimuli; it is obviously a pleasant, regressive experience, which may help the patient to relax physiologically and may give him a certain feeling of security. Or other physical methods may be used. A patient may feel unduly sensitive because of obesity—and the doctor may recommend limitation of food intake. The dermatologist knows very well the tremendous intensity of emotional feeling in the adolescent about acne and how certain measures which bring about improvement in that condition may help. Similarly with problems like strabismus or other distortions or mutilations of the body; correcting them may be of some help in decreasing the sensitivity which they have intensified. It's possible to use drugs. By and large, it's been my experience that it is unwise to use placebos, that eventually patients find out they've been tricked and that the doctor-patient relationship may thus be shattered. It is possible to carry on several types of psychotherapy at the same time. It is also possible to give psychotherapy at the same time one is giving drugs, whether they be digitalis or a sulfa drug or a chemical sedative. Certain drugs may be of value in helping to allay tension or to promote more adequate sleep.

There's another type of psychotherapy. I have spoken of manipulative, educational, supportive therapy, and just now I mentioned relief of emotional tensions. Well, obviously, one means of relief of emotional tension is the interview. The interview certainly is the principal means by which the patient can discharge some of his pent-up feelings, emotions; can at times, with the help of the doctor, see more clearly their source, their origin, their direction; and in so doing get some relief. Whether this is called ventilation, whether it's called aeration, whether it's called catharsis, whether it's given other names doesn't matter; essentially, through the interview the patient is able to discharge some tension and secure some emotional relief. However, one can use other means, too. One can, for example, use work as a means of relieving tension. One can utilize occupational therapy or the development of hobbies or, in respect to certain aggressive feelings, one can utilize athletic sports for this purpose. Similarly one can guide patients into certain types of diversion and entertainment. For these, too, are means by which release of emotional tension may be brought about to a greater or lesser degree.

Finally, a few principles. One is that by and large it is much wiser to err in omission than in commission. In other words, let sleeping dogs lie. If the dogs are actually sleeping, if one has a fairly good idea that the problem is reasonably well compensated and the person has made a pretty good adjustment to his difficulties, it is much wiser to let such people alone or to deal with them in a superficially protective or supportive way.

The second principle for the general practitioner and the internist to follow is to keep to conscious material, not to utilize uncovering techniques unless he knows what to do with the unconscious material when it appears. The third principle is that it is unwise to provoke anxiety in a patient if the provocation of that anxiety has little purpose or value or meaning at the time, or if there is no means of utilizing constructively the provoked anxiety in order to see more clearly a problem which is deep or hidden.

Next, avoid judgmental dictates; avoid moral, prejudicial, dictatorial attitudes. We teach our students to avoid extremes of the pendulum—to avoid being maudlin or mawkish or sentimental but, on the other hand, to avoid being punitive or judgmental. A doctor must try to be objective: that means he must try to be warm, understanding, accepting; it does not mean he should identify blindly with the patient (to use Dr. Murray's term) and lose his objectivity.

Next, when in doubt it's wise to keep your mouth shut. There is danger in premature Pollyannaism, in premature statements to the patient that he's going to be all right, he's going to be perfectly all right this time, and so on, when naturally the patient many times thinks, "Well, how can he say that? I have no evidence that he really knows what's going on in me. And how can he tell that I'm going to be all right?" Such premature statements may result in a break in confidence, a break in the faith that the patient has in the doctor. So avoid premature pronouncements and interpretations.

Next, don't talk too much. This principle is one of the points we've discussed in connection with interviewing; that of trying to give the patient a feeling of lots of time even when you don't have lots of time. Try to give the patient the feeling that you are interested, that you do want to help him; let your attitude, facial expression, your movements generate confidence and generate the feeling that the patient is being understood.

These are some of the points I want to make in this introduction to psychotherapy. As I understand it, Dr. Murray, and next week Dr. Brosin, will continue with other aspects of that subject. Now we'll have a general discussion.

DISCUSSION

STUDENT. I would like to ask when insight is dangerous so far as the particular patient is concerned—for instance, the patient with excoriations of the skin which have been interpreted as representing his unconscious attempt at suicide. If you remove that crutch you expose him, and therefore he has to resort to a more serious mental disturbance.

DR. MURRAY.   I may start on a somewhat narrow point, but the question brings to mind a case we had this morning in our seminar discussion. A fifty-two-year-old woman was childless and was frigid. She had had an inadequate life relationship with her husband because of an infantile emotional component of her own, and she was now approaching mid-life and was on the edge, directly on the brink, of an agitated depression. Now here is the situation par excellence. To show this woman the background of life frustrations upon which her current symptoms are dependent would probably mean to precipitate her into a frank and serious psychosis or, if not, into a situation with no way out except suicide. In other words, merely to face her with the reality of her life situation would be to put her into a blind alley of hopelessness. The treatment technique of choice in practically all circumstances in cases of this kind would necessarily be supportive and environmental.

In other cases the decision might be different. Suppose, for instance, we had known this woman twenty years ago, when the long-time effect of the factors which are responsible for her illness today could have been foreseen, and we had wanted to put her under treatment. At that time it would have been equally dangerous to try to give her insight except in a situation where a prolonged period of treatment was possible. She would have needed this in order to make a gradual transition from her immature emotional development to a more mature phase. If that were not possible, then even if she were only thirty years old we should hesitate to go in and tear down her own defenses only to leave her bare to the breezes of a worse situation. I think this is the kind of situation in which one must exercise the greatest degree of restraint; it illustrates, often dramatically, the point that one must certainly avoid rushing in where angels fear to tread.

DR. KAUFMAN.   I think the fact that the student asked the question proves that he knows the answer. And that is all there is to it. It is a matter of what you are confronting the patient with, with what kind of insight. Take the example he gave. Suppose you find that a skin lesion is an unconscious attempt at suicide and you tell that to the patient. She is left with only one of two alternatives: either she calls you a damned fool and says, "It's all right; if I can't commit suicide this way, I won't commit suicide," or she is driven to actual suicide. You must remember a very simple point: our insight isn't always the patient's knowledge, and a premature confrontation is a very dangerous thing. We must always be sure when we're giving a patient insight, so-called, that we give it in very limited doses and within the patient's capacity to follow. It's much better to have the patient *achieve* insight than it is to *give* insight. When the patient has achieved it, this problem of confrontation doesn't exist any more.

DR. ROMANO.   I think we should mention, too, that one should not provoke anxiety, should not create or intensify anxiety when there is no logical, utilitarian, and productive use for that anxiety. I think that's the fundamental principle of any medical therapy. Before a surgeon operates, he weighs seriously the indications for his procedure. He asks, "What is the possible gain here? Does that gain outweigh the risk that we're taking?" It seems to me that's fundamental in all therapeutic measures. In psychotherapy one should not do anything which may disturb the patient, if the disturbance is of no value or can't be followed through with special skills. Telling your patient, let's say, that her skin manifestations, that her behavior of scratching, and so on, represent a symbolic attack or a self-destructive maneuver is a very harsh indictment and one which could provoke the person to very great distress.

*

I'd like to have Dr. Bauer discuss the utilization of the physical examination as a means of psychotherapy. First, what should be the attitude of the doctor toward data he has collected if they seem to have no relevance to the problem—I mentioned some of them earlier. Should these findings be told the patient? Second, when should laboratory tests be made and how many of them should be made? And third, if patients request certain laboratory procedures they have heard about from the radio or press, should one follow through on these suggestions?

DR. BAUER.   I don't know that I have much to add on the point of the physical examination. There are various ways of proceeding. Many physicians adopt the method of beginning with the part concerned in the chief complaint, and then going on with a complete physical examination. That is the procedure employed by many good psychiatric-minded physicians. Oftentimes it is a comfort to the patient. You've all seen patients who come into the hospital complaining of a pain in the leg and spend anywhere from two to eight weeks in residence and have many things found out about them but still have the pain in the leg, to which no one has paid any attention.

Surely, one should be careful about interpreting minimum physical findings. Perhaps most of them are better left unmentioned. If one refers to them at all, the reason should be very apparent to the patient. Well, it depends on the patient. If you mention them, it should be done so casually that you might just as well not mention them. In some situations, if you're in doubt, you're better off if you forget about these findings even though one of your colleagues may see the patient later and discover them. I think cardiac murmurs are excellent examples here. If even after exercise you can't be sure whether there is a presystolic murmur or not, perhaps it is just as well not to mention it.

I think that through the complete physical examination you have many ways of gaining information about the patient which you suspected in taking the history and that you establish a certain relationship with the patient on this basis. I would like to make a plea for as good a physical examination as your time permits; instead of that half-baked physical or a three-quarter physical, try to make it a habit always to do a complete physical. It isn't very difficult to illuminate sinuses in your examining room or to look at fundi or to end up doing a rectal examination and it doesn't take more than a few additional minutes once it becomes routine. I think you can speak with more assurance, and certainly your patient is more apt to believe that you know what you're talking about, when you have been over him from head to toe.

As for laboratory work, I think it's been overdone and continues to be overdone and that the problem is becoming increasingly worse rather than better. In the Army we saw excellent examples of this day in and day out. I have often told medical officers who were very concerned about the advent of socialized medicine that, with their expensive tests, they themselves were probably doing everything possible to hasten the day. This excessive use of laboratory work is in part our fault. Often we resort to it because we're insecure. We're indecisive.

We're afraid we're going to make a mistake. And there's where the wheels start rolling, and only God knows where they will end in some cases, if the patient has the wherewithal. In the rolling of these wheels one turns up certain findings—BMR of minus 19, blood cholesterol 15 milligrams per cent above the upper limit of normal, and data of that type. Then the physician who is insecure, or who hasn't taken a good history, or who doesn't know how to interpret the good history he did take and has the same reaction toward his physical examination— that physician takes refuge in the diagnostic report.

You've all seen the patient who has been anemic all his life, and has been told repeatedly, "Hemoglobin down a little bit again; have to give you a little iron." We have endless situations of that sort that have their origin in the physician's office. I think when we have finished our history and physical we should try to come to a definite decision. If that is impossible, we shouldn't be afraid either to say or to write on our history sheet that we do not know. Of course, there will be certain laboratory studies that may suggest themselves. For many of the patients that I see, I'm sure that a Wassermann, a hemoglobin, white count, a blood smear, and a urinalysis are all I would want, and I try very hard to stick to these. The piling up of tests may just lead to a lot of misinformation, some of which may be nothing more than mistakes in the laboratory. Say a patient has nocturia three times a night and the history is consistent with acute nephritis sometime back, and you learn that he has albumin in his urine with or without accompanying findings. If the specimen he brings in tomorrow morning has the specific gravity of 1.026, for all practical purposes how far should you go in determining his renal function in great detail? I think we ought to use a fair amount of judgment in such instances. You don't expect this man, who has a normal hemoglobin and the like, to show much in the way of nonprotein nitrogen retention. Yet many a patient would be lucky if that was all he had to pay for in the hands of many physicians. Same way with G.I. complaints. Such patients may have a barium enema, a Graham test, maybe a barium enema of the small bowel—all of which is very time-consuming and extremely costly, and it just prolongs this indecision on the part of the doctor and leaves the patient sitting in a very poor place. We must remember that our indecisions and our making diagnoses on inadequate evidence represent some of the factors that the doctor is responsible for in the production of disease or in the fixation of a set of symptoms which allow the patient to escape certain situations. So unless we are intelligent in the use of the history and the physical examination and make only those laboratory studies that are indicated, we're bound to do harm rather than to help the patient. The patient is usually aware that we are undecided and disturbed and not sure.

Concerning requests of patients for laboratory studies, I often tell a patient that I have his history and as far as I can determine from it he must have a perfectly good heart or he wouldn't be able to do the things he does. His physical examination is normal, but if it would make him feel better to have an electrocardiogram or a seven-foot heart plate at the expense of about $35, we will make it. Now there are some people, I'm sure, for whom you'd just be forced to carry out some of these procedures because they are determined to have them done and will insist on them. But I think, again, that if the history is a reasonably complete one and the physical examination is also, and if we speak with some degree of confidence, many of these patients are willing to accept our interpretation. But don't take refuge in laboratory work. Don't let patients run you; there's no more uncomfortable situation in the world to be in than to have some rich patient who tells you when he can eat white meat and when he can eat dark meat and a few other things. You're the boss of that wagon and you're supposed to drive it, and if you can't drive it better than that, you'd better give up taking care of the patient. You're not going to do him any good. You may be a few dollars better off at the end of the year, but I'm afraid you won't have much satisfaction because he knows all the time that he's getting away with it. And don't forget that these people who sit in our offices know a lot more about us than they ever tell us.

STUDENT. A common complaint I have heard is that a patient comes in and says that he has been to several doctors and they've never told him anything. How much should we tell patients, especially patients who have organic disease?

DR. ROMANO. Suppose a patient does have a structural disease of one kind or the other. It may be important to point out in a very simple way just what the problem is so as to enable him to accept the disability and to live within the boundaries the disability presents. But I think it's very wrong to engage in long and complicated explanations, which may be extremely confusing to the patients, when what they want to hear from you, although they may ask you for details, are words of confidence, words of reassurance that they're going to be all right. So it seems to me that one can err in not telling them anything; I think it is important and wise to give them some idea of what may be basically wrong. But one may err in overdoing that and becoming too detailed. The other point which has been made is that when there are organic findings which are insignificant and have no relevance to the problem it is wiser not to talk about them to the patient. What we should do is to explain simply and in words that the patient understands the significant factors he needs to know in order to live his life more efficiently. I don't think you should go beyond that nor do I think you should fall short of it.

DR. BAUER. I think that you can't emphasize that point too strongly: if you've got a patient with a structural disease, immediately tell him so, but also give him some security about it. That reassurance should come almost in the same sentence, and say it with meaning, for you don't need to lie even if it's a very serious situation. Say, "I know a man who has your difficulty and he's still alive at seventy-five." You aren't telling a lie. And get it in early. Get it in that first sentence. Don't have any lag there. Don't let the patient go home and come back a week later and wonder what this is all about or whether he's going to die of a gastrointestinal hemorrhage day after tomorrow as one of his neighbors did twenty years ago.

DR. JENSEN. I've learned one thing which might be helpful here. After we've made our studies and talked with the patient (though in my case it's mostly with the patient's family) I sit down and attempt to answer the questions I think will be asked. Then as I go through my story, attempting to answer the questions I assume the parents have, I remember that there may be many questions I haven't answered at all. So after I finish I usually turn it back to them and say, "Now do you have any questions?" I have found that many, many times in giving them a chance to ask questions I get in my most effective work. I don't know whether that would do with adult patients. I suspect it would. I do know it works with parents who have come to us for help about their children.

DR. BAUER.   Yes, I think we should always ask patients before they leave the office whether they have any questions or not.

DR. ROMANO.   I think there is danger, as we've all intimated, in giving a somewhat didactic and formal little talk to a patient, one with technical terms which may be very confusing to him and may in turn mobilize even more anxiety. One time I saw a house officer struggling with a fifty-year-old woman who had diabetes. He was trying to explain this, that, and so on. She turned to me afterwards and said, "Look, doctor, tell me—is it good, or is it bad?" I think we have to be realistic. Our mission isn't to explain to people the details of carbohydrate metabolism. The important thing is to talk in simple terms and to answer the universal questions which such persons have. For example, to tell a patient whether he will be able to work. People want to know if they are going to be all right. This is especially true of operations on the genitals or gynecological operations, where, with shyness and all the taboos, the patient, man or woman, may have many inhibitions about asking questions. It may take some time, but it is extremely worth while for the patients and for yourself to speak clearly and to gain their understanding.

STUDENT.   I wonder if someone would say something about the kind of words we use in talking with our patients.

DR. ROMANO.   Some time ago several of us studied the effect of medical words at the bedside of a patient in a teaching hospital. We took a vocabulary of clichés used at the bedside, such as EKG and EEG and words like prognosis and diagnosis and Wassermann, and a great number of other terms, and attempted to find out what the patient understood of these terms. We learned that there was a considerable amount of misunderstanding and ignorance about them. Some of the terms had prestige value because of newspaper, magazine and radio features, and some had unpleasant connotations. For example, the term "degenerative disease" is used very often. To most patients that meant "degenerate" and had moral value. "Nervousness," on the other hand, was a socially acceptable term, much more acceptable than "neurotic" or "psychotic," which meant nuts and screwy and bats in the belfry, and so on. It seems that language always has a few safety valves. It is possible that "nervousness" or "nervous breakdown" may sometimes even have social prestige, because it means being able to go away on a trip or to a sanitarium. At times the words we use have entirely different meaning to the patient. That's why, as Dr. Bauer and Dr. Kaufman have said, it's important to find out just what the patient thinks about the terms that you use.

As to children, as you all know they are much more alert and much more understanding than is generally supposed. Many times doctors, all of us, pediatricians and others, try to use certain terms at the bedside of a child, and of course the expression of the doctor, his averted gaze, his speaking in mumbles may be much more anxiety-provoking than a rather frank discussion at the bedside. So at times it really is not only the words you say but how you say them.

*

STUDENT. Dr. Romano, I'd like to have a discussion on the handling of patients with malignancy.

DR. ROMANO. My experience is somewhat limited, but I can tell you what I think and then I'll ask for the opinions of the others. It seems to me that there are a number of approaches to handling patients with malignancy, particularly moribund patients. One of the things we've noticed about them is that many times the patient asks directly for a dogmatic statement. "Do I have such a thing and am I going to die in a relatively short period of time?" Well, it's been our experience that often when patients say that they're really asking you not to tell them they have a malignancy but to tell them they're not going to die. Sometimes a direct question is a disguise and an indirection; actually they want your reassurance.

What I've done for the most part is never to falter in reassuring the patient. One can do it at times without making a definite statement; you can't say that the patient doesn't have something, but in various ways you can avoid saying that he does have it. And you can use reassuring techniques for a certain period of time to help such a person. Then, of course, as you know, with people dying of malignancy and other diseases, certain defenses may come to the fore, such as denial of illness and at times even feelings of ecstasy and feelings of tremendous well-being; these may occur in dying patients for some period of time right before death. And it's also the maintenance of these defenses that is important. I've seen doctors err sometimes in trying to break them or rather, challenge them, when of course they are useful defense mechanisms.

Dr. Murray, would you care to comment further on what should be told to a patient with a malignancy?

DR. MURRAY. Well, I think that's pretty well covered by your remarks. I was thinking of a somewhat similar situation which has to be handled very delicately. That's in regard to people who adopt this extreme unrealistic, euphoric attitude toward an amputation or toward blindness. In these cases I think one has to bring the reality and the meaning of the handicap to the individual, but one must do it in a decidedly positive way. I saw a man in Boston about two weeks ago who had frozen his feet and had to have two amputations and who was positively euphoric about it. I sat and talked with the man for a while and found he was pushing away the fact that he had had one foot removed and now was going to lose the other one. In this interview I told him about a very interesting chap I had met—a chap who had a bilateral amputation but despite it had been very successful in doing a great many things. He'd been in an airplane accident—I think shells came into the cockpit—and he'd had to have a bilateral amputation but he had prosthetic devices and he got along very well with them. I told the patient that in a casual chat, without making a direct and specific reference to himself and what he was going to have to do. But it gave him something to fall back upon when he became more realistic. I didn't puncture his balloon of unreality, however.

I think that's a practical way to handle a situation of that kind, but I think that if a person is dying and is protecting himself with a shell of euphoria you make a mistake to break through it. That is nature's way of providing something that is badly needed. With our so-called superior understanding or emotional aloofness let's be very careful to be truly understanding and not be deluded about the need for being over-honest.

DR. BOND. I'll hold up the other side of this for some people. There are some people who are greatly relieved by being told that they have an illness, that it is malignant, and that they are going to die. I knew a man who had a malignancy of the skin. He was a physician and he had this thing for about three years before anyone told him what it was. He fussed and fumed about it and was very distinctly worried, and then finally his physician told him that it was a malignancy and that he was going to die. Well, that served a very useful purpose for him. It gave him some limit to his anxiety. It gave him something to plan on and to work on, and he was a very relieved person afterwards. He was told that he was going to live three years, and he lived about twenty after that. But that was all right. I think the important thing is that it's awfully good for some people to come right out and tell them. You have to be a pretty good judge of who they are and how they will take it, however.

DR. ROMANO. Well, I challenge that to a certain degree. Granted, let's say, that a doctor may present special problems. But when you mention it as a small item that this man lived twenty years and not three years I should disagree. It seems to me that although it is necessary to tell some individuals just what the prognosis is, it is important to stress the positive factors as much as one can. I think that when one plays Jehovah in instances like that, many times it is very, very harmful. So it seems to me that when one gives a patient direct information, one should attempt to give with it enough reassurance, protection, support, and stress on the positive aspects to enable the person to master the anxiety and the distress which come with the information. That would be my opinion. Also, you see, with all due professional modesty, it's very difficult for a physician to speak dogmatically concerning the course of many illnesses. It seems to me that one has to err and that it's wiser to err in omission in instances like that—not to be too specific about course, prognosis, eventuality, and to stress the positive aspects.

STUDENT. What about a man with a coronary thrombosis who wants to arrange his affairs and asks you what that diagnosis means? What do you tell a man like that?

DR. BAUER. Well, one doesn't have to tell him the first day he gets his coronary occlusion. I do think, however, that you should explain what happened, very simply, and what you're driving at in the way of treatment. It depends, of course, on the patient as to how positively you can speak and when.

DR. ROMANO.   In continuation of some of Dr. Murray's comments about people with whistling-in-the-dark mechanisms, those who deny their realistic difficulties or have euphoria-like states, we must remember that this is a very common phenomenon and not restricted to amputees. The whole field of chronic disease illustrates this phenomenon and of course it's seen classically in dying people. Now I feel that these mechanisms have value, as Dr. Murray says. It is very wrong to interfere and to take those defenses away unless you have something positive and constructive to offer. In multiple sclerosis, for instance, the euphoric reaction occurs so frequently that it's even been given a name —*spes sclerotica*, the hope of the sclerotic. Here you have an illness of unknown origin, which may occur in early maturity and extend for a number of years, with remissions in between unpredictable recurrences of disability that vary from paraplegia to monosymptomatic disturbances. And many times when you ask these patients how they are, even though they have a paraplegia they say, "All right, I'm fine; I'm wonderful. I'm going to beat this thing; I'm going to be all right." Well, in many instances it's wise to leave them alone. You may think, "I understand that this is going on," and so on. That's fine. But in cases where the patient's attitude keeps him from utilizing what he could utilize within the limits of his disease, then if you're prepared to follow through with something, it may be wise to help him. But in case of doubt, many times it's wiser not to interfere.

DR. RENNIE.   I would very much like to add to this discussion the point that none of us as doctors can control the time element in a person's development. We don't know the time element. Let me start simply with an example of a patient who comes to us in a state of depression. "Will I get well?" he asks. Yes, we know he will in all probability. "When will I get well?" That I cannot tell him. If I say he will be well in a month or two months and he isn't, eventually the patient feels let down and loses confidence. It is the same with a patient with any physical disorder. Human beings can go through a terrible lot of discomfort if they know that at some future time, undefined, they can expect relief. I remember one dermatitis patient who was very uncomfortable and was told by a dermatologist that there wasn't any possibility that he would be over it in six weeks. That was a very devastating thing. The patient could take the discomfort day by day as long as hope was left open and the length of the suffering was indefinite.

I bring up this point because I want to tie it back into what we were talking about previously. I think we as doctors have to be wedded to telling the truth. But we don't have to tell all the truth, for at times that would be too devastating. We can tell as much of the truth as the patient seems to be able to tolerate. There are certainly some human beings who are facing death who have a right to know it, and we would do them an injustice not to let them know it. It is an individual matter, we cannot make a specific statement that one should always do one thing or the other. What to do has to be determined on the basis of the patient with the aid of the relatives who know quite well how he would react. There are many tragic instances of people who had much to do in those last few days or weeks of life and who were denied the right to do it because they weren't told the facts. I think we have to make a highly individual judgment, recognizing the degree of anxiety that is present and the amount of anxiety we might stir up and therefore soft-pedaling and rephrasing but saying frankly, "This is serious but I don't know when it will eventuate; there may be a long period ahead," and so on. But I do think we ought to get on record for telling the truth.

STUDENT. I think to tell the truth to patients who are hopelessly ill is to protect them from being exploited by quacks and other people. You take some patients who have a hopeless illness: if you don't make it clear to them, they may go on spending large sums of money, traveling about, without any hope of improvement. I think it is our duty to protect them from that.

DR. ROMANO. You think that by telling them you would stop them from going around?

STUDENT. I think so. If there is the proper doctor-patient relationship, I think we can.

DR. ROMANO. I personally know of a number of people who know the seriousness of their disease but who resort to all kinds of trips and junketing about for health. However, if the doctor is able to stress the positive aspect, to reassure and help the person live within the limits and boundaries of his disability, some of that might be eliminated.

It's not only the intellectual communication of data in any of these cases that's important. Let's say you have a patient who is dying of carcinoma. In the first place, most such patients know they are dying whether you tell them or not. They have a fairly good idea about it, so it's how you tell them and how much you tell them or how much they can stand at any one particular time that's important. I usually err on the side of not telling them too much at any one particular time, so as to avoid deluging them too suddenly with anxiety.

Essentially, as Dr. Rennie stated, there is no general statement which covers all instances. My feeling would be that the physician's primary responsibility to the patient is to do whatever is best for the patient. In some instances, for legal and economic reasons, or for helping the patient to accept the need for surgery, it will be necessary to tell him directly. In all instances it will be necessary to explain in detail to a responsible member of the family. However, the physician must never lose sight of the emotional readiness or preparation of the patient with whom he is to be frank or direct.

The Meaning of a Psychoneurosis

M. RALPH KAUFMAN, M.D.

I

TODAY we're going to discuss a bit the problem of neurosis and what it means. We've been talking a good deal about neurotic patients. We've told you how to treat them. We've told you how not to treat them. And why not. But we have not discussed the problem of neurosis as such. Dr. Murray, in talking about the normal development of personality, went into some aspects of what we might call neurotic development, and yesterday, in introducing the subject of psychotherapy, Dr. Romano described generally the meaning of neurosis. Today we are going to take up that subject in more detail.

Now there has been a kind of feeling that "a neurosis," "a psychoneurotic," "a psychological factor" (you know, that whole area) is something esoteric, something you can't understand, something that's outside the stream of ordinary medical tradition. The patient has a neurosis, has functional disease, has lack of organic disease, has belly-ache, has various kinds of bizarre thoughts, and so on and so forth. But usually that has not been related to the individual or to the general tradition in medicine. So when you say the patient has vomiting on a functional basis, for instance, you don't know why, you can't find out why. The patient may have a little trouble with her husband, and she vomits. Functional!

Now, suppose I presented you with this kind of case in your practice. The patient has nausea or vomiting, a kind of general pain over the abdomen or a tendency to center down toward the right lower quadrant, tenderness and rigidity, tenderness over McBurney's point, temperature, 10,000 leukocytes. What would you suspect?

STUDENT. Appendicitis.

DR. KAUFMAN. Yes, appendicitis. All right. Now let's break down the signs, symptoms, and complaints of this. What is the rigidity in terms of total organ response? A defense? That's right. What about the vomiting? Yes, perhaps disgust. What kind of disgust? Physiological disgust. What is the vomiting in the case of appendicitis? It's a defense. What about leukocytosis? It's a defense. In other words, this is what Dr. Romano has been talking with you about—it is called part of the homeostasis, part of the total attempt on the part of the individual (biologically, physiologically, and so on) to handle a certain kind of situation. We're accustomed generally in medical tradition to look upon the signs and symptoms of illness as part of the total organism reaction. Now, the same is true in a neurosis. Or in a psychosis.

Now, I just want to make that general analogy. We shall, I think, be able to show you how, in some instances on a rather simple level, one can see that neurotic symptoms and psychotic symptoms, even the hallucinations and delusions that one sees in very sick psychotic patients, are not haphazard. They don't just happen; they are part of a homeostatic, defense, compromise situation. In other words, neurotic symptoms have meaning. And they have meaning in terms of that individual's life experience.

Now let's come back again to Dr. Murray's little boy, Johnny. He showed you in a schematic way the step-by-step development from birth on. He talked to you about the individual's being born a bundle of instinctual energy. That doesn't mean original sin. In other words, the infant as he comes into the world has certain needs and, by and large, these needs are gratified. The needs are rather simple ones—like feeding. He's fed, he's gratified, and he goes to sleep. It's the same way with his bowel function, urine function, and so on. As the infant develops (I'm not going to repeat all that Dr. Murray has said) certain other factors begin to come in—certain relationships. Now let's take the problem of feeding. The child is hungry, is fed. And it's all part of one thing. Now supposing the child is hungry and isn't fed. Those of you who are fathers know what happens when the child is hungry and isn't fed. He cries like hell. He's mad. He wants to be fed. That's all there is to it. That's a perfectly normal response. But if the child is hungry and is fed, is gratified, he establishes a relationship eventually with a person, usually the mother. Over and above the physiological relationship of being hungry and being fed, this person who does the feeding begins to assume a certain kind of significance to the child. An emotional relationship grows up. But if, for one reason or another, the child is frustrated (he wants something and doesn't get it) what happens? He will refuse to eat. And why? Why will a child refuse to eat? Because he's angry. He begins to use the eating or not eating as part of a psychological habit.

Refusal to eat, not eating, is a symptom with which all of you are familiar. All your cases of anorexias, for instance. Dr. Romano (perhaps not in this discussion here) has pointed out that eating or not eating may serve a purpose over and above the one dealing with metabolism. In other words, it may serve some kind of function in a relationship such as that between mother and child. So you can have the infant's refusal to eat as a way of getting things. Now, is there anything neurotic about that? Not necessarily. Children sulk; don't want to eat if they're angry at mother. If they want mother to love them, then they eat. Eating becomes something that one can use to stall, to threaten, to hurt mother, or to be a good little girl or good little boy. Whether one eats or not becomes, symbolically, an important part of the relationship between the child and the mother.

During the course of the development of the child, as Dr. Murray has pointed out, different aspects of the personality appear. There's the part of the personality we've talked about, the part that seeks gratification; there's the part that gradually makes adjustment to reality; and there's the part that embodies all the thou-shalt-nots. Now, what does that mean in terms of the possible neurotic behavior of an individual? If you had only the instinctual part of the personality, didn't have any part which related itself to reality and tested it and knew how far to go, if you didn't have within the personality this conscience, then you would have just Old Man River flowing along without any obstacles. But within the personality there are also the conscience and the ego, which relates itself to reality and tests it. (The ego is perhaps the finger that is put into the water to see whether it is hot, or touches the wet paint when there's a wet-paint sign.) The minute you conceive of three different parts within the individual, then you have the setting for this whole problem of neurosis or neurotic behavior. Namely, the divergent points of view within an individual that provide a setting for a conflict situation.

We have mentioned conflict; you've heard us talk about conflicts. Now what is the significance of conflict for our understanding of neurotics? We have mentioned the needs that the child has, the thing that he wants and for one reason or other cannot or should not have. He shouldn't have it because the parents think that it will be bad for him and so on. Pretty soon the child develops the feeling that if he wants to do this, then father won't like him. Dr. Murray has described to you the mechanism by which the child takes the father into himself and makes him a part of his conscience. As long as the child doesn't do something because father is there and will punish him, or mother is there and will not love him, the conflict situation is between the child himself and his father or mother. However, the result of this very interesting technique the child has of taking father's thou-shalt-not and mother's thou-shalt-not and thousands of other thou-shalt-nots inside himself is that at some time in his development he will stop saying, "I won't do this or that because then mother will spank me or will not love me or father will punish me," and instead will say, "I *should* not do this." This beginning of conscience has an important relation to the conflict. Let me tell you a story of how it happened in one case.

We were kind of modern parents and we said we would never punish our child, but we couldn't help being distressed sometimes by the things Paul did. I've forgotten just what he was doing that particular day, but it was a whole series of things. Every time he did one of these things we'd say to him, "No, Paul." Well, this went on for a little while, and then he did something that caused a bang; we went into the room and there was Paul in the center of it, and as soon as he saw us he began to shake his head. In other words, he didn't wait for us to say "no," he said "no" within himself. Now what happens at that point is that the child may go on and do these things, but something has happened inside himself which says, "You must not do these things." There's still a part of him, however, that says, "I want to do it." Therefore you have the set-up for a conflict situation which has to be solved in one way or another. A person wants to do something. His conscience says "no." He feels a little guilty. He doesn't do it. Another person, or the same individual at another time, if there's something he wants to do (I'm talking of something he wants to do consciously; we'll come to the question of the unconscious in a minute), may feel a little guilty but still want to do it, can't quite come to do it, will get a little drunk. Then he can do this thing he wants, because the part of his personality that says "no" is soluble in alcohol. It's a recognizable phenomenon, isn't it, gentlemen? Now that's one way we have of solving the conflict situation. We can use all kinds of maneuvers to get around our conscience, to get around our sense of guilt, and so to minimize the conflict situation. I can tell you from my personal experience that a hangover isn't always a physiological thing. You know how you feel with a hangover. But you feel worse if you've done something that you're guilty about.

The point I want to make is that one may maneuver, as it were, within oneself in relation to the environment in order to solve these conflict situations. One may solve them in various ways. But one way to solve them is by what we call a neurotic compromise. The child refuses to eat because he's angry with his mother, and there is the immediate situation between child and mother. Now let us take that same child, who knows he's angry and refuses to eat, but suppose that his refusal to eat persists in a situation—in a reality situation—where there is no occasion for anger. In other words, this refusal, which is not a neurotic symptom, may very easily become a neurotic symptom. Suppose the child has laid down a pattern on a normal basis that when he gets angry with mother he doesn't eat. Mother is affectionate to him, tells him to eat, and so on, and the child begins to eat. Now suppose a little brother comes into the picture. The child *may*, in his rivalry with the little brother, solve that problem of anger at his mother, which he may not even be aware of, by a refusal to eat. In other words, to solve a conflict he may use a pattern which was normal in another situation; that is, the refusal to eat when little brother arrives is the child's way of saying, "I am angry at mother," without necessarily being aware of his anger.

I think it's very important to get this general concept in relation to the work that we are doing in the clinic, for there we are looking for information from our patients. We are looking for information that will help us understand why this individual has this or that set of symptoms. We get some information. Sometimes we can see the relationship; sometimes we can't see the relationship. We talk about giving the patient insight into what is wrong with him—into his conflict situation, and so on. Now, if everything that we're talking about were purely conscious, then the individual could be aware of all of these feelings—hostility, anger, resentment, desires, and so on—but part of his personality is at an unconscious level. That's already been discussed with you, and I'm not going into a theoretical discussion of the unconscious. There is a part of us that is unconscious, and when something unpleasant occurs in our life experience we tend to suppress it, we tend to forget about it. We try to tell our patients to forget about it. Now, what happens to this experience that's been unpleasant and forgotten?

Something of this kind happened to me in connection with one medical school and its graduates. I didn't know the school at all, but I wasn't fond of it because I had a single experience with one of its graduates. Just because we have met one bum from such and such a school we shouldn't generalize and say that the whole school is lousy and so on. But I met one of these fellows, had a very unpleasant experience with him, and I developed that kind of reaction. We do, very frequently. We go from a specific thing and generalize. And I forgot about this altogether, as far as I knew. It really wasn't of any very great importance. Once I'd called the fellow lots of names and figured that he wasn't as good a doctor as I was anyway—you know, the way we do these things—I forgot about the experience. About five years later, in a completely different part of the country, I met another fellow. He seemed to be an awfully nice fellow, but I just didn't like him. Being a person of very strong likes and dislikes, I thought this was just another one of the fellows I didn't like. But it still bothered me. I knew there was something about this particular man that was reminiscent of something, but I just didn't know what it was. His air, a certain manner, and so forth. I took a dislike to him at first sight, and that was all there was to it. Well, I had to work with him, and after a time I heard what school he was from. Immediately the thought hit me: he reminded me so much of the bum I'd once hated that right off the bat I hated him too. He has since become one of my very good friends, which is often the kind of thing that happens when you react a little bit over in the other direction. What had happened was simply this. I'd had an unpleasant experience. I'd pushed it aside into the unconscious. That was that. And then I met somebody who reminded me in some way of that particular experience. Automatically, I transferred my hostilities, hatred, and so forth, to this individual who had nothing to do with the original experience.

Now, where was this man, where was this school, where was all this hostility and hatred during these five years? I certainly didn't walk around consciously aware that every time I saw such an individual I was going to feel that way. It was in me. It was brought out very easily. It was in my unconscious. At least, I was unconscious of it.

Well, if this unconscious were a filing-cabinet kind of thing in which you dropped a card, I'd have just forgotten it. But the unconscious, as we think of it, is not that kind of thing. It's a seething sort of thing. It's a part of the personality where there are strong emotions of which we're not aware. But they're there. And they have one characteristic— they are constantly seeking to express themselves. Therefore, when we say something is unconscious, what we mean is not only that it is forgotten but that it is still there with all its emotional drive and tension. If you can understand that, you can begin to understand that you're dealing with a part of the personality in which there are actual drives, actual tensions, and emotional needs, that the experiences which have been repressed have not been killed. Is that clear? If so, then the rest of the explanation of neurosis will be more understandable.

In this unconscious the affect, the emotion that accompanies an experience, is pushed aside, but it's there, it seeks expression. Therefore it is a source of conflict within the personality, for we sometimes are in the position of trying to sit on a boiler with increasing steam. Certain parts of our personality have to act as pressure valves, and other parts have to be under control. But if something is unconscious and seeks expression, a certain amount of energy, a certain amount of inner activity has to be used in the job of holding it down.

Therefore, you've got some things within an individual that are pressing for expression, and you've got external forces and internal forces that are keeping that kind of thing from expressing itself. You've got, then, divergent forces, and very powerful forces. And what happens? What happens is that at times, if the needs are great, the controlling forces have to give way a little bit and allow for the expression of the inner need. But they can't accept the direct expression of tremendous hostility.

For instance, let's say a child is frustrated by his father. He becomes angry. It's dangerous to be angry. If it were just ordinary anger, it would be one thing. But, you see, a child is richly endowed with all kinds of fantasy, too. You all know the make-believe games and the fantasies that you can actually see in children. Dr. Murray drew our attention to fairy tales. Now what kinds of stories are fairy tales? Are they love stories in the ordinary sense? What happens in fairy tales? People are eaten up, they're torn to pieces. Nobody ever dies a normal death in a fairy tale, as far as I know. In fairy tales the kinds of things that happen to people are pretty horrible things, and we sometimes wonder whether we should read them to children, for they really contain a tremendous amount of horror—tearing to pieces, being eaten up, being put in ovens, and so on and so forth. Has that ever struck you as a rather curious kind of phenomenon? The fact is that they're related to the kinds of fantasies a child may have. Let us say that a child is resentful of father, is angry at father, wants to hurt father. We may think of socking pop in the nose. The child may not think of that; he may think of eating him up! That becomes a pretty horrible kind of thing to the child—to eat somebody up. So when we talk of aggression in childhood we have to remember this rich fantasy life and the kinds of fantasies a child has. Then we can see that aggression and resentment in a child are over and above merely hitting somebody. They are associated with fantasies that are pretty dangerous, that have to be repressed, that have to be pushed aside, pushed away. When there is this kind of fantasy, we see why there is great need not to express it and why there will arise a terrific amount of conflict.

But there is a possible solution. The solution for the child who is angry with his new little brother, is angry with his mother, may be to repress completely the hostility—to overreact in the other direction and appear as a passive, submissive child. Dr. Jensen told us yesterday about a two-year-old who was stopped when he was actually on the point of kicking his little brother's skull in. Another child might substitute by taking it out on the dog or developing acute anxiety. Now when you go back to childhood, go back to your own experiences, you'll see that that is the way children function. When they make these compromises, they may make them in relation to those aspects of their physiological functions that have become secondarily emotionalized in the relation with the mother and father. Eating, bowel movement, incontinence, enuresis, and so on may begin to be part of a neurotic picture which is a solution for conflict within that individual and his relationship to the environment. The next step is taking it out of the environment; in other words, the conflict situation arises not because father is right there and will punish him but because father is inside of him now in the form of conscience.

Now when you solve something and get a resultant from the two forces, there are always two sides to it. We see that very clearly in a good many neurotic symptoms. There is the side which says, "Thou shalt not"; one can see this in a neurotic symptom that is an inhibition rather than a function of a particular organ. Let us take the paralysis of the hand. You've seen hysterical paralysis of the hand. Now what happens in hysterical paralysis of the hand? What is its significance? The person doesn't have to use the hand if it is paralyzed. The next question you might ask yourself is what did this man want to do with that hand that made him not want to use it? He may have wanted to sock somebody in the nose. Or, if he were a soldier, he may have been in conflict over the injunction "Thou shalt not kill." During the war we frequently saw soldiers with a paralysis of the right hand or the trigger finger. When we talked to such a soldier and got his confidence, very frequently this came out—the injunction "Thou shalt not kill." He had been given a gun, he was going to kill, it was patriotic, he had to do it for his country, and so on; on the other hand, there were his childhood upbringing and his religious scruples. Now what happened? He developed a paralysis of the hand which inhibited that function and solved that problem. So his behavior had a meaning.

You can see immediately that if a function is inhibited, then it doesn't have to be used, that solves a problem. That's particularly true in the somatic field. For instance, take impotence due to psychoneurotic difficulties. There are many reasons for it. But you can see how the function may have been inhibited because of terrific conflict with guilt. I mean, if a man can't, he can't, and that's all there is to it. There's no problem. But there's another side to this symptom. One is the side that says, "Thou shalt not"; and the other is the side that says, "But damn it, I still want to." So it is with a paralysis of the hand which inhibits one from doing certain things that are bad; it's still the paralysis of a hand that wants to do them. There are always two sides, two aspects, to a neurotic symptom. That's why we tell you that neurotic symptoms have meaning, have some symbolic value.

Take, for another example, a woman who has vomiting as a symptom. If you have an idea that her vomiting is partly psychological, may be part of an attempt to solve some kind of problem, may mean that she is disgusted, you have a hint as to what areas you may have to explore to understand the problem. The woman may fear that she's pregnant. Now one may not want to be pregnant, may not want a child. One may, however, want certain other aspects of the sexual relationship. One may have fantasies of sexual relations, let us say. One may be a spinster in a strict and narrow community and have a strict moral code; in that case one may react to these inner symptoms and fantasies with another fantasy. In the unconscious there has been not only the wish for sexual activity: it has already gone further than that and in the unconscious there is a child. The woman doesn't have the child, but she solves this neurotic conflict within her by the vomiting. In other words, the vomiting to her means pregnancy.

Now, come back again to our child. We can talk about these things—conflict, unconscious, conscious, solution of problems, and so on—but what drives the individual into neurotic conflict? Is it only the fear of punishment? Is it only the lack of love? Is it only a fear of doing this, that, or the other thing? What happens within an individual if something that he wants to do or needs to do threatens him? What is our usual reaction? A psycho-physiological reaction to danger—fear. Now what happens when we're scared? Yes, we feel anxious. And what do we do when we feel anxious? We have certain physiological concomitants.

Now what about fear? I don't want to discuss the question of fear versus anxiety (Dr. Romano is going to do that later) but I want to make one point clear now because I think it's important. You say when one is afraid of something there's an external danger. Now there are lots of external dangers. Automobiles, bullets, bears, women—all kinds of things that are dangerous. Now what do we ordinarily do? Well, some of us run, some stand up and fight, some take cover; in other words, when there is an external danger the individual acts in terms of his own development and his own experience. When there's an external danger one may take certain defensive measures or certain offensive measures, and there may be situations in which one is too scared to do anything. The response to danger is this feeling of fear. Now suppose the danger comes from inside. There are dangers that come from inside. Have any of you ever read *The Temptation of St. Anthony*, by Flaubert? I recommend it very highly. At any rate, there are certain danger situations that may come from inside, not outside. What happens in response to such dangers? Anxiety.

What happens in anxiety? You'll hear about that in detail, but generally we know that some of the physiological aspects of anxiety are rapid heart beat, gastrointestinal upset, pallor, sweating, and so on. Many of our patients come in with those as their chief complaints. When you have that kind of situation, what do you see? When a patient comes in complaining of a fast heart, he may have a hyperthyroid. He may have all the symptoms that have a physical basis. But something else may also be present. The patient may be having anxiety, and he may come to you expressing physiological reverberations of anxiety. We've all seen patients this week whose main complaints are those that develop physically when an individual has anxiety. So you have to be aware of that possibility.

The anxiety itself may be felt or expressed or pushed aside, but it serves a very definite function within the organism. It gives the individual a signal (in the same way that fear does) that something is dangerous and that he must do something about it. So there's the same necessity to an internal danger as there is to an external danger. How the individual handles it depends upon his development.

The child at every step of his development has to face certain kinds of problems which he may solve in what we call the normal way or in a neurotic way or, temporarily, through neurotic symptoms, such as not eating. Then the situation changes externally and internally and this solution is not needed any more. Let us say that at the age of two little Mary develops a non-eating reaction because of her mother's attitude toward her. A psychiatrist treats the child or the mother changes, and the child begins to eat. Little Mary grows up. She's twenty-three. Then something happens that has in it this same implication of loss of love from a mother figure. Mary, who is now big Mary with little Mary inside of her, stops eating: in other words, she uses the same kind of pattern that was laid down early. As one develops, there is a tendency for behavior to repeat itself at times. Part of our character or personality development is just this repetition of patterned behavior. If there are neurotic conflicts and neurotic solutions within this pattern, the individual will have a tendency to repeat it when life situations, external or internal, are met that can't be solved in other ways. But you will remember that I told you that the neurotic pattern is both a solution and a compromise, that it works on the half-a-loaf principle. In other words, if I can't get what I want because of fear of punishment and so on, I'll get at least part of it, even though only symbolically. If I have an urge in my genitals which is forbidden for me, and I develop anxiety because of fear of my own fantasies, and my moral code says I mustn't have sexual fantasies, I must do something about it; then if I develop a pruritus and scratch, I am not to blame. So a pruritus may be a solution of an original sexual tension. We see that pretty frequently.

When a child develops an illness, certain things may happen in the relationship between the child and its parents. It may become the center of attention. Instead of being the last child and perhaps feeling unwanted and unloved, little Mary now has mother paying attention to her; the doctor comes, everybody is centering around her. Every illness has what we call secondary gain. That's a very important point to know about illness. So it is when one has solved problems by means of neurotic compromises; the neurotic illness in itself may begin to give the individual a secondary gain over and above the gains he secured through the neurosis itself. Take, for instance, a neurotic headache in a woman who is using this means to resolve certain conflict situations. Now what happens sometimes when mother has a headache, especially a rather hard-working mother? She gets a lot of attention; she can get out of a lot of things.

We had a case like this yesterday, a rather complicated case whose details we don't have to go into. One aspect of it was that the woman was getting shots for arthritis every two weeks. She lives out-of-town, is a hard-working farm woman, very conscientious and so forth. She comes down to the clinic once every two weeks in order to get some shots which her local doctor could just as well give her. Now, the woman has arthritis and is being treated. Coming down here to be treated for illness is one way for her to get out of a pretty tough job at least once every two weeks. We debated whether we should request the social service to get in touch with her local doctor and see whether he couldn't give her the treatment. But we decided, being kind of gentle souls, that perhaps the best thing to do was to let her come down here, because she had a definite secondary gain out of the trip.

The reason I talk about the secondary gain is that very frequently we can see quite readily what the secondary gain from the illness or from the neurosis is. In much of our treatment of neurotics we work purely in terms of this secondary gain, not with the primary, deep etiological factor. Therefore we have to know in each instance just what the patient gains from his neurotic difficulty; we have to evaluate that gain and see whether we can give the individual a substitute before we take it away from him. So this is by way of a word of caution in regard to what we're talking about in therapy—sometimes the secondary gain becomes a necessary factor in the illness, just as the neurotic difficulty itself becomes something that makes the individual's life tolerable, even though at a certain expense. If the secondary gain does that, and if we can't provide a substitute, we'd better not try to take it away.

We come back again, then, to this question of the neurosis and its meaning. Just one word that goes a little bit deeper on the question. As you know, until relatively recently it was thought even by psychiatrists that there was no sense to the ideas of psychotic and neurotic individuals. Now we have a great deal of evidence from various sources that their symptoms do have meaning and that we can get from them some understanding of what is going on within the individual. Once we grasp that concept we begin to understand the problems to which the symptoms are an answer. Without becoming involved in the highly technical knowledge of symbols, you will find it of interest and value to use this principle in your work with neurotic patients. It is useful, for instance, in your interviews. So many of you have said, "What do we ask for? What do we want to know?" And many of you have been amazed at the facility with which the faculty here are able to talk with patients that you've been working with and in a relatively short period of time to get something that you've been struggling for. The explanation is that all of us are accustomed to size up a symptom picture, take our leads from it, and go in this or that direction. Some of you may think, as you watch us, that we are haphazard birds, taking a little peck here and a little peck there and pretty soon pulling something out. No magic at all! There is nothing up our sleeves. All we do is follow, on the basis of our experience, the principle that symptoms have meaning and allow the patient to disclose that meaning to us.

What I've been talking to you about, therefore, is not only of theoretical importance; it's practical stuff that helps you with your patient. My sketchy kind of talk about the principle isn't going to help you understand symptoms, I know. It just gives an indication of the sort of things you might be looking out for when Mrs. Jones comes to you with symptoms of vomiting, bloating, constipation, or any one of a myriad other somatic complaints. It really is quite an interesting thing purely from an intellectual point of view aside from the inner satisfaction. As one of you said to me yesterday, he had a patient who had a very interesting story. And I said to him, "Did you feel that little inner glow?" And he said, "Yes."

DISCUSSION

STUDENT. When these patients develop neurotic symptoms that are manifested in somatic complaints, do they have a sense of gratification?

DR. KAUFMAN. That's an important question and I'm glad you

asked it, for there are many misconceptions about that. When we say a neurotic is "gratified," don't expect a look of ecstasy. The gratification is a very subtle kind of thing. As a matter of fact, what one sees in a patient is, for the most part, the guilt, the anxiety, the suffering. Unconsciously he may have gratification. But it is an intrinsic part of a neurosis—and of a good many other situations—that before the individual can do what he wants to do he must pay the penalty. So there is gratification, but it isn't a gross kind of thing. Above all, don't accuse the patient of getting gratification. It is so frequently said, "He's just a neurotic; just getting satisfaction out of it." Yes, and he's paying a hell of a price. There is gratification, but it's usually unconscious.

STUDENT. In practice I find that if a person has these neurotic symptoms, and if you're sympathetic with him and agree that he has some of these things, he often feels better. For instance, a person comes in with a burst of pain in the abdomen; he has been kicked around doctors' offices and told he has nothing wrong with him. You make up your mind to agree with him and treat him for something you can cure. For instance, you might tell him he's got something like an ulcer or duodenitis or something else he doesn't understand very well. Tell him you can cure him and put him on treatment. Well, you should see the symptoms disappear! The patient's happier than he's ever been. Now, is it erroneous to do that?

DR. KAUFMAN. Well, it's a question of what you call erroneous. There are two things being confused here. Others have said to the patient, "There's nothing wrong with you, there's nothing to treat." You tell him there's something organically wrong, and you proceed to treat an illusory illness. Now, it isn't true that there's "nothing wrong" with the patient; there is something wrong with him. But you don't have to treat him for duodenitis if the problem is not duodenitis but some kind of psychological conflict situation. In other words, the phrasing isn't quite right. It's perfectly true that with certain patients you can get the results you describe, for you are the first one to say to the patient, "Yes, there is something wrong with you," and so the patient accepts you as the doctor and it is on that basis (not the six weeks that you say it takes to cure the disorder), on the basis of your relation with the patient, that the improvement takes place. On the whole, however, I personally am very much opposed—from the psychological point of view and every other point of view—to telling a patient he has a specific organic illness when you know this is not true.

STUDENT. Do you feel that way because the patients themselves are more or less aware of the fact that they have a psychological disorder?

DR. KAUFMAN. They are all aware of it unconsciously. I think, from a psychological point of view, it's much better never to treat a patient for something you know he hasn't got in order to achieve something which you don't know how to get otherwise. You follow those cases and you'll find that the duodenitis may clear up but that something else will take its place, for the patient still has his problem.

STUDENT. Wouldn't it be a point to try to explain the patient's symptoms, or at least to understand them, on the basis of the physiological difficulties which have resulted, whatever the genetic factors may be?

DR. KAUFMAN. I think that, in a sense, that's what the doctor meant. After all, he didn't choose duodenitis at random. He picked duodenitis as something that's in the general area of the stomach. What he was dealing with may have been the physiological concomitant of the emotional disorder. But that, unfortunately, begs the question.

There are two kinds of pain. One is pain which is related to an organ, and the other is pain which has no relation to an organ as such but is merely localized in an area. There are secondary physiological concomitants to anxiety. Even when we psychiatrists say "gastric neurosis" we are begging the question. What we are saying is that the disorder is functional. It isn't a gastric neurosis; it's a neurotic difficulty which is expressed symptomatically via the stomach, and so we say "gastric neurosis." That doesn't mean that the patient who has diarrhea shouldn't also be treated by chemotherapy. I don't want to go into that question, because the faculty members who are going to discuss therapy will take up the relation between drug therapy and psychotherapy. I am objecting to giving a specific organic diagnosis when you know that you are doing it not for organic reasons but as a kind of psychotherapy. You say to the patient, in effect, "I can't cure what you have, but I can cure the disease we give you. Well, why not? That's what you came for." You see?

II

LET'S continue today with a little further elaboration on the meaning of a neurosis. We played around with various aspects of this problem yesterday and tried to show that neurotic symptoms have significance just as the symptoms of medical disease do. Now there are a number of types of neuroses. We're not particularly interested in classification as such, and actually there has been a good deal of controversy among psychiatrists as to what the categories should be. Most of us think of the psychoneuroses and even psychoses not as disease entities but as reactions and reaction groups. That follows rather logically from the point of view that regards the neurotic syndrome or the neurotic reaction as part of a total reaction in an individual. But we do agree on broad categories. For instance, when I say "hysteria" all psychiatrists know which group I am referring to. When we get down to a discussion of the individual symptoms that fall into that particular group (the limitations of the group, that is) there may be differences of opinion.

Now what do we mean when we say that a person is hysterical? This kind of reaction is very important for the general practitioner to understand, for of all the neurotic patterns of behavior the hysterical syndrome is the most frequently related to the soma, the body. Yesterday I used as an illustration of a paralysis of function a paralysis of the hand. Paralysis belongs in the hysterical group.

The somatic symptoms of hysterical patients have certain common characteristics. One of their characteristics is that they follow non-anatomical lines. For instance, the anesthesias that one sees in hysterical patients—the glove or stocking anesthesia. Perhaps some day we'll discover the exact localization in the brain of an area that will produce a glove anesthesia, but at present we say this doesn't follow any kind of anatomical location. A good many of these anesthesias or somatic involvements, however, are clearly associated with a functional location. Without going into details, I have a feeling, as do some other psychiatrists, that frequently, if one knows what the fantasy of function of any individual is, one can understand why a certain system or group of organs have been involved in an hysterical paralysis or anesthesia.

Paralysis of the hand, for instance, may mean that the individual has an unconscious problem about which he has a good deal of guilt, and the only way for him to solve that particular conflict is to knock the hand out.

There are certain types of psychological techniques which an hysteric uses in solving his or her problems: one of them is repression. Characteristically, the person who has an hysterical paralysis or hysterical neurosis handles the problem of his instinctual life by pushing it aside, by repressing it completely. Now visualize this kind of situation. There is some kind of inner drive which is taboo for one reason or another. It mustn't come to consciousness. It's threatening, it will have certain consequences, and so on. How does the hysteric handle it? He handles it by repressing completely the feeling of anxiety and converting it into an hysterical paralysis. Charcot coined a term *la belle indifférence* to describe the hysterical patient's apparent lack of affect. A woman may have complete paraplegia, be unable to walk, and yet when you come in and see her one thing that strikes you is that she has a madonna-like calmness about her, sometimes even a trace of—well, ecstasy is perhaps too strong a word, but it's certainly a reaction that is quite out of keeping with the fact of her complete disability.

Now what has happened here? What has happened apparently is that the patient has repressed and pushed aside all the instinctual drives that were threatening her, converted them in some way into hysterical paralysis, and then had no more anxiety. Where has the anxiety gone? Has it completely disappeared? Doesn't the conflict exist any more? Don't the drives exist any more? No, the anxiety and the drives have not disappeared, for if through hypnosis or some other method you take the symptom away from such a patient she becomes very tense and anxious. What you have done is to take away her defense and her technique for handling anxiety.

There are other neurotic syndromes relating to anxiety. One of the most characteristic we group as phobias, as fears. You saw in Dr. Murray's little boy, as he was growing up here before you, night fears, nightmares, which represented an anxiety situation. In the psychiatric clinic in Vienna we occasionally had a patient—usually a respectable, middle-aged *Hausfrau*—who had developed a street phobia. And it was surprising how often the street that couldn't be crossed was Kärtnerstrasse, a street that was famous for prostitutes because the police allowed them to operate there. Now what did it mean that a perfectly respectable *Hausfrau* developed a street phobia and that the street happened to be this well-known Kärtnerstrasse? What would you think that meant in terms of what we've been trying to talk about?

STUDENT. Anxiety and the combination of circumstances there.

DR. KAUFMAN. Yes, what kind of combination of what circumstances?

STUDENT. The relationship with those who frequented the street.

DR. KAUFMAN. Yes, the street had a symbolic kind of significance. The phobia would be centered around the impossibility of walking on that street because, on one hand, the woman might be thinking, "That is the kind of woman I would like to be," while, on the other hand, the other forces we've been talking about would say that the wish was taboo. The solution would be a phobia centering around that particular street. All this would be completely unconscious, but the doctor would have a clue as to where the trouble lay.

Now a very interesting thing happens in regard to this handling of anxiety and tension. A street phobia, for instance, may have a logical sequence. The patient may start with a phobia for a particular street; then, as the defenses begin to break down or as the unconscious wish threatens to break into consciousness, it isn't only the street, it's the whole area. Then the phobia may spread to the approaches to that area, and the patient may not be able to leave the house, may not be able to leave his room because he has to have a widening series of defensive measures. Eventually he may be completely incapacitated because that is the only way that he can defend himself against these tendencies.

In another very interesting kind of neurotic difficulty one can see clearly both aspects of the neurotic conflict—compulsions and obsessions. As Dr. Murray pointed out, in all of us, particularly during childhood, magic plays a very important role. All of you will remember that in your own childhood you believed you could do certain things just by thinking about them. Or if you did one thing, something else would happen. Childhood is an age of fantasies and conflict situations, which are handled with a great deal of difficulty. Among the techniques the child develops for handling them are some very interesting ones that many of us may still use. What did you do as a child as you walked along a sidewalk made of wood? You skipped the cracks; if you hit one, something was bound to happen. You didn't quite know what. It was the same in relation to a picket fence. You walked by a picket fence and you touched every one of the pickets, and if you missed one, you didn't know quite why but you felt rather uncomfortable. You'd walk back again and touch it because something would happen if you didn't. Now what does that remind you of in your own clinical practice? What kind of person does that sort of thing? The superstitious person, or one who is obsessionally or compulsively neurotic. You very frequently see individuals who have to do things just a certain way, otherwise they get uncomfortable, anxious, tense. Here is a mechanism used in normal development which also operates in individuals who are neurotic. Now let us take some of these symptoms, and I think you can see their meaning.

You know people who are constantly washing their hands. I don't mean surgeons, who have to do this, but people who are constant handwashers. Every hotel man knows that certain of his guests are going to make demands for a tremendous number of towels. Now what would you think was happening in an individual who constantly kept washing his hands? Washing away guilt? Yes. You know, *Macbeth*. Some of us, who are interested in studying the anxieties experimentally, find that if you prevent an obsessional neurotic from carrying out his compulsions, he immediately becomes very anxious. This symptom complex, then, has the significance of a symbolic cleansing of guilt. This is recognized in our common figures of speech. We "wash our hands" of something. A man comes to us "with clean hands" or "with unclean hands." So we see the symbolic aspects right through our language. These patients actually carry out such ideas as part of their symptom formation.

The main purpose of this lecture is to show you, in terms of your own experiences, that a patient's symptoms may have meaning. I've deliberately chosen rather superficial examples in which one can see relationships easily. Very frequently it's difficult to see these relationships immediately, but if one studies a patient intensively, eventually they can be worked out. This is particularly true with obsessive, compulsive people. I'll describe as an example a case I saw recently.

One of my patients, a business man, developed an obsessive thought, a thought that kept running through his mind, over and over again. He kept thinking as he drove his car, particularly when it was getting a little dark, that he might have hit somebody. That idea kept coming to him. He was a commuter who lived out in one of the suburbs, and he drove his car back and forth from work. When he'd come to his garage in the evening, although he knew perfectly well that he hadn't hit anybody, he would have to retrace his route, saying to himself all the time, "This is foolish; I know it hasn't happened." Still, afraid that perhaps he had hit somebody, he'd turn and retrace his steps to see if somebody was lying there. He'd do it once, four, five, ten times, for each time he'd still have this doubt, which is very characteristic of the obsessional. The more often this happened, the more strongly the thought would come to him that perhaps the injured person had been picked up before he got there. So as soon as he got the morning paper, instead of turning to Li'l Abner, he would look for the accidents. Perhaps somebody had been hurt in the general area in which he lived and he was responsible for it. Eventually, he stopped driving his car. He got his wife to drive him to and from the station. Then he couldn't quite do that, so he'd take a taxi and a train to work and come home the same way.

In trying to discover the reasons for such thoughts, we usually ask when they started. Frequently one gets a hint there as to their meaning, for later, as the patient develops increasing anxiety, he needs more and more symptoms and they go further and further away from the original meaning. It's as if there were a whole series of defenses put up. Now in the case of this particular man, there was a very interesting story as to when he first developed the fear that something would happen in an automobile. He'd been courting a girl for a long time; couldn't make up his mind to marry her, kept putting off the decision in a way that is characteristic of the obsessional neurotic. Finally the prospective mother-in-law got a little fed up with this, and he felt rather forced to give in. Then the man, being a very honorable fellow and always wanting to do the right thing (which is another characteristic of this sort of individual), married the girl. From the church to the hotel he drove his car with his wife and his new mother-in-law in it. They got to the hotel, and there he suddenly went into a panic because it suddenly hit him, "My God, I might have turned this car over and killed my wife and mother-in-law." I think you can see what kind of conflict was going on in this man's mind and what kind of solution he had achieved in his fantasy. Well, he got over that panic but many years later developed the obsession that perhaps he'd killed somebody—not his wife. You can see also why it made him so uncomfortable to have his wife drive.

In this oversimplified story I'm giving you a conflict situation, some of the reasons for it, and the technique which the individual apparently used in handling it. This man developed an obsessive thought which he knew was not true but which nevertheless caused him anxiety. This was one solution—if his wife and mother-in-law were dead then that part of his problem would be solved. But to wish somebody dead—one doesn't do that; it's equivalent to psychological murder. So it is with the obsessional neurotic: his aggressive, hostile desires become too threatening and therefore he has to utilize some kind of neurotic mechanism to handle them.

One can go through a great many of the neurotic syndromes and see that they are not haphazard but fit into the personality pattern of the individual and are the techniques he has utilized throughout life to handle situations. We constantly have to handle situations, environmental and inner ones. When we are confronted with a conflict situation, usually one that is inside rather than outside us (for the outside situation very frequently acts as a last straw and links up with similar kinds of conflict situations within ourselves), if we can't solve the conflict along the lines of normal development, we utilize a neurotic kind of solution. Since there is a tendency for human behavior to repeat itself, the same kind of neurotic solution is used over and over again.

At certain life periods which have both physical and psychological importance these neurotic kinds of behavior are especially likely to appear. For instance, we know that at the time of the menopause there is a tendency for women to get upset in various kinds of ways. They have hot flashes, tenseness, nervousness, feelings of guilt, and so on. The puberty period is another time in an individual's life when there is a tendency for a neurotic kind of behavior to come up. There are many and very complicated reasons why the puberty period is a particularly difficult one. Dr. Murray has indicated to you what generally happens at puberty. It is a period in which choices have to be made, and they may be very difficult choices. So when at puberty you see a boy or girl with neurotic symptoms, remember that puberty is a very difficult period and perhaps the symptoms you see may not have quite the malignancy that they would have later in life.

There's another period, that around the age of five or six, which is also likely to be stormy. So there are three difficult periods in the life of an individual—early childhood, puberty, and the climacterium. When an individual who has had a stormy childhood reaches puberty, he may make the various necessary adjustments in a neurotic manner. If so, his neurotic difficulties will follow the pattern of his childhood. It is for this reason that psychiatrists ask about "neurotic traits in childhood" when getting an individual's history. We want to know a good deal about the individual's childhood, for that is where his pattern was laid down.

I've given you a rather sketchy account of the meaning and significance of neurosis. I've left out a lot of things. Now I'd like you to ask questions or present your point of view.

DISCUSSION

STUDENT. Dr. Kaufman, will you say something about the frequency with which these various types of defenses are used?

DR. KAUFMAN. Dr. Romano is going to talk to you about anxiety later, and perhaps he should be the one to answer this question.

DR. ROMANO. I think that Dr. Kaufman intimated that hysterical conversion phenomena are not so common now as they were in the past, except in cultural groups with rather primitive civilization. I should think the most common neurotic symptom is that of diffuse anxiety which may be nonfocal, such as the cardio-respiratory discharge with motor activity, the tremulousness, and the vasomotor changes that all of you often see. Probably second would be some displacement of anxiety through certain parts of the body: what are technically known as organ neuroses or what today are sometimes called psychosomatic symptoms. Compulsive, obsessive behavior, phobic symptoms, combinations of diffuse anxiety with hysteria occur next most frequently and in that order, while the least frequent today are the hysterical symptoms.

*

STUDENT.   In menopause situations how much danger is there of stirring up things that will turn an anxiety neurosis which is pretty well taken care of into a neurosis we can't do much about?

DR. HASTINGS.   There's a lot of danger at that age period, particularly if in your psychotherapy you quickly uncover many difficulties in the patient's life that have been defended against or buried for many years. I think you have to realize the meaning of the involutional period for any person, sick or well, when you consider how much you are going to bring to the surface, remembering that there is not much point in telling the patient about his mistakes and difficulties unless you have something better to offer him. The involutional period for all of us is a period in which change is much more difficult than earlier. For a woman whose entire life has been her children, it is an age period in which the children are leaving or have left and she is figuratively dead unless she gets other interests. For a man it is a period in which a change of job or even a change of house or city may disturb his defenses. For both it is an age period in which friends are beginning to die. It's the period then, generally, of some storm, a period of insecurity. To deal with a depression at that age by rather quickly removing the cover from a lot of pushed-down memories and disturbances may completely overwhelm the patient. If you try to do that, you have to be sure you are supporting the patient properly and to have definitely in mind why you are doing it.

STUDENT.   What do you mean by supporting the patient?

DR. HASTINGS.   Supporting the patient mainly by your doctor-patient relationship, lending your strength to your patient as he goes through the uncovering period.

STUDENT.   Well, that brings up the matter of the so-called male climacteric. I've heard a lot about it but have never been able to identify it in my own mind. Is there such a thing in the psychological development of a man?

DR. HASTINGS. A psychological picture corresponding to that in a woman? Yes, I think so. I don't think there's much difference whether it occurs in a woman or a man. It's a period, as I have just said, of marked change, of insecurity, of wonder and recognition and realization on the part of the individual that the ideals toward which he has been shooting all his life will now probably never be attained.

DR. KAUFMAN. In the extremes of the reaction that you find in a hospital male patients and female patients have almost identical clinical symptoms. A very important aspect of the question for a physician is that frequently the symptoms are specifically somatic, so it's a temptation to a doctor to use primarily physical techniques or physical diagnoses. We've been kidding a lot about the question of replacement therapy in some of our discussions here, but actually it is a problem that faces one in this sort of case. Perhaps Dr. Bauer, who has discussed this problem with us in our particular group, would say something in relation to that age period.

DR. BAUER. I have nothing much to say other than that in the male we have much less evidence than in the female for explaining the difficulties on the basis of endocrine lack. In both men and women I think the psychological aspects are much more important than the lack of a specific endocrine agent.

DR. ROMANO. It seems to me that most of the errors in the use of estrogens and androgens in the male have been in commission, not in omission. It is our experience that the estrogens are of little or no value in alleviating the emotional aspects of minor depressions in the involutional period. They may be of some value in reducing the intensity and frequency of the vasomotor disturbances, but other than that I know of no particular benefit to be secured from them. My experience with androgens for men is much more limited. Certainly, however, I think it's best to let sleeping dogs lie, if you are sure they are sleeping, and not disturb too much the equilibrium that aging people have reached.

DR. BAUER. I think you ought also to remember in the case of substitution therapy that you are just delaying the situation. It will reappear every time the therapy is stopped, and you will still have the fundamental problem to deal with. Another thing to remember is that the patient is aware of the changes in himself, so it is not much consolation to him to be told, "Why, you're just getting old." It's his problems that he's concerned with, and one ought not to say, "Oh yes, you don't hear quite as well, you don't see quite as well; you're just getting old." He's concerned about those things. He's reminded all too frequently as to what is taking place.

DR. RENNIE.   I want to add a word of caution to another part of this general discussion. The question arose as to whether during the treatment of a person in the involutional period certain features of the personality might tend to overwhelm him. Yes, that is true. Features of the personality can become more insistent when they come nearer to recognition; they can therefore be of greater danger than they were before and may throw the person off balance. But I want to add this note of caution: this can be true at any age period, depending upon the kind of therapy you offer. One can indeed overwhelm a patient by bringing too quickly to the foreground aspects of his personality he is not prepared to cope with. The conclusion to be drawn from that is that therapy is not a process of digging, therapy is not a process of unearthing certain dimly recognized or unrecognized elements in the personality. If you try to do that, the buried material may appear at a time when the patient is utterly unprepared to face it and deal with it, in which case you may overwhelm the patient. Consequently part of the therapeutic procedure is to get the patient ready for the acceptance of material that would earlier have been intolerable to him. It's a help, in such preparation, for you to recognize that many of the things that seem strange are far nearer the normal than you may have previously suspected. But I don't think I can put strongly enough to you as practitioners that the aim is not to do anything to uncover all the unrecognized causes of neuroses. Take plenty of time and be awfully sure that your patient is ready to receive and use such material when it does come into the foreground; otherwise you may have some real difficulties with your patient.

STUDENT.   It seems to me that the period when a young man or woman starts working or having children is a very important one. I

think they have many problems, whereas the person of fifty-five is fi-
nancially established and his children have grown, and so I wonder
whether that first period is not more insecure than the later one.

DR. KAUFMAN. That's a good point you bring up, and it may work
that way for some people. All we can do in our discussion is to make
some kind of generalization, but we always have to come back to this
most important fact—that the human being is not a point in a statistical
curve. Unless you keep that constantly in mind, these generalizations
just won't work, for one man's meat is another man's poison. So always
think of the individual, and think in terms of what life at fifty-five
means to him. What kinds of problems does he have? And in addition
to that, what kind of person has he been? What kind of techniques has
he used all his life for the handling of his difficulties? Then you will
know something about that particular individual.

Perhaps what I'm going to say isn't wholly true, but I want to say it
for effect. In many ways it is unfortunate that physiological change
takes place at the climacterium, for even if it didn't take place, a good
many of our patients would still have their particular problems and
you'd have to handle them in the way I've outlined.

To come back to your other point, I think it is very true that the period in which a man is beginning his career is a very important one. Any
period of life in which an individual has to make serious adjustments—
to the external world and, more important, to his internal demands
—is bound to be important for him. One individual will make these adjustments easily. Another may find that an apparently minor stress will
act as a trigger mechanism to set off a severe explosion.

To state it this way may sound as though we psychiatrists minimize
reality. I think some of you have the feeling that whenever you bring
up something real we say, "That's not of much importance. Look into
the inner man." Now we don't minimize reality. Quite the contrary.
What we try to do is to ask, "What does this reality mean to this individual?" If the reality is tough, the individual's personality assets are
of chief importance, for the same tough situation will leave one man
apparently unscathed and overwhelm another. No, we don't minimize
reality; we have the greatest respect for it. But we are also interested
in what the individual's techniques for handling reality are. That's why

we are so interested in how the person characteristically behaves. The best clues to his character formation, his neurotic tensions and difficulties, are to be found in his past history.

*

STUDENT.   How often do you think the hysteric is conscious of the reason for that behavior? The man with the hand, for instance. Do you think such a person often realizes that his hand isn't paralyzed—really way down inside of himself?

DR. MURRAY.   I think there are variations in that. There may be a more or less conscious effort to evade (this we call suppression) or there may be an evasion by unconscious devices (repression). These evasions run a whole gamut from the very deep ones in which the individual has no awareness at all to those that are very close to the surface. Several of us saw a case of the latter kind yesterday. This patient came to the clinic with the complaint of waking up at four in the morning with palpitations and a feeling of fluttering and tenseness across the chest. We talked with her and found that she had had seven pregnancies and that four of the children had died. They had all been premature births. We talked with her about the heart beat and how difficult life was. That was our first theme: how one had to accept that life is a burden. Following this, we very quickly found out that after the last baby's birth she was afraid of becoming pregnant. She was aware of that, but she would not accept it. I mean, you could just see her wavering between acceptance and nonacceptance of the idea. I left the lady at that point and the student continued with her. She said to him, "Yes, that's very true. I have been afraid. I think of that a great deal. But now for the first time . . ." This is an illustration of a painful situation that was consciously pushed aside.

DR. KAUFMAN.   That question has raised an important point in relation to our attitude toward our patients. If we feel that a patient is consciously aware of the nature of his difficulty, we begin to think, "Why doesn't he stop it? Perhaps he is just putting it on. If he has control and doesn't use it, then he's faking." We saw that attitude so much in the service. Now if you feel that a man is a goldbrick, to use service terms, then your attitude toward him in therapy immediately becomes one of hostility and you think he is really a bad fellow.

I would like to point out that there is a difference between a patient's knowing fundamentally that his condition is not organic and conscious faking. Sometime during our discussion we have mentioned unconscious insight. That doesn't mean that the individual takes responsibility for his condition—responsibility in the sense of consciousness. If we just remember that, it makes it easier for us to treat our patients, for then we get away from the idea that this person is putting it on. As Dr. Murray said, frequently an idea is not so much unconscious as pushed aside, pushed out of proper perspective.

The kind of therapy we've been talking about is that in which more or less conscious ideas are brought out in order to put them into a different perspective. It really is amazing how sometimes one is able to put a series of events into a more or less causal relationship, whereas before that they were isolated by emotional blocks.

DR. BOND.   There is one point I'd like to make about the question that was asked. There are a good many people who come to a doctor using a physical complaint as a calling card. They know very well that that isn't quite what they are coming for, and you can see it very clearly, too, but they don't quite know how to come otherwise, so they bring up some physical symptom and use it that way. One of the best examples I know was a pilot who was on his fourth mission, flying over Germany, when his copilot's head was taken off. He came to the dispensary again and again. Just before he was to go to Berlin again, he came in for the fifteenth time and said to the doctor, "My nose is bad." The doctor took him out and shrank his nose, but the man just sat around and waited and for the fifteenth time told his whole story. At the end of the story the doctor just said, "Well, see you when you come back!" That kind of thing is awfully difficult. You can jump at the conclusion, "The son-of-a-gun is a liar. He can't fool me." In the matter of malingering it is awfully important to realize that if the person is a malingerer, he's going to fool you. You are going to be perplexed. When the person presents a symptom of the sort this man did, he won't fool you; he won't even be trying to fool you. A neurotic ordinarily won't fool you. By a malingerer you will be perplexed; he'll usually do it well enough so that you'll have very serious doubts. But even if the person is a malingerer, what's the difference? He'll usually have enough emotional problems to make him at least very unuseful.

DR. MURRAY.   I think there's one other angle to this point that Dr. Bond mentioned. Sometimes a mother brings her child to you when it's really herself she wants treatment for. She doesn't want to come and say that she is having troubles or that she is worried about her husband. So I think you have to be on the alert to be sure that you don't miss the fact that such a woman really wants to talk about herself.

DR. KAUFMAN.   That brings up a topic, perhaps a little bit beside the point, which is of importance and which already has been implied here a number of times—why does a patient come to a doctor? I mean, we are often in a position of having to ask ourselves just that—"Why does this patient come to see me?" If he comes because he is obviously and grossly sick or you are called to his house, then there usually isn't any such problem. But I'm quite sure that very frequently one wonders, "Here is a patient coming in, just why does he come?" Dr. Bond's man came in to have his nose shrunk. His nose was bad. Well, that was cleared up, but he came back fifteen times. Why? There's always a reason why a patient comes to a doctor.

STUDENT.   You mentioned that at different cultural levels there might be different reaction patterns. A person from some mountainous region in Arkansas might have a typical hysteria, while if that same person lived in Minneapolis or some other city he might have some gastrointestinal symptom. Sometimes such people come in and say, "I have trouble with my stomach, but I think maybe it's nervousness. I've had some difficulty with the family, and it may be related to that." Would you use a different approach and attempt a different solution in therapy with these two kinds of people?

DR. KAUFMAN.   Yes, you've got to treat the man from Arkansas in terms of his knowledge and capacity. If a highly sophisticated, intellectual person comes to you, you can't start your relationship and your therapy with him at the naive level you would use with a person who has a mental age of eight. There again it becomes a matter of the individual evaluation of the person with whom you are working.

You mention a specific situation—the patient comes in and says, "I have this, but I think it is due to nerves." That doesn't necessarily mean that it is due to nervousness. Just as some people will deny that they are nervous (and we've emphasized that so often), a person who is afraid that what is wrong with him has some very mortal implications may sometimes shift to, "There is nothing wrong with me organically. This is functional." I once had an illustration of that which was really very pathetic. A doctor who was a typical Parkinson, postencephalitic Parkinson, was sent in to see me when I was a resident. There was no question about the diagnosis. This man was an internist and, as a kind of hobby, was doing some work in neurology. And he developed Parkinsonism. He was sent in to our hospital, and he knew that I was interested in psychiatry, so he asked to see me. We talked awhile and then he said, "Doctor, you're interested in psychiatry, aren't you?" I said, "Yes, I'm going to be a psychiatrist." He said, "Well, I haven't told this to anybody at all, but what I've got is not Parkinsonism. I've never had encephalitis. There's something in relation to my brother; if I could kill that, this would all clear up. This is all neurotic." This was his perfectly honest evaluation of his problem. Yet he was the crassest kind of encephalitic.

All of us have seen that sort of reaction, and so when a patient says, "I'm nervous and excited," we don't just automatically say, "Look, this patient recognizes that he has a neurotic problem. We don't have to do a physical examination. We don't have to do this, that, or the other thing." Beware of that kind of situation, because there is this obverse of the usual picture of denial of neurotic difficulties. You will find a lot of people who are so afraid of physical illness—especially cardiovascular disorders and mortal diseases—that they may attempt to solve their fear of illness by presenting you with pseudo insight into a pseudoneurotic problem. The technique they use for doing this is in itself neurotic, but beware of it.

DR. RENNIE. I think that question has another implication of great importance, and that is the role that culture may play in the disease picture. Certain disease pictures vary depending upon the culture in which they appear. We used to have examples of that in Baltimore among Negro patients. A foreign doctor would see a Negro patient in the outpatient department and come rushing to us and say, "This man has developed a schizophrenia. He says that he saw the Virgin Mary appear last night in his room." Well, that's a common experience for Negroes in Baltimore to report; the Virgin Mary and all sorts of other figures may appear to them without their being at all psychotic. The cultural setting makes a real difference in the manner in which patients react to disease. In a large city like New York you get a good many leads out of such simple facts as whether the patient comes from the Italian district on one side of town or a family of first-generation Latins in another part of the city.

STUDENT.   Is there such a thing as malingering?

DR. KAUFMAN.   I should imagine that there are malingerers but I have never happened to see one. And in the Army I was on the lookout for them because of the kind of job I had. I just didn't believe that malingering was any kind of problem, and yet, in the line, a lot of medical officers did. So whenever somebody said this case is a malingerer, and I was in that area, I wanted to see the man. Most of the time we could demonstrate that the man was not a malingerer. What we did see very frequently was that the soldier took every advantage of his illness that he thought he could get away with. But in the regular Army, I understand, that was one of the prerogatives a man was given when he joined—the right to swing the lead a little bit and get away with a certain number of things. You know, the fellow who wants to get out of duty—when a new doctor comes to the dispensary what does he do? He makes a try. If it works, fine. If it doesn't, that's all right, too. But when you come to the problem of malingering, that has to be taken into consideration.

I want to reemphasize what Dr. Bond said—suppose a man is a malingerer. What kind of persons are malingerers? I think that immediately carries the problem over and beyond the question of the right or wrong. This is so awfully important in relation to our attitudes. We should never try to put a patient on the spot. Why should we? If a patient comes to you in your practice and you suspect that he is malingering, ask yourself why he wants to do it. There may be compensations. There may be this and there may be that. But at least I want to know why this person does it if he does it. And usually I have found out. Conscious exaggeration? Yes, lots of it. I've been guilty of it myself in the Army. I shouldn't consider that malingering.

You are going to run into that problem now with returning veterans. The question will come up with the men who are applying for a pension. Are they faking? Now if we enter into that problem with the attitude that every man who comes up for a pension *ipso facto* is trying to pull a fast one, then we are going to do a lot of injustice to a lot of people. But if we enter into the problem of what is wrong with this man and then make up our opinion on the basis of that, we may find a certain number of malingerers. The initial attitude is the important thing. And the minute the attitude of suspicion enters into it, the whole relationship with the patient is disturbed.

Clinical Problems

III

1. A FRUSTRATING PATIENT

STUDENT. I'd like to ask what you do when a patient keeps saying no to your questions. Here's this patient of mine, a woman of fifty-nine who complains of bloating, with pain radiating from the abdomen to the left chest and scapula. She is childless, has an adopted son who did not marry the prospective wife she had picked out for him. She professes to have accepted with satisfaction the girl he did marry and gets a good deal of pleasure out of her granddaughter, who lives far away. She has had her symptoms for some twelve years, with variable intensity. They started after a hysterectomy at forty-four, about which she said she was not much disturbed. After telling me this she started in on this childhood business and later said she wouldn't trade her husband off for anything in the world.

DR. KAUFMAN. Don't take quick and unsolicited protestations at their face value.

STUDENT. Then I asked her about her childlessness and got no indication of tension. She said no to all my questions. Am I supposed to turn around and tell her that she is lying or drop the question? If I drop it we haven't gotten anywhere. *What do I do next?*

DR. KAUFMAN. Treat her; give her symptomatic relief. You have already established a relationship. If you aren't impatient and if you don't feel frustrated, you may find that something interesting will happen perhaps three months hence. She will come back to some of your questions, such as the one about not having children, when unconsciously she is ready to. She has created a system of defenses now, and I shouldn't do anything more about her now. If she were a patient in your own practice, you would keep a relationship with her.

STUDENT. But what shall I do at the end of this next interview? Shall I say come back sometime?

DR. KAUFMAN.   Tell her you can't find anything wrong with her physically, but that you know she is troubled by gas and you will give her something to relieve it. Because of the way you have handled her, your treatment is different even if you do give the same medication you would formerly have given. Her relationship to you, symptomatic relief, and reassurance—these are all you can do for her now. You mustn't feel frustrated. The specialist isn't disturbed by his limitations; it is the learner who feels this kind of frustration. You have laid the groundwork with this patient in an area where perhaps nobody has ever worked before. You are going to have a lot of such patients in your practice.

2. THERAPEUTIC LEVELS

DR. RENNIE.   The question has been raised, "What are the goals of this course?"

STUDENT.   It bothered me that people wanted to bring up hypnosis and psychoanalysis. Actually we won't be using that sort of thing. I want to know how much we are to carry from this course and apply to our practice. I think we'll be able to take care of the presenting complaint but we won't be able to cure the patient.

ANOTHER STUDENT.   I am not so much for knowing about the technique employed as something of the type of case that would benefit by psychoanalysis. I am interested, however, in those aspects of psychoanalysis that are applicable in the understanding of human personality.

DR. RENNIE.   I find myself in accord. Do you feel that the didactic material you are getting on the nature of personality is becoming confusing?

FIRST STUDENT.   No, I think it is very interesting. After all, there hasn't been anything revolutionary in what has been said. The lecturers have just given fundamentals that have been proven over the years, facts every doctor should know. The application to our practice is another matter. I think we may do harm in uncovering our patients instead of just giving supportive treatment.

DR. RENNIE.   I agree. It is not your province to do it.

FIRST STUDENT.   That is what we are doing with our patients here.

DR. RENNIE.   Have you gotten into anything very deep? Don't for one minute think that because we are telling you about some of these deeper mechanisms we expect you to handle them. We are telling you about them because we think you ought to know as much as possible about what makes a human being, but with no implication that it is your function to deal with such problems. It is clearly not your function to engage in any kind of therapy aimed at radical upheaval of the personality make-up. Limit your work to making sick people more comfortable, to making them well if you can—that is, free of symptoms. There will be many of them whose symptoms you can touch and probably remove by such procedures as we have discussed. Beyond that I think you should not try to go. Certainly as a result of this work you are going to avoid a lot of errors doctors have made in the past. You won't complicate people's lives by failing to deal with them as persons. You may bring a great deal of comfort and genuine relief to some of them in relatively less complicated neurotic states. Obsessions, compulsions, hysteria are out of your area. I quite agree that any time spent here on hypnosis and psychoanalysis will be time poorly spent. However, these issues have been raised. I think we can get them out in the open and say what things are not your sphere of function.

There is an incredible amount of misconception about what psychoanalysis is. Psychoanalysis is a way of looking at people and it is also a special kind of therapy. It is both a point of view and a technique of treatment. These two aspects of psychoanalysis are fairly distinct although closely related.

The therapeutic use of psychoanalysis does not concern you; it is out of your world and you have nothing to do with it as a therapeutic tool. It is a technique which aims primarily at the uncovering of the powerful, emotional, unconscious conflicts that lie behind the psychoneuroses. Only a few very courageous psychoanalysts feel it should be applied to psychotics. It is a therapy primarily for psychoneuroses, psychosomatic conditions, and certain character disorders. Important motivating conflicts are often unconscious, are not readily available for recall.

When Freud first started, he used hypnosis as a means of uncovering. He abandoned that and devised the technique of free association. In essence, one says to the patient, "For one hour I want you to talk about anything and everything that comes to your mind. All I ask you to do is not to decide whether ideas are unimportant or not but to let every association come." Under this technique, from time to time emotions and thoughts slip through, a dim glimmer of something comes back or the patient makes an interesting slip of the tongue or reports that he had an interesting dream. Then the analyst says to him, "Let's take that dream and tell me what comes into your mind as you think about it." Slowly, in the course of time, the analyst and the patient begin to get a picture of what the important facts are in the genesis of the neurosis.

A psychoanalysis usually requires an hour a day for many months or even years. It is a highly specialized technique that requires long training on the part of the analyst, including a personal analysis. Immediately you begin to see its limitations. It is not synonymous with psychiatry. The important thing is that increasingly psychiatrists are beginning to take, accept, and use these principles that psychoanalysis gave, but to use them in a different fashion.

STUDENT. I think much of that material is very directly applicable in mental hygiene, for example in pediatrics.

FIRST STUDENT. I think the course is going to help us as doctors much more than it is going to help our patients. Indirectly it will help patients, but it isn't going to cure them; they are still going to come back every week or six months.

DR. RENNIE. I think you are going to give your patients better care than you have before.

FIRST STUDENT. I am sure of it.

DR. RENNIE. I think your general handling of patients will be definitely better. If you maintain this point of view and approach, you will touch the lives of very many people more constructively than you might otherwise have done. If you get that out of the course, it is enough.

3. THE MEANING OF PAIN

Complaint. This is a case of a married woman, aged forty-one, whose principal complaint is pain in the back. She describes it as slightly more in the right lumbar region, running down the right leg, the lateral aspect of the leg about halfway down. It is relieved by pressure over her back. It is a sharp pain, worse when stooping and reaching, and very painful in the jerking and jolting of a street car ride. It is worse on sneezing and coughing; it even bothers her on blowing her nose. It bothers her particularly when she leans forward, as when she is sitting at a sewing machine. This pain followed an injury four years ago, when she fell off a ladder. She cannot describe how she fell or tell whether she was unconscious or not. The first thing she remembers is that she was in the first-aid station. After resting for a while, she returned to her work. She can't describe any specific pain that she had immediately after the accident; she just ached all over. Later that evening she passed out while at work, but she can't describe that either. She says the incidents are all blurred; she can't recall them.

So much for the accident. Since that time she has been to various doctors, complaining of pain in her back. She has never improved very much. The matter of compensation came up. She had a hearing on this, but the authorities didn't reach a decision. The spinagram showed a slight defect which could be a disc.

DR. ROMANO. Just a word of caution about spinagrams. In introducing opaque substances into the subarachnoid space and in determining the configuration and contour of the caudal sac, you must be very careful because there are many normal variations.

The orthopedist who was consulted said this patient should be explored. Everything was all set for the appointment for the operation. She and the orthopedist were discussing it. Finally he said, "You don't seem to be very serious about this, do you?" She replied, "No, why should I? It is up to you; I want to get rid of these pains." The orthopedist did not feel satisfied from her attitude that he was justified in intervention and thought it was best to postpone the operation. I think some settlement was made. She seems to have been given a sum of money, but it may have been that she first got a lump sum and then reopened the case. She still insists that she wants to get rid of her pain and she denies that there is any money involved. So her family doctor suggested that she come here for an opinion before going ahead with the operation. She has been seen in Neurology, and the doctor there expresses the opinion that she should not be operated on.

Personal History. This woman's father was a farmer. She has one older brother and two sisters, she being next to the youngest. When Dr. Romano asked her about her siblings, she replied in a rather annoyed way, "I have been over this so many times." Her attitude throughout the interview was one of well-controlled emotion most of the time.

Her father died of a ruptured blood vessel in the heart. His heart trouble began when she was ten years old. He had been downtown shopping and had just stepped off a curb when he felt terrific pain in his chest. Her older sister took him to a doctor, who examined him and said there wasn't anything especially wrong, he could go home. But he continued to have such pain that he couldn't ride in the buggy and had to walk very slowly several miles home. She took care of him for about a week. He was in bed for about two days; after that he was around the house, going back and forth between a chair and the bedroom. She remembers him lying on the davenport, with perspiration on his brow, which she would wipe off. He couldn't lie down very long, had to get up and walk back and forth in the room. Finally he walked into the bedroom, sat down in a chair, and flopped over and died. When I was asking her about this in quite some detail, she said, "Do we have to go through this?" and broke down and cried. She let us believe she was unusually attached to her father, and I could learn no other reason why she, at ten years of age, had so great a part to play in his care.

Shortly after this, I think it was the following year when she was in the sixth grade, she was having difficulty in school. She always had to ask the teacher over again what the questions were. The teacher would read the questions to her, and she would quickly write them down and in answering them get good marks. Finally the teacher asked her why she did this, and they had her eyes examined. A doctor tried out different types of glasses, but she said they weren't the right kind and took them back. When she was in the doctor's office suddenly everything went black and she couldn't see anything at all. This lasted for about three minutes; then she went home. In spite of having glasses, she wasn't able to see, and so she stayed out of school for about a year and a half. When she went back to school her younger sister was in the same grade, and so they let her skip a grade. Apparently her vision was all right for a year, but in her sophomore and junior years in high school the teacher had to repeat all the questions for her and her sister read all her lessons to her. Her only explanation for the eye trouble was that it came on after measles, which is supposed to be hard on the eyes.

The girl finished high school. When she was twenty-two she married a young veteran who was confined to a hospital with a chronic disorder. She said she consulted a number of doctors about it before she married, and they told her she knew what she was doing, there was nothing they could do about it. The husband was in the hospital much of the time for the next five years. At the time of her accident he was just about to have an operation.

DR. ROMANO. If I may digress for a moment—many times a doctor is asked by a woman or a man or by parents shall I marry or shall my daughter marry such a person. It makes considerable difference whether the parents are asking or whether one or the other of the prospective mates is asking. I think, however, it is important for the doctor to realize that it would be wrong for him to assume the role of Jehovah and give dogmatic judgment on whether a person should or should not marry someone. Actually the doctor should try to help the person reach his own decision. The doctor should say objectively, "If you are asking for my professional advice, I shall try to help you to see more clearly what some of the problems are that you are facing, so that you may make as mature and logical a decision as is possible."

The husband had the operation and came home some months later on a stretcher. He has been home and she has been taking care of him ever since that time. He has never worked. The wife has been working off and on at various jobs. She has often had to be sent home from work on account of her pain. Now she has reached the point where she can't get a job; no one will employ her because this happens so often. She has to get rid of this pain in order to get a job. She and her husband have some compensation from the government. It was originally $100 a month but was cut down to nothing for a long period of time and is now about $87 a month.

There is one other point that came out in the discussion. Besides having pain in the back she has pains in the chest up around the scapula, right side; she also has numbness in her right arm and she has had a "parlysis," as she calls it, of the wrist, so that she had difficulty in handling glasses. A number of doctors examined her wrist but couldn't find anything wrong with it. She insists there was a little bit of a bump there. Only a few weeks ago she went to a doctor she calls her Uncle Dudley (she wouldn't say what his name is), and he said, "Oh, I'll fix that all right," and manipulated it a little bit. Since then she has had no trouble and has been able to handle a glass.

Together with the pain that she has in her right side she has a feeling like cold water running around. I tried to learn a bit more about her hand. In talking about the death of her mother, which occurred two years ago, she said the nurse asked her to take care of the "hypodermoclysis intravenous."

She said she would stay there and hold her mother's hand; she used to hold it for hours and hours until her hand was numb. I asked her which hand. She thought a bit and said it was her left hand. She is right-handed, I think.

DR. ROMANO. Well, let's go back for a moment, Dr. H. Here's a forty-one-year-old woman who was next to the youngest in the family with two above her. Did you get any feeling at all as to what kind of childhood she had before the death of her father?

DR. H. (STUDENT). I couldn't get any information about that from her. She got along fine with everybody, she said.

DR. ROMANO. The second thing is that her father died when she was about ten. What was your feeling about the significance of that event to her?

DR. H. It seems to have a very strong meaning to her at present, for that was the first time she cried. Her lip quivered and the tears ran down her face, and she said, "Do we have to go into this?"

DR. ROMANO. After her father's death she began having difficulty in school. She had trouble seeing the blackboard, had trouble reading, and this amounted eventually to the teacher's reading to her, and then to her staying out of school for more than a year, and later having her sister read to her. That was a rather drastic procedure for a girl who at most was somewhat myopic. Rather unusual, wasn't it? A lot of kids are myopic and they have their sensitivities and difficulties over not knowing it, but when it is found out it is easy to get glasses and they can see all right. Of course, glasses in a little girl present a problem, too, and they did much more so years ago than they do now. A little girl can wear glasses now without being stigmatized. But this girl had the teacher read to her. In other words, she became a very dependent person, cared for almost like a little baby. We don't know why she remained home for over a year; it may have been the doctor's advice; but regardless of the motive she was cared for and protected like a baby instead of an eleven- or twelve-year-old girl. So this whole period of some years before and during pubescence was characterized by an exaggerated amount of dependence.

Following graduation from school there are four or five years we know little about. It would be important to know about her adjustment then, for it would give some inkling of her flexibility. Was she able to leave home? Was she able to work? Was she able to have friends? Did she date? Just what was she doing all that time?

DR. H. I assume that she was working.

DR. ROMANO. Now comes this next step. She marries a man who is chronically ill and hospitalized at the time she marries him. She had some doubts about the marriage. We don't know what her motivations were. Many times when patients ask, "Shall I marry?" what they are saying in plain English is, "Please tell me that I should or should not marry." They want you to confirm what they feel. That is why it is very dangerous sometimes to be dogmatic. You have to find out what is going on in a person to know how you can help a person best.

What significance would this marriage have? Marriage of a woman to an invalid—in a wider sense, to a man who is not a man, a depreciated, devaluated, sick man. Who is going to support her? A hospitalized man—one considers what their sexual relations are to be. Are they going to have children? Who would support the children? What was she going to do if he was in the hospital? What would you think some of the motives, some of the thoughts of a girl who married such a person would be?

DR. H. Well, it seems to me to be the exact opposite of what her life had been before that. She had always been dependent on someone, and now it would be the very opposite.

DR. ROMANO. That's right. Almost a reversal. But we don't know what it may mean. Certain very dependent people get into positions like this for a number of reasons.

Let's consider for a moment what other possible interpretations there may be. If a woman marries a man like this, in one way it is like not being married. She doesn't sleep with her husband. It is like being married and yet not being married. Maybe that was the only type of marriage that she could wish for and that she could achieve. I think it is a very significant item in the life history of this woman. What has her life been since she married?

DR. H. She's been working to support her husband all this time. He has been in the hospital much of the time and home part of the time. I asked her, "Under these circumstances do you live a normal life as far as your husband is concerned?" She replied that she didn't care much about having sexual relations with him. Lack of that didn't seem to bother her very much one way or the other. And since her accident her back has been so painful that she couldn't possibly do that, she said.

DR. ROMANO. And how old was she when she married—twenty-two? In the fifteen years before her accident how much did she work? That fact is really going to help us, I think. What did she do? Did she support him, I mean? He has been getting $100 a month, hasn't he?

DR. H. Yes. He is a veteran. He got $100 a month. That $100 a month couldn't have supported them, and later he didn't get anything for a long while and it was necessary for her to work. As I understand it, most of her work was as a clerk in various places.

DR. ROMANO. Well, my hunch is this. I don't think this woman has ever assumed any realistically independent life. I don't think she has assumed the burden of this man. I think there is another interpretation possible here. Granted that we don't have all the data, in many instances marriage to a disabled man may at least minimize the threat of sexuality. The woman may identify with this man who is sick and cared for, and through the identification be cared for, too. From what I could see of her in the few minutes I was there, I have a feeling she has never made any really serious overture with respect to assuming responsibility. That would be my hunch about it, but we must have more data as we go on to confirm it.

I think that thus far we seem to be dealing with a woman who for various reasons had considerable difficulty in growing up and was probably a quite dependent, immature person. She married this man, and in marrying such a man attempted to solve some of her anxieties, some of her difficulties in meeting the normal social and sexual demands of marriage. There is no better criterion of normality than of being able to live with another person, being able to love another person, being able to assume responsibility. Those things are indices of being adult and capable. I have a feeling that this girl has never been able to give, and I think we shall see that in certain of her defenses which will come up later.

She has tried, indeed has gone out of her way at times, to participate in community activities. She says, too, she has always wanted to keep an open house for kids. She never had children, she says, and yet over and over again she feels she really did have them because she opened her doors to them and they came in. Remember when I asked her the question, "Do you have children?" she said no. "Weren't you able to or were you sick?" I asked. "Would you care to talk about it?" Later on she accused me of feeling that she was being selfish in not having children. You remember how defensive she became about the whole question of children? She had to explain to us over and over again, defensively and almost aggressively, that she did do these things, that she did give of herself.

And now with this accident. It happened at a time when the question of the husband's operation came up and there was therefore some possibility of change in the situation. In this accident she fell, was bruised, and then came the period of repetitive physical examinations, including films, spinagrams, and so on. Now this is an object lesson for all of us. You see here the danger of unnecessary repetitive examinations. You see here the danger of a doctor's not making a courageous decision. You see here the danger of not knowing the setting in which an accident takes place—the setting, the emotional preparation this woman had for injury.

Now, what does this injury mean? Actually this woman is crying out, "Please take care of me; please be good to me. Here I am working like this. Take care of me." You may ask if that is so why does it happen that she has pain? Is she suffering? The question comes up, what is the economy, the utilization of pain for purposes of that sort? "I have done my best with this man," the woman says. "I have given him my all. But I'm sick now, too."

There is something else, also. What are some of the feelings a person has toward an invalid he has to take care of? What are some of the normal feelings? Let's say your wife became ill, you were in circumstances in which you couldn't afford a hospital or a nurse, and had to do both your own work and take care of her and all the household chores. What would be some of your feelings? You would be very ashamed of resenting it, you would feel terrible, you couldn't think about it, much less talk about it, but sometimes these thoughts would break through. That is a normal experience when one has to sacrifice certain things and become slavishly attentive to a loved person. Now, don't you think that this woman may have had some such feelings about the life she has led? She arranged her destiny and unconsciously she chose this role of suffering. She has been a long-suffering, self-punishing woman. This accident allows her to say what she has felt many times. Now she can say, "I want to be cared for, too; someone has to take care of me." She can say that if she has pain and is suffering. If she is suffering, she can ask for something. If she suffers and pays the price, she may have the love.

You remember, too, how defensive she was when we talked to her about her backache. She began to cry again and she looked at me and said, "Oh, you doctors, you think it has to do with that compensation. I don't care whether I get the compensation or not." What's the significance of that? I hadn't talked about that. I didn't even know there was a matter of compensation in it. I said, "Perhaps you are a little bit sensitive about it." She said, "Well, the other doctors have accused me and they said that I want it, but I don't. All I want is to be rid of this pain." And then she winced. Then she showed hostility to us and said, "Well, I'll get the money somewhere. I'll get $75 and go down to another clinic." You can see what was going on there—what that meant was, "Look! You aren't as attentive as you should be. You are not getting to the point on this thing. You aren't going to help me, I see. I feel that; I am going to go somewhere else where they will help, where they will take care of me, where they will appreciate me." Did you sense that? You remember we asked her to come back Monday, and she toyed with the idea and finally she said yes—very much like a little girl who wants you to win her over.

Of course there are many areas in this case we don't know anything about. Her relationship to her mother, for instance—her mother's illness. One sees many times in such a person, in a self-punishing woman, that the relation to the mother and the feelings toward her are involved in the problem.

What we have done a few times with problems like this is to hospitalize the patient on the psychiatric service and, during the initial period, gratify a number of his very dependent needs by the use of various devices, such as hydrotherapy and massage. We instruct our nurses to be quite giving and pleasant and accepting of this person. This is after we have made the necessary diagnostic tests and physical examinations. After this initial period, we begin with interviews and help the patient to understand in a very minor way his present situation. Then we use a case worker and others to find out what can be done realistically in re-arranging the environment—for instance, to get an adequate income to maintain the family and to return the person to work if that is neces-sary. We have done that with some long-term compensation neuroses. We use suggestion a great deal. Many times the patient's accessibility to insight therapy isn't very good, so one must be very careful how far one goes in interpretation. Whenever there is long-continued pain in a person, you are usually dealing with a very deep and definitive type of emotional need. If you are not equipped—and even when you are equipped—you must go slowly in giving any broad interpretation of underlying hostility.

STUDENT.   May I ask a practical question? Why do you hospitalize them on a psychiatric service?

DR. ROMANO.   There are a lot of dangers in putting them in a psy-chiatric hospital, of course. It may frighten them. It all depends on how you do it. What I'd do with a patient like this would be to see her a number of times, to get more data, so that I could have a clear under-standing of what was going on. That would be the first thing. If com-petent physicians had already examined her, as they seem to have done, I would accept their findings. I would not repeat anything that wasn't necessary. I would examine her physically (sometimes that's necessary and sometimes it isn't), and I would say definitely and dogmatically that there is no need at this time for an operation; it is not necessary—period. However, I wouldn't deny her pains or argue with her about them. Any remark about the pain being imaginary or unreal would provoke tremendous hostility in her and defeat any program that you have in mind.

DR. H.   What do you do if she says directly, "Do you think my pain is imaginary?" Do you say it is due to emotional circumstances?

DR. ROMANO.   If you are asked that question, you can say, "There is no imaginary pain. I do know that there is no need for you to be oper-ated upon. People who have had injuries in the past sometimes have pain that lasts a bit longer, and sometimes when the pain does last longer it may be due to being worried or being upset or being anxious about something." Go that far right there.

DR. COTTRELL. I think the usual proper answer to "Do you think this pain is imaginary?" is that it may not be directly. The point is that in saying "imaginary pain" the patient means you think he has no pain. In the wider sense perhaps it is imaginary, but to imply that you do not believe that he has pain is certainly the wrong thing to do. Isn't that right?

DR. ROMANO. I would go even further than that. I never use the term "imaginary." The pain that a person has is real to him. We may be able to explain some types of pain through our knowledge of neuroanatomy, but neuroanatomy isn't the complete answer to pain. There are many types of pain. There are many things about pain we don't know. The whole concept of pain is obscure. We know something about the afferent pain tracts in the cord. Does this answer the whole question of pain? No. Pain is real, whether we can demonstrate its anatomic basis or not.

The question is, What is the meaning of a pain to the person? Anna Freud, in taking care of English children during the war, did some experiments with hypodermic injections in very young infants. The infant would cry as long as there was a wheal. In other words, the infant would cry as long as there was pressure on an intradermal pain nerve-ending. As soon as the wheal disappeared, the crying would stop. In the older infants, when you did that, crying did not stop when the wheal disappeared but continued indefinitely. In other words, the emotional meaning of pain was entirely different. Pain may mean something in respect to punishment, in respect to feelings of guilt or hostility. The whole idea of pain is so wrapped up in our emotions and our emotional experiences, relates so much to feelings of love and hate and so on, that we never use the term "imaginary." As Dr. Cottrell said, you are giving a moral indictment when you do so. To the patient it means "You don't believe I am suffering."

To come back to the question of hospitalization for this patient, you would have to be very, very cautious as an internist in hospitalizing a patient like this because you might entrench dependence and invalidism and you might create new symptoms. Actually, I wouldn't hospitalize her if I were you. I would be hospitalizing her as a psychiatrist and not as an internist. As an internist, if you don't have facilities to carry on the various procedures I spoke of, I wouldn't hospitalize her. That would only entrench further some of her difficulties. I think this should be done only if you have a skilled team ready to do a special job.

DR. H. How would further examinations be dangerous? Is it that they would increase this dependence, that she would become more and more dependent all the time as you do more examinations?

DR. ROMANO. Obviously there are dangers at either extreme. If the doctor attempts to reassure the patient and reach a diagnostic conclusion before he has examined the patient adequately, particularly if the patient has been seen by other doctors and given various diagnoses, the patient is apt to distrust the doctor and not come back. At the other extreme is the danger of doing repetitive examinations and keeping a sword of Damocles over the head of the patient for a long period of time. The doctor's indecision and insecurity may be quite infectious and therefore increase the patient's anxiety.

It may be easier for this woman to deal with her pain and her suffering and so on than to face these very deep needs that she has. To face them she might have to say to her husband, "You are an old man of the sea on my shoulders, you are a burden that I can't take; I am not prepared to take this burden; I want to be taken care of myself. If I give all this to you, who is going to take care of me?" You can see how a neurotic symptom is an attempted solution in such a situation. Never satisfactory, never completely satisfactory, but it is partially satisfactory. Many doctors take a moral attitude; they say, "Oh, these damned neurotics, all they want is this and that." One must remember that every neurotic patient suffers. Neurotic behavior essentially is inappropriate behavior. It is also regressive behavior, that is, an attempt to deal with a problem at an earlier and usually less efficient level of adaptation. For this regression the patient must pay a price. This price is the suffering which the patient experiences.

STUDENT. What are the mechanics of transferring a case like this from a general physician to a psychiatrist? It would be, I suppose, to give him all the information you could in a letter, but there is a lot you can't transfer that you yourself know.

DR. ROMANO. That is an extremely important point—not only who should be sent but how they should be sent. Many times I have had patients whose doctors have said, "Well, I can't do anything more for you. As far as I can see, there is nothing wrong with you." Some doctors say, "Maybe I should send you to a psychiatrist, but you are not yet quite bad enough." Many doctors feel jealous; they think they ought to treat the patient. The proper preparation for referral of a person to a psychiatrist is the same as for any other special investigation. Talk over some of these problems with the person to a certain degree, sense what is going on, and then say, "There are doctors who have special skills, such as surgeons. If there were something wrong with your eye or your ear or your nose or your chest, I would ask for help from a doctor who had had special training in those areas. There are doctors who have had special training in understanding problems like yours where emotional factors are involved. You ought to think about that, and I can name someone that you might go to see and have a chat with him and talk over your problems."

"I don't see this as a special problem," the patient may reply. "They ask all those funny questions, and I don't see that I am crazy." You can say, "The psychiatrist is a doctor who has gained special knowledge and skills so that he can understand and treat more effectively many people who are emotionally disturbed. This is an illness like any other type of illness. It doesn't mean that you are crazy. He will ask you to talk about your symptoms and your troubles, and he will wish to know from you what some of your life experiences are."

You have an important responsibility as family doctors to help people understand what psychiatry is, what it is not, and what it can do at the present time. Ignorance lies less in the fact of not knowing things than in knowing a great many things which are not true. The family doctor, because of his pivotal position in society, must be one of the important means through which the general public corrects its prejudices and learns to understand what the goals and scope of modern psychiatry are.

Any more questions about this patient and the problem of pain? To clarify this recommendation of hospitalization: this is a specific therapeutic suggestion, not one to be used indiscriminately by internists and general practitioners.

STUDENT. I chiefly wanted to ask what are you going to do about the pain?

DR. ROMANO. We are going to see her again and try to learn more about her pain and, more particularly, what special meanings the pain may have. At this stage of my knowledge of this patient, I feel that she is one I would like to refer to a psychiatrist for further and more detailed investigation.

STUDENT. I have a question about something we see in our general practice. Patients come in and say, "I have a pain in here, and I am nervous." Does that indicate that there is just a little more latitude for you there, that they already have a lot of insight?

DR. ROMANO. Dr. Kaufman spoke of that today. Nervousness and statements by the patient that he is nervous may mean a great number of things. Naturally there is a wide range of capacity to be able to be aware of, understand, and deal with emotional problems in one's self and in others. For the lack of a better term, it has been called psychological-mindedness, and you can see its manifestations in patients, in medical students, doctors, case workers, and others who deal intimately with sick or disabled people. It is very difficult to define. To many it usually means the capacity to experience and feel what others are feeling without losing one's own identity in the process. It is indispensable for those who have to deal with anxious, frightened, demanding, angry, and helpless people. Patients, too, vary in their ability to be psychologically minded. Some are able in a short period of time, with or without direct help, to have some understanding of what is going on within them. Others have a very thick cellophane layer of intellectual rationalizations that are very difficult to penetrate. In the latter instances, it is wiser for the doctor to err in omission than in commission. There is a fundamental principle in all medical therapy and that is that the principal and only indication of therapy should be to help the patient. In psychotherapy one could say that one should never provoke anxiety or disturb a patient unless one is prepared with knowledge and method to use the anxiety which is provoked toward constructive ends.

STUDENT. I wonder about this patient. If her picture is that of a dependent person, if you try too hard to eradicate this particular situation, may she not pop up with a worse one?

DR. ROMANO. A person like this—as I suggested by mentioning material-giving and case-work help—is apt to be a dependent person the greater part of her life, and she may need your help and support for a long time. You must expect it, just as you would expect to give long attention to a patient with chronic glomerular nephritis or to a patient with repetitive cardiac decompensation. There are many patients that a case worker and a doctor or psychiatrist have to see supportively, almost as a good parent to a child—be kind to them, be good to them, and give to them. They need that to carry on. If you know that and can deal with it objectively, without getting mad or without identifying blindly with the patient and his problem, your efficiency as a doctor will be very much greater. It does require emotional maturity to be a doctor, a nurse, or a social worker. It requires a higher degree of maturity to want to continue to help people even though you know you are very much limited by certain internal personality or external environmental factors. Medical students have to learn that there are some people who are going to die in spite of everything that medical science has to offer them. Psychiatrists and social case workers learn that there are many emotionally sick people whose problems cannot be measurably changed. However, even in these instances it is possible to help. To recognize one's limitations and operating efficiency within these zones is the mark of a good doctor and a good social case worker.

DR. COTTRELL. May I give one practical suggestion? If the first doctor a patient sees gets a complete list of all the complaints that that person presents, it often saves a great deal. The doctor who took the history about this patient got the facts that there were dripping sensations around here, weakness of the hands, that there were crying spells, and so on. If you just keep on saying, "What else bothers you; is there anything else? If you didn't have these things would you be perfectly happy?" A few little questions like that and you get the list down to something more than backache and pain down the side. Oftentimes it saves you and gives you the clue. You may not want to follow everything up but you get insight that may direct you what to do.

DR. ROMANO. To repeat briefly, the doctor must have interest in dealing with the emotional problems of his patients. It must be a reasonably mature interest, fortified with knowledge of what the more or less normal emotional experiences of men and women are in our society. He must have some knowledge of certain methods which one uses to obtain information about the patient and his problem. With repetitive experience he will learn to use judgment in dealing with the knowledge that he has obtained and with the relationship that has been established between him and the patient.

Diagnosis of Psychoneurosis

JOHN ROMANO, M.D.

THIS afternoon we're going to discuss some of the points concerning the diagnosis of a neurosis, and later we'll continue our consideration of psychotherapy.

As you probably know, the most common error made in the diagnosis of neurotic people is that the diagnosis is made by the exclusion of pertinent structural disease. Now, obviously, it is as important to obtain positive data in the diagnosis of a neurosis as it is to obtain positive data in the diagnosis of any other condition, whether it be malaria or subacute bacterial endocarditis or a broken bone. One must learn to accumulate the pertinent data and to aggregate them and interpret them so that one may weigh their relative positiveness or negativeness.

The first point to take into consideration is the presenting complaint. The very nature of the complaint may be significant—a certain type of headache, such as a crown of thorns, a certain type of blindness, or a sudden paralysis of a limb. Such complaints may in themselves constitute presumptive evidence of psychological disturbance. This is particularly true of hysterical symptoms, where the pertinent points may be a sudden dramatic onset or a sudden dramatic relief. There are certain hysterical symptoms which have been experienced by people through the ages. The *globus hystericus* is one such symptom. A certain type of binding headache is another. Paralysis, hemianesthesia, hemihypalgesia, hysterical gait are others. Such symptoms constitute presumptive evidence of a neurosis, but they are presumptive, not complete or confirmatory.

The next point is the onset. The onset may help us to obtain positive data with respect to the precipitating factor. The precipitating factor itself may be quite cursory, trivial, something of which the doctor or friends might say, "Well, that's nothing. I've had things much worse than that and I have not been troubled." The event may have special meaning to the patient, however, so that one should find out whether the patient had any special feeling about what was happening at the time his symptoms appeared, whether the situation was similar to anything that had occurred before. In other words, get some idea of the setting in which the event occurred—what the patient was doing, who was with him at the time, what he had been doing shortly before that. Then, what was his emotional state at that time; that is, what was his preparation for the incident?

Age is the next point to consider. As was pointed out in a previous lecture, there are certain critical periods in personality development—early childhood, pubescence, and the climacteric—when there is relative weakening of psychological equilibrium, a need to strive for balance, and the person is accordingly more vulnerable than at other times. Hysterical disturbances in adolescent girls are fairly frequent, as are emotional disturbances in the menopausal period. So age plays some part. Age is particularly pertinent in those cases in which the history shows a person who has been relatively healthy and well balanced and then has a sudden onset of what appears to be an hysterical condition at age fifty or fifty-five. One should be very cautious about this interpretation in the absence of pertinent precipitating factors.

Next, the current behavior of the person, the appropriateness of his behavior to his disability is to be considered. In the hysterical person, for instance, there is likely to be a disparity between the complaint and the general behavior. The patient may have a daily headache which is very severe and yet say that he's able to sleep and eat and walk all right. In other words, get some idea of the severity of the problem and how it has affected and influenced the individual's daily life pattern.

The physical examination and the behavior of the person during it may give further clues. Note whether the patient has any unusual reactions, any undue modesty, any particular or exaggerated concern about one or another part of the body. In connection with the physical examination you will, of course, obtain the necessary laboratory tests and from all this reach a diagnostic conclusion as to whether the physical findings explain the problem which the patient presents. Here, however, is a possible source of great error in the diagnosis of neurotic people—namely, that random physical or laboratory findings may be found and then assigned as the cause or reason for the patient's behavior. If the patient is told this, a secondary elaboration of new symptoms or an entrenchment of the previously experienced symptoms often takes place.

So much for the current scene, for the behavior of the patient as he or she comes to you. One next obtains, through the medium of the interview, certain data as to who this person is and what kind of situation he finds himself in. Go back to the critical periods of early childhood and adolescence and get some idea of how emotionally healthy the person was, what kind of social adjustment he made, something of his relationship to his parents, siblings, and friends, what was the gross personality pattern with which he combatted his everyday anxieties. Did he have a tendency to utilize extremes? Was he too quiet, too restrained, too passive, too inhibited, too good? Was he perpetually aggressive and antisocial? Or did he utilize modifications of one extreme or the other? In other words, get some idea of what his behavior was not only in a quantitative sense but also qualitatively—what psychologic defenses he has had to use and how effectively he has used them.

Along with that, of course, get data concerning the patient's adjustment in school, in relation to work, in relation to fellow employees and employers, whether he has repeatedly had difficulties with people in authority. Similarly with health—get not only a record of previous illnesses and their nature, hospitalization, sequelae, and so on, but also the patient's attitudes toward health and disease and his parents' attitudes toward him during his childhood illnesses. How able was he, as a child or adult, to reach out in convalescence to normal independence? Did he ever before the present episode have neurotic symptoms or other disturbances of an emotional nature? If so, what were they? Find out also about the sexual adjustment of the patient. As you probably know, modern psychology pays much attention to sexuality, because a good sexual adjustment is one of the best criteria of normality and maturity. Choosing a member of the opposite sex, experiencing love and tenderness toward him or her, loving children, all these are indices of maturity—that is, of having grown up and become able to love someone besides yourself.

Next, to make a positive diagnosis of a neurosis, one must obtain evidence of a conflict situation, for the symptoms of neurosis are the means

of compromise between opposing forces. One set of forces seeks gratification. Another set attempts to control or deny this gratification. The
conscious part of our personality attempts to keep a state of balance. It
is when the balance is upset that symptoms occur and the patient becomes sick. This is the fundamental basis of the neurosis. One must attempt to learn what these conflicting forces may be.

Another point to be considered in diagnosing a neurosis is the determinants of the choice of the symptom. Why, for example, does one
person who is emotionally upset become blind, hysterically blind? A
second person may utilize symptoms which indicate a certain isolation
from himself, such as hand-washing rituals or thoughts that are very
disagreeable and unpleasant. Another person may have a diffuse type
of anxiety, a catastrophic anxiety. What are the determinants of the
choice? What are the determinants of the site and the nature of the
symptom? Many times it's not possible to work this out in detail and
certainly the general practitioner and internist may not be able to discover why a specific symptom is utilized. But many times, for example
in hysterical blindness, you are dealing with the person's conflict about
seeing something, and the blindness serves to prevent him from seeing
something. This is a point to which Dr. Kaufman has directed many of
his remarks in the past two sessions. We'll talk a little more about it in
a few minutes.

There is another point in respect to making a positive diagnosis of a
neurosis, and that is that when any complaint is given, one tries to find
out whether the patient ever had any experience with anything like
this before. Has anyone he knows had anything like this before—
mother or father or brother or sister or friends? Has he ever read about
it in a "doctor book" or seen it in a moving picture? In other words, the
complaint may be related to a previous experience of the patient, or it
may represent what we call identification with some person in the
patient's life; hence we pay particular attention to what are called
pseudo-hereditary factors. Many times it's important to find out what
the patient's parents died of, what their symptoms were, when they
died, and similarly for his brothers and sisters or other close associates.
These facts may provide a lead to the specificity of the presenting
symptom or complaint.

When these data are accumulated and one begins to interpret them, the precipitating factors may seem quite trivial and of no great importance. Nevertheless, the precipitating factor may be extremely important, for it may touch off, as a trigger, certain unresolved emotional tensions in the patient. The setting and the preparation of the patient are extremely important, for they give you some conception of the host factor, the patient.

We have to deal not only with the stimulus factor but with the host factor—how ready the patient was, what his state of excitation was when this experience happened. Here again previous experience, the age of the patient, all the specific points we have mentioned, must be taken into consideration. Data concerning childhood are particularly important. In the case of most neurotic patients there was a period in childhood when normal satisfactions and normal securities were not obtained. Usually there are exaggerations of psychologic defenses, and there may be a repetition of certain disabilities from time to time in relation to mental stresses and sexual adjustment. Finally, and most important probably to accumulate, is the evidence of conflictual factors, those opposing forces which bring about the conflict situation.

In general, then, our premise is that one should not make the diagnosis of a neurotic person or a neurotic symptom on the basis of negative data. One should make it by determining the relative importance and significance of physical factors, and by obtaining positive data—as much as one can—as to the emotional disturbance. Neurotic persons may have physical disturbances; many times they do. There is no rigid division or mutually exclusive separation between organic disease and neurosis.

DISCUSSION

STUDENT. Dr. Romano, do you think of emotional disturbances in the relatively normal person, the psychoneurotic, and the psychotic as being at least to a great extent a difference in degree?

DR. ROMANO. I think there are both quantitative and qualitative factors at play. It depends on whether you have a reasonably healthy person—emotionally and physically—who has been subjected to an unpredicted and unprepared-for shock. Let's say he's had an auto accident in which he has been badly bruised. His car has been shattered. He is apt to be jittery and tremulous; there may be changes in the ebb and flow of his speech; he may show the picture of exaggerated motor discharge with his jitteriness. He may have repetitive dreams for a night or two. But he'll recover and become balanced again within a reasonably short period of time. That, you would say, is a more or less normal reaction.

But now suppose this accident happened to a person who was in the midst of considerable turmoil; let's say he was harboring a considerable amount of hostility and anger toward people in authority, perhaps toward his foreman, and had had difficulty in resolving his feelings toward authoritarian figures in his life. The very same accident might have quite a different meaning for him. It might mobilize a great number of these feelings of anger and hostility and the ensuing fright and guilt which might be associated with them. So instead of recovering soon, he might experience pain from his bruise for two or three weeks or months, particularly if there was a great deal of diagnostic indecision and medical insecurity and repetitive tests, together with legal compensatory complications. Those things might add fuel to the fire of his own inner feeling. The prolongation and intensity of the experience depend not only on the stimulus factor, you see, but on the host factor —what the preparation was at that time for that experience to occur, what capacity the host had to digest, to assimilate the stimulus factor. A stimulus factor may be so overpowering, so deluging, that it goes beyond the homeostatic adaptiveness of any biological organism. It's been seen in combat, in earthquakes, in fires, and instances like that. But many times the intensity of the response depends on the specific capacity of the individual to assimilate or digest or adapt to it.

Now, to come again to the determinants of choice. Many times one asks why this person with this emotional conflict has this specific symptom; why not another? There are a number of theories about that. One is that it is purely coincidental, there is no logical connection. A second is the weak-link-of-the-chain hypothesis, sometimes called constitutional, sometimes called two-strikes-on-the-ball, sometimes called weakling. In other words, the theory is that at a time of stress one breaks at the weakest link. A third explanation is the Pavlovian concept of conditioning. Certain parts of the body, certain areas of the body, may be associated frequently with deep and meaningful emotional experiences. They are heavily invested and charged with emotion, so that later on, when the person experiences a similar emotion or is in a similar conflict situation, that part of his body is affected through this past conditioning.

Recently there has been accumulated a body of data which seem to support what may be called a configurational theory. Most of it has been accumulated by people who use psychoanalytic techniques and methods. They have shown that there may be a mosaic arrangement of drives and attitudes and emotional defenses which are related to certain organs or parts of the body. For example, the work of Franz Alexander and his associates and others on peptic ulcers. We'll speak in more detail about that in other lectures. The supposition in peptic ulcer, in a word, is that it relates to an axis of dependence-independence. In peptic ulcer patients one often sees a considerable inability to express even normal dependency needs; they have a compensatory, overdetermined reaction to be big shots. The big businessman, for instance, does all sorts of things to sort of prove to himself that he is not dependent. Other axes are used to explain certain other phenomena, such as bronchial asthma, certain skin conditions, hypertension, migraine, fainting.

Now the criticism of this theory is that, granted it is possible to accumulate data to indicate such connections, when you're dealing with as ambiguous an emotion or human drive as dependence-independence in a civilization such as ours, you are apt to find conflicts on this subject in every person you see. In other words, every human being in our civilization has the problem of how to take care of his dependency needs and how much to achieve from success. So how specific these factors may be in the production of peptic ulcer is a question. The fact remains, however, that there has been collected in the past fifteen years information which is valuable and which seems to have been checked by a number of people in other fields.

The peptic ulcer picture, for example, has been known for many years. Westphal and Bergmann mentioned it at the turn of the century. Gastroenterologists have pointed it out. General practitioners have pointed it out. Psychiatrists not using psychoanalytic techniques have pointed it out. With psychoanalytic techniques a more penetrating analysis of the total problem has been made.

*

DR. BOND. I'd like for a moment to get back where we started on the positive diagnosis of a neurosis. There are one or two more points, I think, to be brought out about that. I'll start with an example regarding ruling out a neurotic illness. The reverse of what is usually done is sometimes awfully useful.

We had a girl brought into our hospital who had symptoms of fatigue and uncomfortableness in the back of her neck. She had developed a post-lumbar headache that was of great severity, so great that her local doctor had put her on rather large doses of morphine for a period of eight weeks. I walked into her room and she greeted me with, "I hate you; get out of here!" I told her she couldn't hate me that much because she didn't know me well enough. Then I sat down, and she told me really quite a story—some secret suicidal attempts, how much she hated her oldest child, how fond she was of her husband's best friend, and she went 'way back into her life. She had been forced to go into a convent, and she had a great many problems that weren't easy for her. So I listened to that and I left her. The next morning I went back, and her headache was exactly the same.

Well, now, that's not what you'd expect; that's not the way things work. If you know they don't work that way, then you know you'd better look somewhere else. Consequently we did an EEG on her just as a preliminary step, and we found she had a lot of fast activity all over her head. We did a spinal tap that afternoon and found she had 3,000 cells per cubic millimeter. How she got them I don't know; but in any case that's what she had. She had a very serious and stormy course of illness, recovered, and returned to being a very neurotic, difficult, immature girl during her convalescence.

Don't just jump to the conclusion that because the patient has some emotional problems they are necessarily the cause of his symptoms. Work on the symptoms and continue to tie them in together and see whether you can find some meaning for the symptoms in terms of the emotional problem. You can get tricked badly. People do have, very frequently, two kinds of trouble, organic and inorganic.

There is one other possibility that I'd like to say something about, of which head injuries and similar conditions are beautiful examples. This is the situation in which there may be a blending of emotional and organic disease with a confusing conglomeration of symptoms. There's an awful lot that we do not know about the relationship of the brain and its organic structure to its function. There's a big gap in there. But the emotional and functional side of a person's disability has an enormous amount to do with how much use he makes of what he's got. In a disorder like a headache, a trauma, it's a fine thing to go ahead on the basis of straightening out the emotional problem as much as possible, for that will let the patient function at his maximum. There are almost always very important emotional factors connected with head injuries. You certainly don't need to say that you're going to get the patient back to perfect health. You will, however, get rather surprising results if you help the patient handle that part of his trouble that is related to his emotions.

DR. ROMANO.   One may cite, too, many instances in which patients were considered neurotic on the basis of excluding physical disease, while actually there might have been some suspicion about physical disease because we could exclude neurosis. Recently we saw a girl of fifteen who had been treated by a number of physicians. She was considered neurotic because she had difficulty in going to school, and it was felt that this was a clear instance of a wish not to go to school, of rebellion and antisocial activity. We could find no evidence of neurotic conflict, and upon closer scrutiny it was learned that this girl had difficulty in climbing up the two steps of the school bus. When she was examined we found that she had unmistakable signs of myasthenia gravis. This girl's nervousness, her anxiety, was related to the fact that no one would believe that she was disabled, no one would accept the fact that she was unable to meet the demands of her society because of her physical disease.   *

STUDENT.   What is the relationship of fatigue and neurosis? Take a child with a pseudo-hypotrophic muscular dystrophy. The factor of fa-

tigue has not been recognized. That child can have all kinds of problems and difficulties, he can be irritable, combative. He can have many
emotional tie-ups, too, like the child who couldn't get up the steps.
When a diagnosis is made the parents are told not to push that child;
but the father still wants him to walk, and therefore they try to make
him walk. The child is extremely fatigued all the time. When you stop
that, stop the fatigue, the child is no longer irritable. Isn't fatigue a distinct factor in neurosis?

DR. ROMANO.   I think you've answered the question in part. Here is
a child who is not able to do certain things; that's equivalent to being
unable to adapt to certain stimuli, and so in that state of excitation the
child experiences distress. This is a clear and unambiguous situation
that you see whenever you push children too quickly or too aggressively, whether you push them intellectually or physically. In the field
of any organic disability or any restriction of function, whether it be
motor or sensory, you may provoke distress when the human being is
flooded with stimuli to which it cannot adapt.

You speak of neurotic fatigue. People will say, "I don't know why
I'm tired. I haven't done a damned thing all day long. Yet, I feel tired
all the time." Fatigue is a cliché. Fatigue is used in a tremendous number of ways. There's the fatigue of muscular aches from playing golf
for the first time in the spring. There's the fatigue related to ennui or
boredom from doing repetitive, monotonous tasks without adequate
motivation or without adequate periods of recuperation. Then there's a
third kind of fatigue, which statistically is by far the most common and
has nothing to do with muscular aches or with monotonous tasks. It has
to do with emotional factors. You may ask what produces it. I think
the clue to that is that in the neurotic person there is a tremendous battle going on inside all the time, a tremendous tug-of-war which takes
so much energy in itself. The fight of the forces wishing to express
themselves and the repressing forces related to conscience, with the poor
ego trying to meet the environment and control these forces at the same
time, causes the fatigue which so many neurotic patients experience.

DR. BOND.   I would like to say something about fatigue as an etiologic
factor in the production of neurosis. The best study I know is the one
that we were able to do in the Eighth Air Force. A lot of boys got aw-

fully tired and had to go off flying for three, four, or five days. Their chief complaint was, "I'm tired. I'm so tired I can hardly see." A good many thousand boys were taken off for that tiredness. That occurred around D-Day and at one other period when they flew them seven out of eight days. Those were the times of great effort. They were not the times of high losses. It was a very different thing with boys who broke up, who had a neurosis from combat. Difficulties of that kind appeared at the times of the greatest losses, and there was a very close statistical correlation with the losses. The striking thing is that there was a qualitative difference in being tired and in being neurotic, a difference which ordinarily is not clearly recognized.

DR. ROMANO. Perhaps fatigue is a provocative factor in releasing certain neurotic symptoms. I think the mechanism is essentially that fatigue weakens the controlling strength of the ego, thus producing an imbalance.

Summary of the First Week

THOMAS A. C. RENNIE, M.D.

AT this mid-point of the course it may be worth while to try to sum up what the experience of the week has been and what we have aimed at. The first few days were filled with new vistas opening up. I hope and suspect that as the course goes on we'll come a bit closer to earthy reality. Perhaps we have talked over your heads: we may have missed what you really want to get out of this course. We urge you to pull us back to earth any time we seem to be getting into flights that take us too far away from you.

By this time you've seen a number of patients over in the hospital. It is the interest that centers around such patients that I think should be the primary focus in this course. These patients are sick human beings representing a great variety of conditions. We have made no very deliberate effort to select patients that would show you easily and in typical form examples of neurotic difficulties. When we first planned this course we had an idea that we might try to find psychoneurotic patients that would demonstrate in rather pure culture some of the points we would talk about in the lectures. We abandoned that idea—I think very wisely—in favor of showing you sick people as they come through a medical clinic. It is true that the director of the clinic has scrutinized patients to some extent and has selected for you some in whom he thought emotional factors were operating in a significant fashion or who might have personality problems that would be rather easily available to you for study and understanding. In the main, however, there has been little selection of material, and so I think the patients you have been examining must represent to a considerable extent the run-of-the-mine kind of sick human beings who come to you as practicing physicians.

You've discovered a lot of interesting things about these patients. That's partly because you have a new orientation to the problems of sick people. You've had some patients who found it very difficult to share with you, in one or two interviews, significant emotional material that bore on their illness. A few of you have been fortunate enough to have patients who spoke readily and easily about emotional matters. There have been patients with problems apparently so deep or so ingrained or of such long standing that very little information was immediately available to you, and you began to suspect it would take a long time to work out any essential emotional material in a therapeutic way. In any case, however, I am certain that you have become convinced that emotions play a vitally important part in all illness.

I would like to tell you that we feel the same way as you do about some of the more complicated cases you have seen. There is no member of the teaching staff who feels that he could elicit from all these patients the kind of material we have been talking about in our didactic work. There is no member of the teaching staff who believes that he, as a psychiatrist, could cure all these individuals. I want you to have no feeling of pessimism about what might be expected in the psychotherapeutic treatment of some of those individuals. We're not primarily concerned about that anyway. It would be a disconcerting and sad fact if any of you left this course with the idea that you were psychiatrists or pseudo psychiatrists or budding psychiatrists or anything of the kind. That is not the aim of the course.

The course has two aims: first, to sensitize you to human beings who are sick and, second, to give you some conception of how you, as practitioners, might work more effectively toward the relief of these sick human beings. The first objective I think we have accomplished to a considerable extent. I think you are sensitive to and aware of many aspects of human beings which you may have known something about before but which have now become more important to you. A word of warning about that. It is very easy in one's psychotherapeutic zeal to go chasing down that particular line of attack to the neglect of the everyday experience you have had for years in dealing with the somatic issues involved. I am quite confident, however, that as soon as you are back in practice the old habits of working will reassert themselves and you will give all the necessary and due attention to somatic problems. I venture to say and hope, however, that henceforth, even in taking a medical history, you will do your work with a different orientation and will seek from each patient certain facts that previously may have seemed unimportant to you, for you will have a new attitude toward sick people.

During the coming week I hope you will find that there are some concrete and specific things that you can do in psychotherapy. These perhaps have not as yet been made real enough or practical enough to you, although you will recall that Dr. Romano made a rather specific statement as to the kinds of therapy you as practitioners might be able to carry on. Next week his statement will be elaborated at length, both in seminars and in your individual discussions with the instructors.

In talking with the patients in the clinic, you have started, as always, with the main complaint, the patient's primary reason for coming to the hospital. More often than not the patient has given you this on a somatic basis, but you, in eliciting its development and chronology, have begun to pay some attention to the total human setting. As you listened to the patients' descriptions of their lives, you were probably aware of two large areas of possible influence. First, there were the life events, the circumstances of the life which might constitute a particularly noxious or difficult or stressful influence and so have a bearing on the disease. Second, you began to realize that just knowing the external events told you only part of the story; in addition, you had to know a great deal about the inside of the person—what he was like, what his attitudes and feelings were, what his emotional relations were, and what was the general set of the personality which rendered that person vulnerable to the environmental circumstances he described. You had to consider both of these aspects. The latter aspect you approached in a number of ways. You watched the patient, looked at him, observed the emotional reactions that were at play. You learned something of how to judge the anxiety or other emotional responses exhibited by the patient at the very moment the examination was proceeding. You began to see how those responses can be used as clues to the understanding of what is going on inside the patient. Then you gave the patient an opportunity to talk and share with you and tell you some of his feelings and attitudes about his illness as such or about the external circumstances that have been difficult for him.

This is the procedure you will follow next week and, I hope, all the rest of your lives. As busy practitioners, you may have to do this in a somewhat abbreviated way. We recognize that. Nonetheless, with this new orientation, you will do a number of things that will be helpful to patients, whether you have time for much eliciting of the internal feelings of the patient or not. I think, too, you will make fewer of the unnecessary examinations that some doctors are prone to fall back upon because they are anxious or uncertain or hardly know how to interpret a patient's illness. In consequence, you will traumatize fewer people by ill-spoken statements or premature interpretations, and fewer patients will have to go running to other doctors and clinics in a vain search for help.

We set up this course with a view to giving you thorough insight into these matters. We started off by giving you a description of the biographic development of human beings—what goes into the making of human temperament and personality, what are the crucial dynamic experiences from childhood through maturity that lead to its ultimate development. As you know, we touched only very briefly on constitution and heredity. We did this because, for one thing, we know so little about it and, for another, it is an area about which we can do nothing anyway. Moreover, we are convinced that it is the experiences of the individual and his feelings and emotional reactions thereto that are of predominant influence in personality development. Hence we have chosen to focus on that which we know more about and which is more amenable to change through therapy.

We have told you that all human beings go through a certain biographic development which has multiple aspects, that this development is infinitely varied and colored, depending on many individual circumstances, but that there are certain crucial experiences which are especially important. We've told you what those experiences are in the development of the child. We've told you of many other emotional factors which come into play and which contribute to the adult personality make-up, frequently without his awareness or knowledge. We have given you some insight into the fact that we all function in terms of conscious awareness but are motivated also by powerful emotional factors which frequently are beyond the power of consciousness and must therefore be considered repressed or essentially unconscious.

I hope we've made it clear that the unraveling of unconscious factors is a job for the thoroughly trained expert. It is a job which frequently takes a long time. We want you to know those things are there so that you may understand what goes into the make-up of people, so that you may know what children are going through and what the implications may be for their future development. This, however, is not the material you will usually be dealing with as practitioners doing psychotherapy. Of course, you will have some patients who talk easily and freely and in whom some of these matters come readily to the foreground of awareness. In such cases you obviously would do a disservice by keeping the patient from expressing these feelings and thereby getting some understanding of what they mean. In general, however, your practice will not deal with the unconscious.

After describing various stages of human emotional development, we went on to what constitutes a psychoneurosis and what kind of imbalance or conflict commonly lies behind such a disorder. Dr. Kaufman told you, so persuasively, that the organism is always in a state of relative balance. Always there are certain strong emotional attitudes struggling for expression; always there are certain forces of repression attempting to keep them in line. So we see in a neurotic person an individual who is out of balance because some elements of personality are not working smoothly and harmoniously within him.

From there we went somewhat further along the road of understanding what conflict means—what it derives from, how the human being tries to reach a balance, and how when he fails he gets characteristic symptoms that you have learned to recognize. In addition, we have given you some introduction to common methods of therapy. We have told you that your function, in the main, can be reasonably delimited. Dr. Romano told you that you deal with all kinds of complex environmental circumstances in whose alleviation you may play a vitally important role. You have heard a bit about social workers and the part they can play in the understanding and alleviation of environmental stresses. We have told you, in addition, that you can work not only with external stresses, although such work may be very important in bringing relief to the individual, but with certain of the internal emotional stresses as well.

Your primary function, it has been said, lies in the relationship between you and the patient. I think you know something of the nature of that relationship now. You know something about its tremendous power for good in therapy, and you have intimations also that this relationship has inadvertent inherent dangers and that one can misuse it. You understand something now of what the patient brings to you as a physician, the kind of feelings and attitudes that he invests you with.

Sick people are essentially dependent people looking for security, and they find that security primarily in their feelings and attitudes toward you as a doctor. Consequently just being the kind of doctor who understands those feelings and attitudes is tremendously helpful to many sick and troubled and uncertain people. More than that, you give these people an opportunity. You do this best when you listen and say as little as possible and permit the patient all the freedom he may need to share his troubles with you, for it is in this talking and sharing that a large part of therapeutic usefulness lies. The patient is relieved of anxiety by the mere fact that for the first time he can talk freely about some things. Most of you have had the experience of having a patient say, "This is the first time that I've really been able to talk freely about this." Don't underrate that as therapy. That is very important therapy. It may seem relatively casual to you, but it is the very crux of therapy. It is an important function you are filling in just doing that.

You will go beyond that in dealing with some individuals and their internal problems. You have already learned that as patients discuss these things you find that they have strange attitudes, misinformed attitudes, that they've been frightened, that they are completely at sea about what their illness means. Part of your job, then, is the explanation of what these things really mean in their lives. This can be very surprising, very new to the patient but it can also be tremendously valuable therapeutically, for in so doing you take all the anxiety and the sting away from the somatic or organic interpretation and put it where it rightfully belongs, in the area of the patient's personality. That very frequently brings an immediate relief.

Dr. B. will tell you, for example, that during this week he has been seeing a patient who for some two and a half years has had overwhelming states of anxiety expressed as feelings of numbness that come on her quickly and wake her up at night. Within the week this patient, who is a very intelligent person, has said to him, "Well, you know, I am finally convinced that it is not my body that is sick; this is the expression of my emotional or mental reactions." With that insight this woman has gained a new kind of courage or comfort or ability to handle her symptoms. Yesterday she said to the doctor, "Last night I felt one of those things coming on, and then I remembered what I had learned from you, and for the first time I was able to handle it."

I dwell on this point at some length because I have had one or two of you say, "Well, this is all very well. Perhaps I can get the patient over his anxiety. But I haven't really treated him because I haven't dealt with those unconscious dynamic factors that you people have been talking about." Well, I think you do yourselves a great injustice; you fail to give yourselves credit for what you are doing. I hope, therefore, that as the course goes on next week more and more of you will ask for specific information and help in how to deal with these things that you are now beginning to see with considerable clarity.

Briefly, then, the course thus far has taught you something of how human beings are made up and how they come to be that way. It has taught you what illness in terms of psychoneurosis means—a failure to bring harmony out of certain conflicts. It has given you a specific tool for interviewing, for understanding, for listening. It has taught you something of what your function as a doctor is in relation to sick people, and it has given you a beginning understanding of some concrete things that you can do without feeling that you have to be a psychiatrist and deal with unconscious conflict material. Perhaps I overrate or underrate or quite misunderstand what has happened this week. But that's my summing up of the experience. It would be surprising indeed if it wasn't exciting and gratifying to you, for I can't help feeling that a whole new vista in the understanding of sick people is at least beginning to be opened up to you.

DISCUSSION

STUDENT. We've been offered certain do's and don't's during the past week. On the *do* side we have a certain stirring within us; we want to probe and explore. On the other hand, certain *don't's* have been brought out. Don't take the cork out of the bottle and parade a lot of this stuff and traumatize the patient unnecessarily. Don't remove a prop unless you have another to put in its place. Now what practical advice can you give us as to where the red light comes in, so that in our inept way we're not going to blunder?

DR. RENNIE. Very good. The purpose of this meeting is to let the neophytes answer questions. Let's have your expressions of opinion on that.

STUDENT. All week I have been trying to define what illness is, and I have just this morning decided that it is a patient who needs help and who, so far as we are concerned, comes to us for help. The green light, then, is our recognition of the need for help and, I suppose, how within our limitations we can offer that help. If we always look at the patient and ask, "What help does this patient need? What help can I give him?" I don't think we'll run into any trouble.

DR. RENNIE. Who would like to formulate the *do's* that you've learned?

STUDENT. I'd say the first of the *do's* is the ventilation that comes very easily on the part of the patient, or with not too much effort on your part, that allows the patient to tell you his or her story. In other words, just the telling of the story often helps. The next is, well, first get information that does not touch too much on a sensitive area in the patient's life and that takes relatively little probing on your part. If the patient blocks too much, lay off. Maybe another *do* would be to find out whether there are external stresses which you can be of some help with.

STUDENT. There's another aspect, too, that's important. The minute you start setting up questions you tend to channelize the patient's thinking and condition him to the answer you want to get. Probably it's much better to have the patient proceed spontaneously. While the material may seem irrelevant to me, it may be relevant to the patient in the development of a coherent and cogent pattern. What I've got to do is place it in the proper relationship to other material.

STUDENT. You have to size the patient up and get the whole individual. Don't specifically center your interest on one symptom, one complaint the patient has.

STUDENT. And don't forget the somatic. I had a patient who, three hours after seeing me, went into a fulminating meningitis.

DR. RENNIE. Any other *do's* you think should be added?

STUDENT. I would like to add some *be's*. Be honest with yourself. Be sympathetic with your patient. And be as unprejudiced as you possibly can.

STUDENT. Haven't we got a long way away from the question? Wasn't the question "How far can we go, where should we stop?"

DR. RENNIE. We are coming to the *don't's* pretty soon, which may include that.

STUDENT. In reviewing the patients I have seen, I find that most of them can go just so far, and I feel sure that with future interviews they can go only a little farther. But in getting into their story, I am wondering whether with our limited knowledge we should stir into those subterranean conflicts?

STUDENT. Well, I think the ventilation must always be voluntary on the part of the patient if we are to stay out of trouble.

STUDENT. It seems to me that if we touch on some of the sensitive areas where the patient seems to hesitate or block or show some evidence of stopping, we might ask a question or two; that's perfectly within our province. If we do this and it doesn't produce any results, I think we shouldn't continue to hammer away. But it may be in how we do it. I've seen a few cases and I've elaborated the history and the patient has ventilated the more or less conscious things on his mind. Then Dr. Rennie has come in. He looks at the patient in that dreamy kind of way—always with a certain gesture—he holds his glasses in his hands and is very solemn. He touches on some of the points I've been touching on, but for some reason or other the steam valve opens and out comes the material. I think that material was not buried very deeply, and I don't think it's very far out of my province to try to make things easy for the patient. I think they do go away feeling better, and certainly they must go away with a certain transference toward the doctor. I think this is within our province. We're not delving too deeply when we do that, and we are giving the patient a good bit of therapy when he lets off that steam.

STUDENT. A little matter of mechanics has occurred to me. I think sometimes it's not well to work too continuously with a patient if he's been balking on something, so to speak. If you go out of your office and take care of another patient or two and then come back, he's been thinking in the meantime and sometimes he comes through easily with something that you've been trying to get out for a long time. That's one way we busy practitioners can find a lot more time to do these things. We don't have to keep so many other patients waiting. It may be that being away from the patient for a while will give an opportunity for something to happen that would take maybe a week or so otherwise.

DR. RENNIE. That's very important; you have to give patients time. They may have told you something that was pretty disturbing. Sometimes it would be a great mistake to go back the next day and pursue that. It is important to have a day or two days in between before you again approach anything in that fashion.

STUDENT. I'd like to know something about the way these other psychiatrists work.

STUDENT. Well, I can tell you. Frankly I had wondered, too. But I am sure that the patient whom Dr. Kaufman saw with me yesterday realized that she had a personal friend. I don't think he hurt her at any time. When she needed a bit of quiet, he gave it to her. She was an individual asserting herself with a little help. When she didn't know what to say, he didn't embarrass her by silence but brought up another phase of her personality. Of all the impressions I shall carry away with me from this course, one of the strongest is that hour I spent watching Dr. Kaufman interviewing.

DR. KAUFMAN. Let me add a word here which I think is awfully important. Don't run out and buy yourself glasses. Don't develop a technique of dreamy eyes. Don't try to pattern yourself on me or on Rennie or on Jock Murray. We've got certain kinds of personality, and we work in relation to our personality. Don't try to develop an artificial kind of an approach within yourself. There is that tendency. When you are in medical school you tend to identify yourself with one or another teacher. But in this work the essence is to develop what you yourself are in relation to the occasion. Don't feel that a technique consists of this or that kind of thing we've been doing here, that it is a kind of a pattern which you've got to fit into.

Another thing that has been brought up here is that your relationship to your patient should be free and easy. With increasing experience you are going to be less apprehensive—not about what you are getting but about your inability to get certain things out of it. That you've got to learn by experience. Nobody can tell you what to get out of a patient.

In answer to the question how far you should go, go only as far as the patient will allow you. Sometimes the patient has a tendency to want to go into a lot of things that are rather deep but you'll learn what these things are as you begin to understand people, not from what we've been telling you, but from your own experience. The danger is to go too far. We've always told you that. But we can't say for Mrs. X that she can only go just so far, for we don't know Mrs. X. You have to learn that kind of thing.

We've given you a series of *don't's*. Perhaps we have overemphasized them a little bit. We've given you those *don't's* because we've tried to present general broad principles. The chances are that with the knowledge that caution is necessary—as long as it doesn't inhibit you so much that you don't get anything from the patient—you'll find that you'll know the level to which it's safe to go with a patient. That's something that your own experience is going to teach you.

Now, every one of us in this room, we psychiatrists, have made errors. And sometimes we've made errors that have been pretty bad. Sometimes an error is inevitable, so don't let's inhibit ourselves and get scared to death by the possibility that we'll make a mistake. What you need to know is that caution is necessary, but the minute you begin to be too cautious, then you inhibit what you are trying to do. I appeal to your own experiences and to your own knowledge of what you do about diagnosing appendicitis. You can make a mistake in the diagnosis of appendicitis. How do you *not* make a mistake in diagnosis? On the basis of what you learn about appendicitis plus your clinical experience. So our *don't's* were, in a sense, telling you that you can go too far. We didn't at any time intend to say, "Now you must not under any circumstances do this, that, or the other thing." We can't tell you that; we don't know the patient, we don't know your personality, and we don't know just how much free flow you will learn.

Some of you undoubtedly have already gained a lot of self-assurance in relation to your patients. You can see that from one day to another your approach to patients has been so much easier. On the first day everybody was just a little bit rigid; nobody knew just exactly what to do. As soon as you saw that some of these things can come out more or less automatically, you began to find your level. I think that's been your experience. I think there was much less feeling on Tuesday than there was on Monday, much less on Wednesday than there was on Tuesday, of the fear of going too far. That doesn't mean that you are going too far; it's just that you begin to develop a little bit of assurance in relation to what it is that you want to know.

There's another thing—this question of identification. The worst thing to do is to identify yourself with your patient, if by that you mean you want the patient to do what you would do under the circumstances. But from the point of view of understanding, how do we understand other people except by trying consciously or unconsciously to put ourselves in their place? One of the techniques that I personally use very frequently when it's difficult for the patient to say something and yet I want that particular thing said is to talk with him very casually and tell him what I know he has felt. That's a technique which I have learned and have developed, so don't be afraid of identifying yourself with a patient in that way. That's what we call empathy. We depend a good deal on empathy; what we *don't* want to do in this business of identification is to try to make the patient do what we would do under the circumstances. That's a bit dangerous.

STUDENT. Dr. Rennie, I've noticed the friendliness you psychiatrists have when you come in to see a patient. Many times I've seen the patient's face light up; he seems to be glad that you've come in. He says, "Here's a friend." He's probably gone to doctors and sort of felt the doctor was thinking, "Well, if I can get rid of this patient, the easiest and quickest way is the best way." Lots of times you have come in and talked to a patient about nothing much at all just to get personally acquainted. For instance, you ask about certain things that he'd like to do, and so forth, and the patient seems to feel that he wants to open up. He has nothing to hold back: "Here's a friend. Here's someone I can talk to who won't make fun of me and won't laugh at me inside." I think a lot of patients feel that way about doctors.

And there is another thing that patients feel about you. They think, "Here's somebody that's my friend, he's got lots of time, and I'm the only person concerned. As far as he's concerned, he's not thinking about running to another patient. It's just as if he's got all afternoon and I'm the only patient that he's got on his slate." I know lots of patients seem to feel that way. They are in no hurry to leave. I think that we men can carry that back to our private practice. When we go in to see a patient, if we really want to help him and he is a vital concern of ours, I think we'll do much better.

STUDENT. That's more or less what I had in mind. The thing I'm thinking of is the period of silence. Sometimes just sitting and saying nothing may be useful. I find that somewhat difficult and I'm likely to start shuffling my feet or something like that. I think that out of actually seeing the interview carried on by some of these experts, we get something of an evolving pattern, the silence and the not moving around too much. That certainly must be disquieting to the patient.

DR. RENNIE. What have the rest of you observed about these instructors?

STUDENT. Don't you think that perhaps we expect miracles when we are starting this kind of work? It isn't only that you look with dreamy eyes or somebody else does something else, but that the minute you come in, you men who have had experience, the patient unconsciously senses that you know your business. It's just as if we were taking care of some condition such as a fracture. A doctor walks in and the patient knows whether he knows his business pretty well. The fact that you people can get immediately things that we can't shouldn't discourage us too much. As time goes on, we'll develop not only a little more ability but a little more confidence, and as we develop more confidence in what we are doing the patient will sense it and will tell us more. I think that the patients have an unconscious feeling of security when you men walk in on the job that they don't have when we enter, and therefore they will tell you more than they will us.

STUDENT. I definitely noticed the tension relax when my instructor came in. I particularly noticed that both the patient and I were very sedate and serious and that my instructor always managed to get a smiling set-up, so that there was a feeling of relaxation on the part of the patient.

STUDENT. There's something else, too. I don't know the term that would apply, but when Dr. Rennie was talking to a patient who brought out how hard a life she had had, he said, "Well, you really have been an unhappy person, haven't you?" The recognition of the patient's feeling, not letting it stand just at the patient's telling him these things, that was what helped. You turn around and say, "Well, you really have been unhappy!" or "You really have had a tough time!"

DR. RENNIE. If I may add to that, this was a very interesting situation in which a patient had an extraordinarily difficult reality situation to deal with day in and day out. She seemed pretty tense as she was talking, and she probably talked for at least forty or fifty minutes, largely just verbalizing this fact. When I made one rather casual remark, "I suppose this must have been pretty difficult for you," she was able to express it emotionally. Her feeling came out then in a burst of tears. She had *talked* about the situation for some time and then she ended up by *feeling* about it—releasing the feelings she had.

DR. MURRAY. It is very interesting to listen to this discussion, and very satisfactory. I think you are grasping the ideas very well. Now, in the first place, we gave you a word of caution about psychotherapy— don't be a bull in a china shop. Psychotherapy is effective; that you've seen. But there isn't any effective drug that isn't poison in improper dosage. The scalpel itself—it is effective as an instrument but it must be used properly. But doctors make mistakes with drugs, they make mistakes with the scalpel, and by making those mistakes they learn: they learn not to make the same mistake again. That's the important thing.

Second, psychotherapy is like a drug: if we give too much of it the patient's going to vomit. If you tear in like a bull in a china shop, making interpretations about things you shouldn't, the patient will say, "That's a lot of baloney." And you simply will not get within his arc. You've given him an emetic and you have removed yourself from the sphere of influence.

You have seen, all of you, the one thing that is important—that you really are in empathy with your patient and that your patient senses it. You'll acquire that ability after a while, after you've had experience. You will learn to become easy and relaxed and to use your conscious functions less actively, so that your own innate humaneness responds to the patient on his own wave length. In this relationship you will be absorbing automatically and naturally what's going on and you will have an automatic, empathetic understanding rather than a highly intellectual interpretation of the patient's problems.

I can give you, in closing, one last point about technical activity; that is if you know why you are doing something, if you know what you want to accomplish by what you're doing, you are usually safe in doing it.

DR. RENNIE. Have you come yet to any particular way of phrasing questions that you've found particularly helpful? You certainly are going to have to ask some questions, and the manner in which you ask those questions can make all the difference in the world. What's been your experience?

STUDENT. It seems that the best way is to rephrase what the patient has said. For instance, if a person says, "My mother is domineering," you phrase that in the form of a question and she'll probably tell you all about it.

DR. RENNIE. That's an important point. You will find that device very useful. You can use almost verbatim at times the statement that the patient has made to you, for then you haven't changed it or given a different implication to it at all; you're going right back to the material that the patient gave you. This will enable you to avoid the error of asking the kind of question which makes a patient feel rushed or hurried or makes him give you an answer which may or may not be the one he wanted to give. It will enable you to avoid ever forcing a patient to give an answer that puts him on a spot so that he has to hang on to it and can't relinquish it for a long while. As much as possible, talk in terms of the language the patient himself has given.

Are there any other particularly helpful ways of phrasing questions that you've discovered?

STUDENT. I think there's some value in concluding an interview by asking a patient, "Well, what do you think of all this? What's your reaction to all this conversation?" I think one can learn a lot about the patient just from his attitude toward the whole interview.

STUDENT. I think you can also find that out from a subsequent interview by asking the patient, "Well, how do you feel? How have you been doing?" The way they answer that is an indication of what you have done.

STUDENT. Dr. Rennie, that is the particular area in which I have the greatest insecurity in my interviews—how to terminate an interview. I still haven't thought of a graceful way of parting with a patient.

DR. RENNIE. Suppose at the end of your allotted time you just said frankly, "Well, now, I'm sorry—our time's up for today, but I'm very much interested in these things you've been telling me about and I would like it if you would come back another day and let us continue talking about these things." Anything wrong with that in closing an interview?

STUDENT. I think that would be very graceful.

DR. RENNIE. Do many of you find it difficult to say frankly to a patient, "Well, at this point I really can't tell you the cause of these things, but we will look into it further"?

STUDENT. I think some people like that idea. I have seen a lot of people who don't like to have you tell them that particular day what's wrong with them. Lots of these people come and seem to want you to say, "Well, now you come back tomorrow and we'll go over this thing. We're not quite finished, we're not quite ready to reach a decision." A lot of them seem to say, "Oh! Well, that's just fine! Gosh! I'll be glad to come back tomorrow!"

DR. SCHIELE. I try to use what I call a positive approach. I credit the patient with the termination of the interview. I've done this in a number of cases, and I change my tactics to fit the situation. For instance, I want to credit the patient with the fact that he's done a pretty good job in recalling something that may have been lying dormant for quite a long spell of time, so I say, "Now that you've told me all these things, you'll want to go home and think them over. When you do, you might recall to your mind other things that will help fill in the picture a little more completely. I'd appreciate it if you would come back and tell me some of the things that at our first meeting didn't stand out largely in your mind." In other words, I've left the door open for a return and a reconsideration of the problem.

STUDENT. There is another aim in closing an interview, an important part of therapeusis. I think it's of value to review what has taken place during the interview, for often during the course of an hour not only I but the patient is so confused with the numerous things that have been discussed that a review of the high lights can be extremely important. As an illustration of that, a patient I just saw presented something rather common—fear of losing her mind. In the course of the interview I attempted deviously to reassure her, but after an hour or so we'd gotten away from that point several times. I wanted to make sure that that reassurance remained uppermost in her mind, so as a parting shot I went over the point with her and made certain that she grasped it.

DR. ROMANO. I think there are a number of variables in terminating an interview. Is it a first, second, third, or eighth visit? Then, has there been some prearrangement as to how long the interview should last? With these two variables in mind, I think your central points have been made: that is, first, to indicate the ground which has been covered and certain factors the patient can take away; second, to indicate whether there are areas still to be covered and, if so, to direct thinking toward them. Third, it is important not to give the impression of undue, Pollyanna-like optimism or to suggest to the patient that all problems are solved, for this may arouse anxiety and perplexity on the part of the patient as to whether you know what you are talking about. Fourth, allow an opportunity for a return visit. Indicate your own interest and your own continuation of thinking about the patient's problems; that helps sometimes.

DR. RENNIE. Dr. Bauer, have you anything to say in summing up this week?

DR. BAUER. Well, I've had the very distinct impression this morning that this all-important phase of the practice of medicine is being assimilated. Perhaps some of you have at times failed to realize that you probably are in a much more advantageous position than a consultant to whom you refer patients, particularly those of you who come from smaller towns, in that you know an awful lot about your patients and their environment. That, I'm sure, is of tremendous help to you in taking care of patients, whether it's an acute medical illness or some type of neurotic problem. Perhaps, too, you fail to appreciate that psychiatrists do not usually see their patients every day but prefer to have an interval of two to five days, not only to give the patient time to mull things over but also to give the doctor an opportunity to decide the possible significance of some of the things that he has observed.

As Dr. Kaufman said, be yourselves, not Rennie, not Murray. You can't be any one of these fellows; your personality is not the same. But you've all been successful in medicine and you should have a certain degree of confidence that with the passage of time, with more acute awareness of what this is all about, with willingness to try to understand your patients, you'll have success in this direction, too.

I'm sure you'll recognize where not to go. I think it's very important for you to realize that you can do a lot more than you've done. Most important to you personally will be the fact that many of your patients will be less disturbing to you, will cause you less anger. You won't come home at night and throw your hat down on the table in the front hall and say, "Damn it! If I see another neurotic again I'll go crazy!"

The patients you approach in the way we've discussed this week will soon gain some insight as to what you're driving at. Even though you're treating them without any medication, the patients will come back to you. They may still have the same symptoms when you see them for the eighth time, but they will now realize that the situation is different from what it was when they went to see the last doctor. They stuck with the last doctor for three years, and they got thirty-six prescriptions. You, in contrast, have been kind and very frank and have given them some insight as to what's going on. Success has not been apparent up to the moment, but they realize for the first time that they are partly at fault, that it is not all the doctor's fault, and you get a much, much better therapeutic relationship. If you bear that in mind in the handling of long-standing situations, it will be much easier for you and much less frustrating, and you'll obtain better therapeutic results. There are much bigger dividends in taking care of some of these patients than in taking care of an acute medical emergency, for if you're effective in even a partial degree you are apt to be influencing the lives and happiness of many other people in addition to the patient himself.

Anxiety

JOHN ROMANO, M.D.

I

I SHALL have two mornings to present to you data and clinical illustrations of the problem of anxiety. The first morning I shall talk about various uses of the term "anxiety" and pay particular attention to the anxieties of patients who have demonstrable physical disease, to the problems of convalescence, and the reactions to chronic disease. In the second lecture I shall consider anxiety as it is experienced in a neurotic manner and discuss the various adaptive devices utilized to relieve one of anxiety.

You know that the word "anxiety" is used very loosely to denote anxiousness, apprehension, fearfulness, fright, fear. These terms are used interchangeably and it is important to know the special meaning the patient attaches to the term with which he describes his experiences. Anxiety may be defined most simply as an emotion, an unpleasant emotion. It is an emotion generated by a conflict of forces in the economy of the person and used by the ego (the conscious part of the personality) as a warning signal that in some way or other the personality has been threatened. The threat may come either from outside the body, from some noxious influence in the external environment, or from forces that seem to rise from within the personality.

In the older literature and in popular usage, fear is contrasted with anxiety. The term "fear" is used to describe anxiety which results from or is associated with some obvious external force or event, while "anxiety" is restricted to the situations in which the threats to the integrity of the person come from within the personality.

It was pointed out in a lecture a few days ago that the degree of anxiety, its onset, and certainly its course are determined not only by the precipitating external events, but also by the characteristics of the person who is made anxious: namely, his readiness for anxiety, his capacity to deal with new excitations, his capacity for maintaining a homeostatic equilibrium. All of us can remember experiences which illustrate in its simplest form the onset, development, and course of anxiety. Academic examinations may be used to illustrate in a simple way the problem of anxiety. The degree of anxiety (the degree of unrest and excitation) you may have in anticipating an examination is dependent upon how well trained you are, how well prepared you are, the severity of the approaching examination or your fantasies about its severity. In such a situation one may experience the more traditional aspects of anxiety, those that relate to cardio-respiratory function and motor discharge. It has been known for a long time that certain changes take place in the cardio-respiratory and skeletal muscle functions at such a time, as evidenced by changes in pulse, blood pressure, breathing, sweating, tremor, weakness, etc.

The other day I used as illustration a man who had had an auto accident. I pointed out that if a person is more or less normal, reasonably resilient emotionally, able to take on new experiences without being too much disturbed by them, if such a person has a bad accident, it is normal for him to experience anxiety for some time afterwards, to have a continuous feeling of jitteriness, tremulousness, even affecting the timbre of his voice. He may even experience one or two disturbing dreams at night, in which accidents or injuries and his taking an active part in destruction or injury predominate. This is the normal reparative process of working through a frightening experience; through this the more or less healthy person is able to recover in a short period of time with no significant residual. However, if the accident happens to a person whose homeostatic balance or emotional equilibrium is at the breaking point, or to a person whose capacity to deal with new or intense experiences is limited, there may follow a prolongation or an increased intensity of the experience far beyond what the situation warrants.

*

For the most part this morning I want to talk about some of the normal anxieties of sick people as you see them as general practitioners and internists. I want to point out some of the normal emotional experiences and some of the normal psychological defenses of sick people. Granted that the variations on the theme are dependent upon who is sick and on the intensity of the sickness, there are some fundamental facts regarding the understanding and management of sick people that general practitioners and internists should be aware of. An adult normally has a great number of interests beyond his personal self-interest in friends, family, work, community affairs, national problems—in other words, much of his emotional force and intellectual interest is directed outward. With the onset of acute illness there occurs a phenomenon which is more or less universal. Acute illness is a threat to the security of the person; it is an experience that provokes anxiety. The ego becomes aware that in some way or other the balance of the personality is threatened, and the individual experiences anxiety. The nature of this anxiety is dependent on the two groups of variables we spoke of before: namely, the person's readiness for anxiety, and the acuteness, intensity, and duration of the illness. In acute illnesses that come with no preparation, such as an acute coronary occlusion, the anxiety experienced may be tremendous because the experience is sudden. The noxious stimulus may be so sudden or so strong that it deluges the balancing forces of the personality, with the result that the person is unable to use adaptive devices successfully. Many times in such cases one sees panic or terror of one kind or another. On the other hand, if the person has had a disturbance over a period of time and then has an exacerbation of the illness, he is apt to be less tense, and the anxiety is apt to be better controlled.

Now let's get back to the more or less healthy person who experiences an acute illness without much preparation for this threat to his security. The first thing that happens is that the person withdraws his interest from the outside world and turns it back into his personality. Because of his illness he becomes less able to meet the demands of his environment. He becomes more dependent and, being more dependent, he needs more help. This phenomenon is popularly called retirement from reality; more technically, it is called a regression—a regression to an earlier form of adjustment. It is a regression to early childhood, where the emotional needs were great because of the child's inadequacy to meet the external world. The regression occurs because the personality needs all of its resources in order to cope with the problem that it faces.

In this setting, particularly in acute illness, one sees the significance of the doctor and the nurse. Since the patient is dependent and anxious, he needs support and help from people in his environment. Naturally, then, the doctor and the nurse play not only the realistic role we have spoken of (persons with special knowledge and skills that are able to give help), but also the role of substitute parents. For the relationship of a patient in acute illness with his doctor and nurse is not unlike the child's relationship to his parent. Both are in a state of dependence; both are anxious; both need support from without to help them through this period of danger, to help them grow up. Consequently, as Dr. Kaufman and Dr. Murray have been pointing out, the patient is likely to overvalue the doctor and the nurse.

Now there are many ways in which patients may experience acute illness. I have been describing the most common. At the other extreme there is the patient whose predominant pattern has been that of an overdetermined need to be independent, to be a big shot. His behavior when sick, even with an acute illness, may reveal a great number of interesting facts about his personality. He may become extremely dependent. Or he may use other defenses, one of which is the denial that he is sick. "I will not go to bed," he may say. "I am all right. No doctor shall put his hands on me." He may deny his illness because of the difficulties he has in experiencing the dependent, helpless feelings of illness.

If we have this conception of the emotional aspects of illness in mind, we can understand more clearly what convalescence may mean. Convalescence, in many ways, is like adolescence. It is essentially the growing up of a patient who has been helpless and dependent and who has had an increased need for love and protection and support from those about him. In convalescence the person again reaches out for the normal goals of his adult life, becomes interested in the people about him, and channels his emotional interest away from himself and onto the objects to which it had been attached before.

You can see, then, some of the practical problems that arise in the management of sick people; where the possible points of error may be; and how a positive approach may be used successfully with patients. In sickness the patient needs care and attention which are proportionate

not only to the illness but also to his own emotional needs. In convalescence the doctor and nurse should try to help the patient return
to his previous interests and should avoid measures that may entrench
the symptoms of invalidism or delay the growing-up period.

For example, how long should a patient remain in a hospital? The
principle should be that the person should remain in bed only as long
as it is necessary for reparative processes to get under way; he should
be started on the road to recovery, emotionally as well as physiologically, as soon as the physiological factors permit. Here I think we
should say a word about rest. Rest is a therapeutic agent which is prescribed very often and at times indiscriminately and without due knowledge of its dangers. Granted that rest as a means of bringing about recuperation of forces is a very important phenomenon, nevertheless the
prescribing of rest for long periods of time may provoke considerable
anxiety in a patient and prevent him from reaching for and achieving
normal and mature goals again.

So with the problem of acute illness—the anxieties that are experienced by patients who are sick depend on one hand on the forces of the
illness. What preparation has the person had for this illness; have
there been any prodromal symptoms? Has he been aware that he may
be quite sick? Has he been able to work through his anxieties about this
illness? How acute was it? How intense was it? How overpowering?
We know that an overpowering symptom in illness may deluge and
make impossible any compromise or defense arrangement. On the other
hand, we are dealing not only with the illness in itself; we are dealing
also with the person who is sick—his capacity to maintain balance, his
capacity to maintain homeostasis, his readiness for illness, his need for
illness, his conscious and unconscious utilization of illness. All of these
factors must be kept in mind in understanding the nature of the anxiety
that is experienced by the patient and the forms it takes.

A patient I knew comes to mind. A young girl, aged sixteen, was
brought into our hospital some years ago with pain in the abdomen.
This pain later went to the right lower quadrant, with rigidity of the
rectus muscle, nausea, and an increased white count, and it seemed unmistakable that she had acute appendicitis. She was operated upon, and
she did have acute appendicitis. In the postoperative course her wound

healed well. She was afebrile, her abdomen was soft, she had no signs or symptoms of any complications of any kind. Yet she felt weak and unable to get out of bed, so she remained in bed for a considerable period of time, baffling everyone as to just what was going on. Well, very briefly, the problem was this. She was the youngest child of three, had been the darling of the family, and later had felt quite deprived and rejected when all the members of her family either left home or became very busy with outside activities. She was a girl who was very immature and dependent and who needed much support. When, as a result of severe illness, she reexperienced attention and love, it was difficult for her to relinquish them and grow up again. This feeling was accentuated by the therapeutic program in the hospital, which injudiciously allowed for a long period of bed rest without any attempt to help her convalesce and grow up again. I am sure all of you have had many experiences with patients of this kind.

In summary, then, anxiety is an emotional experience that is useful —useful and normal. It serves the purpose of bringing to the awareness of the conscious part of the personality a serious danger. The anxiety indicates that the personality is being threatened in some way, and it mobilizes certain defenses, some of them being retirement, regression, a pulling-in of emotional forces, and an increase in dependency. These defenses are of value in helping the person assimilate and digest the emotional experience of the acute illness.

In chronic illness the nature of the anxiety and the nature of the defenses may vary considerably from this, though again they are related to the duration of the illness and the various means the person has used in the past to take care of illness. Patients with multiple sclerosis, with chronic arthritis, with repetitive, disabling episodes in their lives, oftentimes use other mechanisms, which are essentially those of denial. These mechanisms are similar to those seen in very seriously ill patients, such as a dying patient, where there is a direct or indirect denial of the severity and implications of the illness. Many years ago Hippocrates described this reaction on the part of the tuberculous, calling it *spes phthisica,* the hope of the tuberculous. Some of the German literature calls the reaction in multiple sclerosis *spes sclerotica,* and recently some of us have noted something that could be called *spes polio* in poliomyelitis patients. This hope is a device used by the personality to assimilate, digest, and work through the anxieties which are engendered by these disabilities. Similarly, in amputations we have the phenomenon of the phantom limb. In studying the dreams of patients with disabilities such as polio or amputation, we have found that rarely does the person dream of himself as mutilated, though he may dream of being weak or walking with crutches and then achieving normal strength and throwing the crutches away. Among children with polio, dreams of walking, running, jumping, playing football, are very common. One has the feeling that in patients with parts of their bodies removed the personality is trying to keep together as much of the body as it can. It is trying to forget or deny that something has been taken away. However, in many instances there remains, even with this defense mechanism, considerable anxiety and distress.

Now to go back to the problem of anxiety. I have said that anxiety is that unpleasant emotion which comes from the depths of the personality, which comes to the awareness of the conscious part of the personality and is used by it to indicate that there is danger and that the resources and the forces of the personality should be mobilized to meet the danger. In this sense it is a valuable, useful emotional experience which helps not only to signal warning but also to prepare defenses. In the older literature the term "anxiety" and the cardio-respiratory motor discharge are used to describe preparation for fight or flight. Actually in clinical experience one rarely meets instances where that phenomenon is illustrated clearly. Most types of anxiety that we see are responses not to external forces but to inner forces.

As Dr. Murray and Dr. Kaufman and others have said in previous lectures, anxiety is probably a nuclear factor in all neurotic symptoms and is caused by a conflict of opposing forces. On the one hand, there is an aggregate of forces within the personality which seek expression and which the child has learned may bring danger with them, such as aggressive needs, the need to be loved, or envy, or hostilities of one kind or the other. This aggregate, as Dr. Murray told you, is called the id, the impersonal aspect of our personality. On the other hand, there is the incorporation of the do's and don't's of society, which is technically called the super-ego and which we call conscience. There is constantly a struggle between these two forces—the id seeking satisfaction for certain needs, the super-ego denying these satisfactions. Between them is the ego, the conscious part of the personality, a Janus-like structure with two faces, trying to satisfy the strivings of the id and trying to meet the demands of the super-ego, at the same time facing the external world and trying to adapt itself successfully to it. Most of the anxiety that is experienced in adult life, aside from the anxiety that accompanies sickness (and it, too, is colored by conflict)—most of the anxieties of adult life come from conflicts within the personality, from dangers within the personality, and not from dangers from without—although an external danger may provoke or qualify the anxiety arising from within.

Neurotic behavior, neurotic symptoms are compromises, attempts at homeostatic balance between these two forces. Neurotic behavior occurs when there is lack of control of these forces within the personality, when the ego is no longer able to control these forces so as to allow for certain gratification and yet keep within bounds the demands of all the parts of the personality. Neurotic behavior is inappropriate behavior in the sense that the current stimulus factor is not proportionate or in a direct ratio to the behavior which it provokes. (Actually, it is only seemingly inappropriate; inner tensions may be far more threatening than appears on the surface.)

This, then, is anxiety in the broad sense of the term. The term "anxiety" is sometimes used to indicate an eager anticipation or a morbid anticipation of something about to happen; it may be confused with fear, terror, apprehension, and so on. But essentially what we mean by anxiety, what doctors should understand as anxiety, is this unpleasant emotion whose function is that of mobilizing the individual's defenses to deal with danger.

Clear examples of various types of anxiety are described by Anna Freud and Dorothy Burlingham in their study of "blitzed" children in London. They point out four types of anxiety. One is anxiety which comes as a result of an external threat to the body. This has been called "real" or objective anxiety or fear. Now, as you probably know, the real anxiety of a child may be very slight because he doesn't have the intellectual or perceptive ability to know enough to be frightened.

These researchers found that many times the actual presence of an un-exploded bomb which might have been very disturbing to an adult did not disturb the child. The degree of real anxiety experienced by any person is dependent upon his ability to understand the nature of the danger which threatens him.

The second type of anxiety is what may be called conscience anxiety. In children it refers to the bogey man. Essentially the bogey man is the child's creation of a person who will punish him if he is naughty. It is the first step in the incorporation into his personality of the do's and don't's of society. Instead of direct incorporation of his mother, father, and the other members of the family, there is this displacement to certain magical factors like the bogey man. So when a child experiences guilt or fear that if he is aggressive or does not do certain things he will be punished, he utilizes the bogey man. In the children studied in this London nursery—and in all children—one sees the anxiety related to conscience.

The third type of anxiety related to the destruction which was going on around the child in the war. The normal child in growing up learns to channelize or to sublimate his destructive feelings and direct them to positive ends. In the setting of destruction and killing and war, some children became very confused, for the behavior of adults seemed to condone and accept destructive feelings which the child was trying to repress and utilize constructively.

The fourth was what may be called infectious anxiety, the anxiety related to the mother. There were children who went through literal hell in being bombed and hurt—buried under debris for days without food. If the mother was able to withstand this experience and be relatively free from exaggerated anxiety, the children too were free from anxiety. On the other hand, even in our own country, far away geographically from war, the anxiety and tension which a mother experienced was found to be readily communicated to her child.

There are other types of anxiety which derive from the nature of the inner forces. These we'll talk about in the next lecture, when we'll also talk about the defenses which the personality uses to ward off anxiety and to digest and assimilate it.

DISCUSSION

After a recapitulation of the varieties of anxiety seen in the study of London children, discussion turned on the question of bed rest after surgery, as follows:

STUDENT. What about the situation in which a patient with a catastrophic illness is taken to surgery and the surgeon is a strong believer in getting out of bed the next day? What are the emotional potentialities involved?

DR. ROMANO. You mean the patient hasn't had any time to work through his anxiety at all?

STUDENT. And the surgeon says the best thing for him is to get out of bed the day after the appendectomy. We are by-passing so much.

DR. ROMANO. Well, it depends, of course, on who it is that is sick, and what balance he may be in. Usually with an acute illness, which is sudden and which has not been prepared for, there is some need to work through and reexperience the anxiety which in itself brings about certain defenses. One may err either way, obviously. Statistically the greatest error is in commission, isn't it, in medical practice?

Dr. Bauer, I wonder if you would say a few words about the needs of the patient acutely ill and the dangers of indiscriminate prescription of rest as it relates to acute medical illnesses, catastrophic and otherwise, and the ways in which a doctor may help a patient utilize the positive things that he has left.

DR. BAUER. I think whether he is treating an acute or chronic illness the physician must be aware that he is always dealing with two situations: one, the patient, the personality of the patient who is ill; and the other, the disease from which the patient is suffering. It is for that reason that treatment of the patient must be varied greatly from one individual to another. If we adopt a routine method of therapy, it stands to reason we shall be in error because, as we go from patient to patient, we are conscious of the fact that therapy has to be individualized and that what is good for one man may be very bad for another. In one instance it may be exactly what the patient needs and in another it may be a gilt-edged invitation to a flight from reality. In recent years many people have been interested in the ill effects of long-continued bed rest after various acute medical and surgical illnesses. I think in many instances it is because of organic complications that the surgeon or obstetrician or internist has advised that the period of rest be shortened—for example, to avoid thrombophlebitis and thereby lessen the number of cases with pulmonary embolism and the number of deaths that might occur from such a medical accident. At the present time we have physicians advocating the shortest possible period of bed rest for patients with true structural abnormalities, with such prevention in mind, not for the reasons that Dr. Romano outlined this morning. Unless we know the person who is ill, how he grew up, how he matured, how well balanced he is, we aren't going to treat him as intelligently as we should.

DR. WOLFF.   In an analysis of about five hundred medical and surgical patients in general hospitals, from the point of view of the presence of personality disturbance and the severity of the disturbance, we were able to find out that at least thirty per cent of the patients with ordinary medical or surgical problems had personality disturbances that were serious enough to modify the course of the illness or to interfere with the patient's return to his working life. The duration of convalescence in this group with significant personality disturbances was increased up to three hundred per cent; that is to say, some of them remained at least three times as long in the hospital as patients without such disturbances.

I also want to say a word about the cultural aspects of illness. The doctor, of course, decides how ill a man is, and this changes from time to time depending upon the pressure of the society in which the fellow lives. For example, when I was a student and during my early days of teaching, it was a dictum that a man unconscious as a result of a head injury stayed in bed a week for every hour of unconsciousness. Under those circumstances many patients stayed in bed in a hospital for eight, ten, twelve weeks, usually flat on their backs, and when they got upright they had a good deal of trouble adjusting themselves to the new position and the implications of that position. Now during the last war, owing to the pressure of circumstances and the need of men to get going again, they were urged to get out of bed shortly after they were conscious, or at least as soon as they felt able to get up again, and as far as could be ascertained the sequelae of that short bed rest were fewer and the patients returned to their work lives much sooner. When illness becomes an opportunity for a man in our society temporarily to give up his responsibilities and to receive a great deal of care, attention, and affection which he doesn't get under ordinary circumstances, it obviously becomes attractive to remain that way. When the attitude at home and at work and in society changes so that it isn't the way to get these things, an individual will very often get going sooner.

*

DR. ROMANO. I think it may be important to say, in conclusion, that the doctor should avoid error in two directions. He should avoid error in becoming maudlin—that is, in identifying with the patient and accepting the patient's dependency needs uncritically. In other words, the doctor and the nurse should utilize this intense emotional relationship to help wean the patient gradually back from dependence to his normal, realistic life. But some doctors have handled this situation in a punitive fashion and have pushed people too fast. One can err in either direction. The premise we gave you, the principle we have talked about a number of times, is that each therapeutic step should be taken with full recognition of what has gone before and the patient's preparation and his readiness for the next step. If one goes too fast or pushes too fervently, one may cause increased anxiety and further regression. The lesson, then, is not to delay this growing-up process, nor to retard it by indecision or oversolicitude of a maudlin nature, but to help the patient recognize what resources he does have and how he can utilize them most effectively.

II

YESTERDAY morning we presented to you certain data related to the general problem of anxiety. Attention was paid to certain popular conceptions of the term anxiety and a definition was given. Anxiety in its simplest essence was said to be an emotion—an unpleasant emotion, and one which is experienced when the personality seems threatened. Threat, I told you, can come from outside the person (that is, from the environment, from external forces) or from within the personality. I also mentioned that with this unpleasant emotion there are certain physiologic changes, and that the traditional physiologic changes are those connected with certain discharges related to the cardio-respiratory system, the skeletal-motor system, and certain vasomotor changes.

I then went on to point out that there are three or four types of anxiety. One relates to external forces and may be called real anxiety or fear. Then there are anxieties related to instinct and to conscience. In these anxieties (understandable only on the basis of knowledge of the emotional maturation of the child) opposing forces in the personality endanger or threaten the integrity of the person. The fourth type of anxiety is that which was seen in children during the war—the anxiety of the protecting person, which seems to be contagious to the child.

Most of the morning was spent in a review of the more or less normal anxieties of the sick person, the person who has a demonstrable physical disease. As an example, a person who is acutely ill, who has a sudden, unprepared, unpredictable illness, was cited. The emotional experiences of such a person were described—the withdrawal of many of his previous interests, his retrenchment of the resources and forces within himself in order better to protect himself, and his need, in this newly dependent, less mature state of development, for intensification of a helpful relationship with his doctor and nurse. Then certain points were made with respect to understanding the normal emotional experiences of illnesses which are not acute but which may be repetitive, as in multiple sclerosis, or chronic, as in certain disabling conditions such as arthritis, where other emotions are experienced and other defenses are used. Then something was said of the normal experience of convalescence—how, like adolescence, it means a reaching out for realistic living and maturity and achievement, losing the dependent state, reaching out for the more independent, more adult state.

In the discussion which followed there was pointed out the tremendous range of variables and the need to avoid the pitfalls of the two extremes of attitudes on the part of doctors toward patients. One extreme is a maudlin, mawkish, sentimental point of view in which the doctor identifies too completely with the patient, in which the doctor loses his objectivity, entrenches the patient's dependence, and prevents a return to maturity. The other extreme is a too punitive attitude that insists on patients' doing too much too quickly or fails to give them the gratifications they need in order to grow up again.

This morning we are to continue our discussion of the theoretical and practical aspects of anxiety as they relate not only to real anxiety (that is, anxiety due to external forces) but also to neurotic anxiety. As Dr. Murray and others have pointed out, here the theoretical structure, the actual events, the one, two, three of what happens in the traumatic neurosis can be used as an illustration of what happens in all anxieties. The sequence of events can be seen more clearly in this neurosis than in others because the provoking or precipitating or external forces are more demonstrable and more readily understandable. For that reason we have asked Dr. Murray to tell us the story of one of his patients whose experiences in air combat illustrate, I think, very clearly some of the fundamental points in traumatic neurosis. After he has described that case I shall give you certain clinical examples of neuroses as one sees them in civilian life, neuroses without a precipitating factor of any great magnitude, and then I shall describe some of the defenses that we as human beings use to help combat and channelize anxiety-provoking stimuli and adapt ourselves to them.

DR. MURRAY. Ben was a twenty-four-year-old waist gunner who had had a high school education and a year in college. He liked mechanics. He loved flying. When the war began he was a top-notch rotary engine mechanic in the Pensacola Naval Air Base. He had a good berth there, one in which he could have ridden through the war if he had so chosen. He didn't want to do that; he wanted to fly. So he gave up his job, and he applied to be an aviation cadet. As his vision in one eye was not good enough, he was refused. But he still wanted to fly, and so he went in training for gunner and radio man. Presently he went to the Mediterranean theater and flew out of Italy five missions over Yugoslavia and Austria and Bavaria. He really loved the first five missions; some of them were hot but that didn't bother him any. He loved them; he loved to fly.

On the sixth mission he and his crew had been flying over Wiener Neustadt, where they dropped their bombs. On their way back to Italy, over Zagreb, one of the waist gunners went forward to transfer gas from the reserve tanks to the wing tanks, and instructions had been given that the bombardier was to come back and cover the waist gun during that period. The bombardier was the weak man in the crew; apparently he was scared for some reason or other and did not come back as he was told. Then the plane was jumped by a couple of Messerschmitts which poured some incendiary bullets in and which had apparently come in from an uncovered angle. Ben looked around, a little bit angry at the bombardier because he hadn't come back; he had had trouble with that man previously. When he looked around, he saw that the tail of the plane was in flames.

This story came out very, very clearly, sharply chiseled in the subsequent pentothal interview. As Ben looked around and saw that the tail of the plane was a blazing inferno, an overwhelming attack of acute anxiety immediately hit him. "Oh, my God!" he said. But he was a sharp fellow, and he immediately thought, "Well, I'm all right; I'll get my parachute." So he went for his parachute—there over on top of the radio where he always put it and where he definitely remembered putting it before he got in the plane. But it wasn't there. Wham! Another attack of anxiety hit him. "My God, to be in a plane like this with no parachute!" Not good. So he looked around some more but couldn't see it. Finally he did see it. It was on the back of the other waist gunner, who was his buddy. He was sure the parachute was his, and now another attack of anxiety hit him. "What the hell will I do about this?" Remember, I told you he was a good boy. So he said to his buddy, "I can't find my parachute; help me find it, will you?" So they went looking.

About this time there was a lot of to-do. The captain had said to abandon ship and there was a lot of commotion about it, for the bombardier had apparently gone berserk or frozen. They had to get him and throw him out, push him out of the plane. By this time Ben was madder than hell at the bombardier. He was kept busy helping to push him out of the plane; then he turned to look again for a parachute—he and his buddy—couldn't find one —and there was more anxiety. But they kept on looking, and finally they found one down under the flight deck, and his buddy stood there helping him get into the parachute. Just about the time he got his parachute strapped on, the tail broke off the ship and the ship went into a spiral dive, straight down, round and round and round. The centrifugal force was enough to plaster all the men up against the skin of the ship; nobody could move, and there they were.

It was curious. We have told you about regression, but you will never see it any more clearly than in what Ben said under pentothal about what he was thinking when that ship was spinning round and round on its way down, and he believed it was just a question of a few moments until inevitable death. What he thought about was this. "Oh, my God, what terrible sin I must have committed in my life that a thing like this should happen to me!" You see the regression to the simple attitude of the child—rewards and punishment. When anything bad happens to you, that means you have been a naughty child and this is the just punishment. But, of course, the fact is that Ben was just tremendously loaded with anxiety, for as he now thought he was spinning down to his inevitable death.

The later story, as nearly as the natives of the locality could tell him, was that three thousand feet up the fire had got down into the gas fumes and the plane exploded. Ben and most of the rest of the crew were tossed clear. Ben was knocked about, but apparently he woke up with just enough sense to pull his ripcord, for about a thousand feet up, observers told him, his parachute opened and he descended to the ground. He was badly burned—had first and minor second-degree burns about the face, and his clothing was completely burned off him. He landed, however, found that he was in an island of Partisans, about eight miles in diameter, surrounded by Germans. A group of Partisans picked him up immediately and took him to a hospital they had in an underground cave, where Ben was treated for seventy-four days. By the end of that time the men had built a runway, working at night and camouflaging it by day. When that was finished, a couple of C-54's were flown in by some Russians and the men were evacuated to Italy.

Now there are very important points to remember about Ben. First, he was a normal lad when he went into the Air Force and a good sort of fellow, and, second, he had an anxiety attack as a result of an overwhelming experience. At first he struggled to master the anxiety by activity, and then suddenly, with the tail burning off and the plane spinning down, he was completely helpless and his anxiety became overwhelming. That you can see. Now he was in the hospital; the danger was all over. Ben, however, continued to have anxiety attacks. He held the anxiety off at arm's length with these ideas, "I'll get out of this God-damned place pretty soon and I'll get home, and when I get home with my mother and my girl, I'll be all right; I won't have any more trouble then."

So, at the end of the seventy-four days, Ben got out, and he went back to the Bronx, his home town, but unfortunately his wishes about his trouble being over did not come true. The anxiety began to come back, and he was irritable with his girl and with his mother because he did not find in them the omnipotence which in his childish state—due to his anxiety—he was seeking. He got angry with his mother and his girl and fussed at them; that bothered him terribly and increased his anxiety. This went on in a moderate way until one day the anxiety hit him so severely that he really fell into a fugue-like state, a state where the boundaries of reality were extremely indistinct.

He lay in his bed, thrashing around and crying and, of course, his family became very much frightened. They sent him to Halloran General Hospital, where he stayed for three or four days and was given sedatives. When he quieted down a little bit, he was hurried off to the Army Air Force Convalescent Hospital at Nashville, and that was where I ran into him.

I asked Dr. Murray to present this very colorful and dramatic story because the traumatic neurosis, the neurosis which seems to be provoked by external forces of certain magnitude, may help us to understand more clearly what happens in the personality when it is faced with such a noxious force, a dangerous force of great strength. When one reduces this story to its fundamental emotional factors, the essential points are as follows: First, this man had a stimulus of overwhelming magnitude that deluged his personality and made mastery or control of it, at the time, impossible. In other words, human beings may have experiences that the normal capacity for control or mastery or assimilation cannot deal with—experiences that the ego cannot handle. Second, the ego in this condition may be compared with the ego of a child, which is weak because it has not received through growth and experience the forces to strengthen it, or to the ego of the acutely sick person, who is not the same mature, strong person he was before the illness. Third, this man made repetitive attempts to master his situation. What one sees over and over and over again in the traumatic neurosis are the repetition of the experience—small doses of it, sometimes in dreams and sometimes in the waking state, and renewed attacks of anxiety—and the utilization of many defenses, such as this man's illusion of relative invulnerability and more particularly his illusion of fantasy that everything was going to be all right once he had reached his goal of being at home with his mother and his girl.

I think it would be safe to say that in civilian life one rarely sees traumatic neuroses of this clarity or of this magnitude; that, with the exception of the occasional catastrophe, such as earthquakes or fires or railroad accidents, man does not face dangerous forces so great as those seen in wartime. A great number of the patients we see in civilian life seem to experience anxiety—at times even overwhelming anxiety—but these cases show two essential differences: first, the precipitating factor often seems to be trivial or cursory, and, second, the patient seems to be

aware of little connection between the precipitating factor and the resultant anxiety. As we said yesterday and the days before, most of the
adult neuroses in civilian life have to do not with the management of
strong, dangerous external forces but with opposing forces within the
personality.

Some time ago I examined a man about thirty-five years old who was
referred to me by an internist in Columbus. His presenting complaint
was that he experienced periods of considerable distress marked by
palpitation, some anticipatory hand-sweating, some changes in breathing, oppression in the chest, and a feeling that he was going to die or that
something awful was going to happen to him. At times he would feel
faint, and on one occasion he almost fainted. In reviewing his history
it was found that these episodes of anxiety started one evening when
he returned home from a trip and went to his office late at night. On
getting off the elevator at the third or fourth floor of his office building,
he suddenly experienced this strange feeling. He had no idea why it
came or what it meant. He was frightened and called a physician immediately. The physician examined him and assured him that he would
be all right. He revisited the physician the next day, was examined, was
found to have no demonstrable structural disease, and was again told
that he would be all right. But his attacks recurred; his sleep became
broken; he had some restless, frightening dreams in which there
seemed to be a great deal of activity and in which he was injured many
times or injured someone else.

I saw this man two or three times a week for fifty-minute periods for
a number of months. It turned out that he was an only son and that his
father was a very autocratic, almost Prussian kind of person, who had
constantly depreciated him. In every attempt the patient made to reach
out for certain goals early in life, and particularly in adolescence, his
father would attack him, so to speak, by either depreciating what he
was doing or threatening that if he did it certain things would happen.
For instance, the father forbade the boy to play football, and when the
boy (to tell the story briefly) did play football, he broke his nose in the
very first game. There were many such instances in which the father's
threats and the father's attitudes seemed to be confirmed by the boy's
actual experiences. What one saw in the façade of this man, what one

would call his character or his total personality picture, was a submissive, quiet, passive person, whom everybody regarded as being very gentle, who seemed to be quiet spoken and without any great need, at least consciously, to exert himself or to demand certain masculine goals that are normal in our culture.

It so happened that this man's father was a banker. As a boy he had wished at one time to go into engineering, but his father had insisted that he go into banking and he had been able to adjust to this demand and had gone into investment brokerage. On the day of his first attack he had made a trip to a small town in another state and had negotiated a very significant sale of municipal bonds and, in doing so, had for the first time reached maturity, so to speak, in the economic field. With this sale of bonds he was able to consider breaking away from his father's support; it allowed him to think for the first time of starting his own brokerage office, of being able to go on in business alone, and to break away from the control of his father. As I have said, this was the occasion of the first attack. The second attack occurred two mornings later, when the patient was waiting for his father in the automobile; one of the things the father insisted upon was that his son chauffeur him to and from work daily. This arrangement cut in on the patient's time and made it impossible for him to see certain clients; it was a source of tremendous annoyance to him. In that setting, while waiting for his father, who was unusually late, he had the second attack.

The anxiety that this man felt was not traumatic in the sense of being occasioned by an external force or danger, but it threatened his compensatory defenses, which had up to that time been fairly satisfactory. To be more explicit, we are dealing here with a man whose basic feeling toward his father was essentially that of considerable rage, anger, resentment in having been kept down, having been depreciated, having been treated like a little boy. He was able to handle this rage, anger, resentment by the adoption of a defense mechanism which we call a reaction formation. This is essentially the use of a system of behavior that is the opposite of the presenting emotion: instead of showing anger, rage, resentment, he became submissive, passive, dependent, and quiet. For a long time this man was able to maintain adequately his homeostatic balance as it related to his father. He became decompensated when his defenses were threatened; in other words, with the sale of the municipal bonds he was able to become an economically independent person, to break away from his father's support and control, and now, in his new setting, he was flooded with anxiety because that meant the equivalent of becoming angry with his father, competing with him, breaking through the defenses he had used before.

To understand completely the adult civilian neurosis as it relates to the formation of anxiety one must always go back to what has happened in childhood. As Dr. Murray pointed out in his lectures on the development of the personality, the little child's anxieties (and the same anxieties extend into adult life) are those which relate to fear of loss of love, fear of punishment. Many times those two fears may mean the same thing. The child is a dependent, helpless biological organism. He has to be loved to be able to mature; he has to be loved to be able to grow up and to reach out for adult goals. Any threat in respect to the protecting, loving source mobilizes anxiety—anxiety that he may lose his parents' love or that he may be punished. The child learns that there may be danger associated with the gratification of certain of his instinctual drives, his anger or rage or certain types of sexual feelings and intentions. The child then uses a defense we have spoken of, namely, that of repression, the unconsciously purposeful forgetting of things which may endanger his position in his relationship to his parents. Repression occurs in childhood because the child does not have the intellectual and perceptive apparatus with which to perceive danger, understand it, and use compromises or certain other adaptive devices. Repression is, accordingly, a very archaic, simple means of handling dangerous matters. ("I will never think of these matters; I won't allow them to come into consciousness; that is the easiest way to handle them.")

In this patient, then, we are dealing essentially with the prolongation of a child's conscience. This man and most other neurotic people have the consciences of children, and their relationships to people are often the prolongation of some of the anxieties which they had as children in relation to their parents—tremendous fear of loss of love and of punishment. In this instance the decompensation occurred when the man's defenses were broken by the sale of the bonds and his reaching toward achievement and independence. So rage or the handling of anger toward loved people is, many times, the motive or the force which precipitates or provokes the anxiety attack. Another great force is that of sexual excitation. Ethical codes in civilization are concerned principally with attempts to control rage and sexual excitation.

The second patient I want to describe was a young woman, about twenty years old, recently married. I won't give you all the details of her past life. She was an exhibitionistic, immature young woman, who had never been able to reach complete maturity, in the sense of being able to tolerate a reasonable degree of frustration and in being able to establish adult friendship. She seemed to have an exaggerated dependence on certain people and a certain lack of control. Her husband, who entered military service shortly after their marriage, worried about his wife's remaining sexually continent during his absence. He felt, to be more specific, that his brother had roving eyes, and he warned his wife against possible overtures on the brother's part. After the patient had been alone for a few months, she quarreled with her parents-in-law, which led to estrangement and an increase in her loneliness. In this setting she was asked details of sexual experiences by a young woman friend who was about to be married. This conversation excited her sexually. Soon afterwards the girl and her parents-in-law were reconciled. The brother-in-law made certain advances to her, which she repulsed but which left her excited. He told her he was going to visit her some night and that she shouldn't be surprised if she were to find him in her apartment. A night or two later, after she had gone to bed and was reading, she heard a noise in the kitchen. She wondered who it was or what it was, and finally she got up and went to the door and found that it was a cat. She thought nothing more about it at that time, but when she awakened in the morning she was unable to move either arm or either leg. However, she was still able to speak, and from time to time called out for help; finally, some hours later in the morning, the landlady knocked at the door, came in, found her, and, becoming very alarmed, sent her to the hospital where we saw her.

Our examinations showed a young woman who seemed to be remarkably free of anxiety but who appeared to be unable to move her left or right arm or her left or right leg. On neurological examination, the reflexes were present and the plantar signs were flexor. In other words, there was no structural disturbance of the central nervous system that we could discover. There were some changes in sensory modalities in that she was unable to feel pin pricks over certain areas of her body. In the interviews which followed we found that she had been anxious and excited the night before when she heard the noise in the kitchen, but it wasn't a very marked anxiety; she was unable to tell us the dream she had the night she awakened with this paralysis. Now, I am going to ask some of you if you are able to interpret what the paralysis may have meant.

STUDENT.   Well, possibly, it's a—she felt her brother-in-law was coming to her apartment and the paralysis may have meant to her her inability to protect herself against advances from this brother-in-law.

DR. ROMANO.   Anything else?

STUDENT.   It might have indicated, too, some acquiescence on her part to the advances.

DR. ROMANO.   That is the essential point. In other words, the symptom served both purposes, didn't it? On one hand, she could say, "I am powerless to resist"; on the other, "I cannot and should not take any initiative." In other words, she couldn't help it if such a thing happened and she couldn't be blamed. That essentially—we will speak more of it later in a lecture on psychopathology—that essentially is what happens in the hysterical symptom: there is a partial gratification, partial relief of the repressed wish at the same time that there is a rejection of the repressed wish. "Partial release" in that if she were paralyzed she could not resist such an overture, such an attack; at the same time she rejected the wish by saying, "I have nothing to do with it because I am helpless and I have done nothing to invite it."

Now in the present instance probably two defense mechanisms were used. One sees in hysterical people, classically, the mechanism of repression—that is, unconscious, purposeful forgetting. This girl, when she came to the hospital, had no memory of the series of sexually exciting episodes I described to you. The second mechanism (which isn't so much a mechanism as a symptom formation in itself) is conversion. The anxiety concerning sexual excitation, concerning the do's and don't's of that behavior, was converted into physical symptoms and the anxiety seemed to be bound, so that when one looked at this girl one was struck by her complacent, indifferent attitude rather than by any aspect of anxiety.

*

Let's consider next some of the defenses which all of us use from time to time to handle anxiety, when we experience threats to the balance within us. One defense which we have spoken of before is that of *regression*. This means that when faced with a threat, when faced with a need for growth, when faced with a need to meet certain demands, there is within all of us, and more particularly in neurotic people, a tendency to return to a lower level, an earlier level of adjustment where life was probably more satisfactory. Dr. Alexander, in the book of which Dr. Brosin spoke yesterday, spends a great deal of time on this concept and uses the concepts "inertia" and "economy" in connection with it. Man resists change; whenever change from one level of adjustment to another is indicated, especially to a more complicated one or one that is new and that may give fewer gratifications, there is a tendency to retain the *status quo*, not to move, and more particularly at times even to revert to earlier levels of emotional maturity. We spoke of this in connection with acute illness. It may occur in a four- or five-year-old child when he has a new brother or sister; he may begin to wet the bed, to have temper tantrums; his speech may regress to a much earlier, lower, more immature level. Such regression is a rather universal, ubiquitous experience; one sees it constantly in all neurotic patients.

Repression is a second type of defense: namely, unconscious, purposeful forgetting, the censorship of ideas and wishes which pertain to objectionable or dangerous instinctual demands or those which the child thinks may be dangerous to him. The child feels, "If I do these things, or if I allow myself to think about these things, I may lose the love of my mother; I may be punished by my father." This is the concept "repression."

Identification is another defense mechanism. One may use this term in at least two ways, probably in many more. One is the identification Dr. Murray spoke to you about in the maturation of the child; the capacity of the child to identify with, let's say, his father or with father-like figures so that he may act like them. This is healthy identification, some of which is conscious, some of which may be unconscious, and which may be similar in part to emulation. There is also a rather morbid, rather unhealthy type of identification which occurs many times, as when a person seems to identify with an aggressor or with a noxious force. There are many stories of little Jewish boys playing games in which one will become Hitler, the premise being "If I am Hitler, then how can Hitler hurt me because I already am Hitler?" With this defense, if you are identified with a force of which you are afraid, you can no longer be hurt because you are the force.

We spoke in the past few days about the fourth defense, that of *denial*, and said that it is used extensively. One sees it, for example, in illness. I spoke of our experience with patients with polio and the nature of their dreams, the concept of the phantom limb, the psychological point of view. In war there are the denial of danger and the using of illusory devices such as "this is just a game" and "the better man will win." These illusory devices consist of denying the gravity, of denying the danger of the situation. Then, some of us may know people who characterize themselves as wearing a heavy coat of armor about them—everything must be wonderful to them all the time. They are unable to meet realistically the difficulties or deprivations or frustrations that all of us have to face in our daily lives. They have to insist that everything is wonderful; they are true Pollyannas, with an armor coating of insistence that all is wonderful, when actually it may be quite lousy.

Then there is another mechanism which is called *displacement*. In this the anxiety, the original or initial anxiety, may be displaced to some other object. One sees this classically in the animal phobias of children and of adults, where the anxiety related, let's say, to a cruel father or to fear that the father may hurt or punish the child is displaced to an animal.

Next is the defense of *condensation*, where anxieties over a number of areas may be condensed or concentrated in one specific experience, such as a phobia of one thing or the other. Condensation is one of the structural factors in dreams.

Symbolization is another defense. You who have had military experience know about the tremendous use of amulets, of charms. People who wore them utilized a number of mechanisms—certainly regression, magic, and special symbols—in order to have their invulnerability guaranteed. Then, of course, symbolization is seen in certain compulsions, such as hand-washing; some persons continually have to wash their hands over and over and over again, symbolizing their need to prove to themselves that they are clean and innocent and not dirty, sinful, or guilty.

The mechanism which may be called *devaluation* is seen in our daily lives (as are all of these); in this, essentially, one depreciates the threatening force, one minimizes the magnitude of the external force. This defense is seen many times in a very broad sense in the person with a sour-grapes concept and in the martinet—in the Army, in industry, or in the school or the hospital—the person who must be rigid, attacking, punishing toward other people because in that way he keeps them down and attacks them first so that he will not be attacked.

The mechanism of *projection* consists of attributing one's inadequacies, one's anxieties, one's feelings to other people. "That so and so; he feels that way, he feels this way!" One sees this mechanism at work in a broad cultural sense with respect to minority religious, national, and racial groups. I often quote to my students the statement of the King of Denmark when asked by the Nazi what he did with the Jews. He replied, "What do you mean?" The Nazi said, "Well, how do you handle the Jewish problem?" The King of Denmark is said to have answered, "We have no Jewish problem. You see, we don't feel inferior to the Jews." Projection may be seen in its most classic form, probably, in the type of mental illness called schizophrenia, where there is a considerable break between reality and nonreality, and the ideas and concepts of the patient are not only projected upon others but their influence is felt sometimes within the patient's body, such as in bowel function, breathing, genital feelings, and so on.

Next is what may be called *isolation,* the mechanism of isolation. In this defense the connection between certain events is lost, though not completely forgotten, and the emotional feeling seems to be separated from its normal context. One of the best examples I know of occurs in a fairy tale of the good mother and the wicked stepmother. There the child's feelings of loving his mother and being loved and his feelings of being angry with the mother at times for not giving him what he wants are isolated, are separated into the good mother and the bad, wicked stepmother. It is easy to isolate badness from the good mother, to hate the stepmother, to hate the witch, and so on, and thereby not endanger the relationship with the mother. Again, the institution of prostitution is based essentially on this mechanism of isolation. Many people are unable to equate tenderness and love and giving, in the psychological sense, with the sexual act. In fact, they may find it necessary not only to be free from these tender emotions, but even to be contemptuous of or to attack the woman with whom they have sexual intercourse—thus prostitution, which allows for the isolation of tenderness and loving from the sexual act.

Another mechanism is that of *undoing*. This mechanism goes further than that of reaction formation. You remember the example of reaction formation I told you about—the man whose whole life was spent in doing just the opposite of what he felt about his father, being passive, submissive, dependent, and quiet. If this man had used the mechanism of undoing, he would have gone even further than that. He would have done something positive to prove that he did not want to hurt his father. For example, he might have developed the symptom of stopping his car frequently to be sure the engine was all right. In other words, this person who really wished to hurt his father, instead of being merely passive and submissive might have developed some repetitive act to prove to his father not only that he did not want to hurt him but that he wanted to save him from harm.

There are still other types of defense mechanisms. One is seen in the blocking of certain emotions or the postponement of certain reactions. This defense occurs frequently in grief, about which Dr. Bond and Dr. Brosin will tell you later. In such instances the grief may not be experienced immediately but may be postponed and may be reproduced, perhaps in an exaggerated or disguised form, later on when some experience catalyzes it or brings it to the fore.

Then, too, there may be combinations of mechanisms. I have in mind a young woman who developed a street phobia. This young girl, about to be married, found rather suddenly, to her great distress, that she was unable to walk more than a block or two away from her house. Once she got a block or two away she would develop tremendous anxiety and would have the feeling that she was going to die. She said, "I know it's silly; it just doesn't make sense. The whole thing is nonsense, but I just can't do it. I feel awfully silly. The whole thing is nuts." "The funny part of it," she continued, "is I can't go downtown in the daytime. I know it's perfectly safe, but I just can't go downtown. But if someone goes with me beyond the two blocks, even if it's only my little brother, why, I seem to be all right; I can get along."

Now, essentially, what the phobia meant in this case was, first of all, a displacement of anxiety. This girl's basic anxiety concerned marriage —reaching out and achieving social, sexual, economic independence. In this scene, in this setting, the anxiety was displaced to this street phobia. It was also condensed, in the sense that the whole area of anxiety relating to maturity, responsibility of marriage and all its connotations was condensed to this specific phobia and was symbolic of many things —symbolic first of all of what walking and staying at home meant. If she were at home, she was a child; if she were a child, she shouldn't get married, she wouldn't have to get married; if she were a child, she could remain at home. There was also the mechanism of identification —identification with her little brother who was comforting her; he was a child and therefore didn't have to be married. Then, too, the street had symbolic significance, for, as you know, in many countries even today in Europe an unmarried woman is not allowed to walk alone on the street, and there is a sexual significance to a woman walking alone on the street, the connection with prostitution, the cognate term of the "street walker." So there were many defenses—symbolization, condensation, displacement, identification—that played a part in this girl's specific street phobia.

There is another defense mechanism, which really isn't so much one defense as a combination of many defenses and which utilizes many of the defenses which we have spoken of. This we call *sublimation*. Sublimation is the utilization of a number of defenses in such a way that impulses are gratified in a socially acceptable manner.

Sublimation as a way of dealing with difficulties may be contrasted with other attempts at solution. We know, as Dr. Murray and others have told you, that every boy's problem is to work out a way of relating himself to his father without being intimidated or having to be too aggressive toward or too denying of his father; to be able in adult life to look at his father not as a child does but as a mature person does—not having to be dependent on him but still being able to love him. This is a goal a boy arrives at in the course of normal development. In the course of arriving there he uses a number of defenses in such a way that his pent-up feelings about his father find outlet and more or less normal gratification in creative actions.

The problem may not be solved so satisfactorily, however. One boy may—let's say, in adolescence—develop a phobia about knives, a phobia that represents symbolization, displacement, condensation, and many other defenses. That boy, in his inability to meet the demands of growing up and relating to his father, says through this phobia of sharp instruments, "I am afraid of what I may do, or I am afraid of what may happen to me if I become angry or too independent in my relationship with my father. I may be punished for thinking certain things or for wishing to do certain things." This is a neurotic solution to the problem of relationship to the father. A second boy may try to find a solution to the problem by repetitive, stereotyped, self-destructive, anti-social behavior—getting into trouble with all figures of authority, teachers, ministers, priests, doctors, policemen, judges, employers. This kind of attempted solution, in our present nomenclature, we call psychopathy or the neurotic character. The attempted solution is a constant acting out of certain rebellious attitudes. It is unlike the neurotic solution, which used a phobia, or the normal solution, in which the boy sublimates and directs his normal feelings into creative outlets and channels. Another attempted solution to the problem of growing up is that which uses psychotic means. In the psychotic solution the boy's relationship with his father may be that of a complete break with reality; the boy's delusion may be, "My father is dead."

Sublimation, then, is the phenomenon in which impulses are gratified in socially acceptable and creative activities.

All of these mechanisms we have spoken of today we see in frequent operation in our own daily lives. There is a quantitative and a qualitative difference—but principally only a quantitative difference—between the ways in which we use many of these defenses and their occurrence in neurotic and psychotic patients.

To review briefly today's lecture, Dr. Murray told you the story of a boy who experienced repetitive, intolerable anxiety—one, two, three, four times at least—and after a period of seventy-four days in caves at Zagreb returned home. There, with the disappointment of reality, with the bubble of illusion burst, he had to work through repetitively his anxiety concerning his undigested emotional experience. We pointed out, first, the overwhelming nature of that stimulus, the intolerableness of it; second, the shattering of the ego, the inability of the ego to assimilate or digest the experience; and third, the working through of the experience by repetition, by small doses.

We jumped from there to civilian life and told you the story of the man who had an acute anxiety attack getting off the elevator. A reaction formation had been his defense. He had become decompensated psychologically by his business achievement, and with that the man thought, "My God, what will happen to me now that I am a man and now that I'm going to be independent of father? What will my father do to me if I do such a thing?" That caused the onset of his anxiety. Then there was the girl with the direct conflict situation of "I wish this but I cannot have it." She developed a conversion symptom that meant, "If I am paralyzed, and this happens to me, then I did not take the initiative." It was a compromise.

Then, utilizing the first instance, reaction formation, and the second, repression and the binding of anxiety to the conversion symptom, we described the various mechanisms of defense that all of us use from time to time to handle the anxieties of everyday life. We explained that they can be used singly or in combination, in varying degree, and that when seen in certain exaggerated forms they comprise the essential symptomatology of the clinical neurosis. In the next lectures Drs. Brosin and Bond will point out to you how these specific defenses are used in certain neuroses and, possibly, in some psychoses. They will show that the meaningfulness, the alphabet of the neuroses, lies in the neurotic symptoms, and that the clinical syndrome is dependent on which mechanisms are used for which purposes.

DISCUSSION

STUDENT. Is rationalization a separate mechanism or is it related to several of the other mechanisms?

DR. ROMANO. I think rationalization is a specific mechanism, though actually it may consist of a number of mechanisms. Dr. Brosin, would you care to discuss the relation of rationalization to any one of the mechanisms?

DR. BROSIN. I think it is customary to consider rationalization a separate mechanism. It might well be considered in combination, however, for purposes of discussion. Perhaps one should begin by reemphasizing that probably very few of these mechanisms are found in pure culture in life. It is only for ease in thinking about them that we discuss them separately. What are the common rationalizations? Negroes are considered inferior people for a great many reasons by those who find it necessary to believe this. It is the same with any other racial myth— Jews are aggressive; Germans are orderly; French are insidious. Now what is that but displacement also? It also involves a good deal of mythology, symbolization, power and prestige drives, and probably other mechanisms that I can't think of in this hurried review. Rationalization is a good example of combination; it is useful as an entity only for purposes of instruction.

STUDENT. Is fatalistic thinking a form of that?

DR. ROMANO. Will you explain what you mean by fatalistic thinking?

STUDENT. The individual who gets over his anxiety about a danger by saying it isn't going to happen to me unless my number is up.

DR. ROMANO. Well, the men who have had more experience with the military can answer that. In my experience the illusion of invulnerability was extremely common. To a certain degree this is a normal and useful defense. When it is used in an exaggerated form, it comes in the field of pathogenesis. I would like to have Dr. Bond speak on that point because he has had much more experience than I have had.

DR. BOND. Yes, I think that is a very good example of defense by rationalization, but it is a little more complicated. It is the breaking of fatalistic thinking that is the first step toward trouble, when the feel-

ing that "It's going to happen to the other guy, not me," suddenly becomes "It's going to happen to me, not the other guy." What Dr. Romano said is also true—that some people build fatalism up to an enormous degree. I know one boy who went through thirty-five missions
but would never speak of a single one and who didn't keep track of the
number of missions, with the result that he had to be told when to
quit. Instead of discussing his experience, rehashing it, going through
every detail of it, and thereby mastering it a little bit, as soon as he got
out of his ship he would go off into the woods by himself so that he
wouldn't hear anybody else talk about it. Now that was a very primitive form of defense. It worked for him for thirty-five missions; it probably wouldn't have worked for many people that long. And when it
crashes, it is likely to crash entirely.

DR. BROSIN.   Can we impose on Dr. Bond some more to discuss
superstitions? They all illustrate magical thinking and defenses.

DR. BOND.   Well, there were a lot of superstitions in the Air Force
that were connected with charms. I remember one man who had a
champagne cork wrapped in wire and who wouldn't move without the
thing. Many men wouldn't move without a certain piece of clothing—
particularly an old, outmoded piece of clothing—just as a little boy or
little girl, three or four years of age, won't go to bed without his toy
animal. A very primitive thing!

The superstitions of playing the game were most marked in some
phases of the war. It wasn't right to shoot anyone who parachuted out.
It was a most unhappy occasion when somebody got mad enough to
machine gun a bailed-out German. I remember one gunner who did it.
He became a pariah; no one would fly with him; everybody felt that
he was, well, a little beyond the pale. The idea was to keep death far
away, to keep it on a nice, clean basis.

Then there were superstitions about commanders, about groups.
There was one group called the Bloody Hunters. It was a terrible
group to get put into, for the superstition was that if you went up you
got killed. Actually, this group had no greater losses than other groups,
but when they got their losses they really got them—they were wiped
out three times in a period of a year. There were also superstitions

about the effect of oxygen on the body, about the effect of high altitude flying. All these were protective devices, and they are often displacements as well.

DR. ROMANO. If I understand correctly, the wearing of amulets and charms increases tremendously in any war. There was nothing peculiar in that respect about the experiences in this war. It seems that Dr. Bond has touched on the basic consideration: the similarity between the child taking a doll or animal or other toy to bed as a means of protection and the man in combat using such magical means to protect himself. Both use animistic, magic means to buttress and support their security.

*

DR. ROMANO. I would like to ask Dr. Jensen to tell us about some of the practical considerations doctors could keep in mind in taking care of sick people, especially sick children.

DR. JENSEN. I think we have too long neglected this very important subject of anxiety in children. In our experience over the past seven or eight years we have been impressed by several facts. One is many doctors' total disregard of anxiety as it affects children. It is rather distressing to have a parent come in and say that on the advice of a physician she has very severely punished her child in order to make him behave. Then there is the fact that in dealing with anxiety in children you have to deal with an intermediate person, usually the mother, and that that person also has anxieties. In illustration of this, I well remember a mother who brought her nine- or ten-year-old boy in for study and evaluation. He had suffered a very severe and sudden illness at the time he was about three years old. She said, "You know I was so upset that I didn't dare leave my boy's bedside for two and a half weeks. Then when I knew he was going to get well, the doctor had to give me morphine to get me to relax." There was no indication that the doctor in that particular situation had been aware of the tremendous influence that the mother's anxiety had on the child. Interestingly enough, seven years later that mother and child were snarled up in a situation that simulated the original illness.

I think the first thing that we have learned in dealing with the anxieties of children is that they develop when the limits the child can tolerate have been exceeded. There are a number of circumstances which, when added together, press the child beyond his limits, and so he develops anxiety. Perhaps the basic one is that of interference with or disruption of the parent-child relationship.

The problem of anxiety in children is one of the biggest ones we are called upon to deal with. It is very subtle, but as we sensitize ourselves to it we can do a great deal in helping children and families of children in expediting illnesses. In connection with this I would like to call your attention to an interesting paper that appeared within the course of the last year, which emphasizes something that we have all too long neglected—that is, the development of anxiety states following certain operations in childhood. I refer to the excellent paper that Dr. David Levy presented at one of the meetings of the American Psychiatric Association several years ago. It appeared, I think, in the *American Journal of Diseases of Children.**

STUDENT.   About organ neurosis—is this thought of as a defense mechanism in itself? If so, is there any particular type of gain, say, in having a skin eruption or something involving the heart?

DR. ROMANO.   If you remember, we spoke briefly the other day about some of the determinants of "choice" of neurotic symptoms. We spoke of why in some instances anxiety is expressed through certain channels, while in others it may be bound, as in the hysterical conversion symptom; why one person may develop a phobia while in other cases there may be somatization of symptoms.

Then, in respect to somatization, we reviewed the possible determinants of why certain parts of the body were used rather than others. As we said, this is a controversial point. One theory holds that it is fortuitous; a second that there has been a weak link in the chain, and that the weakest link breaks with stress. A third theory is the Pavlovian concept with respect to conditioning—emotional conditioning of a certain part of the body or certain system of the body with certain emotional experiences. A fourth theory is the one probably most widely accepted today among psychiatrists: the configurational concept that certain parts of the body have to do with certain basic emotional needs. For example, eating has to do fundamentally with being protected and

* David M. Levy. Psychic trauma of operations in children and a note on combat neurosis. *American Journal of Diseases of Children*, 69: 7–25, January 1945.

being loved, the infant's means of being loved is to be fed by the mother's breast; hence eating and retention of food may have something to do with that. Biting may be related to certain emotional needs in respect to attacking and displaying aggression. Vomiting may be related to disgust or, on the other hand, to attacking or rejecting something. These data refer to the organ neuroses or psychogenic organ diseases. Actually, there appear to be many determinants for the "choice of symptom" in the organ neuroses.

DR. MURRAY. I think if we first formulate the mechanisms of defense and what they are trying to do, we can show the organ neurosis as a special type of response to the anxiety situation. We have been hearing of a series of mechanisms of defense—mechanisms of defense which cannot stand at all by the criteria that intellectual judgment brings. In other words, here is a system of logic of the inner emotional life which is quite distinct from the system of logic of the intellect. That's the first thing you want to understand about the body of defense mechanisms. The second is that the regression to the utilization of this system of unconscious logic has been forced by a tremendous, overwhelming experience. The individual has been driven back from the high aim of meeting life with the logic of intelligence to dealing with it on a more primitive basis, with the logic of the emotions. As Dr. Brosin showed you yesterday in a wavy line,* a man goes down and then he goes up in his ability to meet life on these various levels. If you have that broad over-all concept of the meaning of these defenses, then you begin to see more clearly what goes on in the neurosis.

DR. ROMANO. I think it is safe to say, Dr. Murray, that there is a considerable difference between various types of somatization experiences. We have studied fainting, which is a very common and terrifying human experience, and have tried to distinguish between hysterical fainting and vasodepressor syncope. As you probably know, fainting is due to a great number of conditions; it may be due to a loss of blood volume, it may be due to a great number of factors which prevent an adequate supply of blood from going to the brain. We also know that by far the most common cause of fainting is some emotional disturbance. When one studies patients who seem to faint because of emo-

* See page 281.

tional conditions, there seem to be two mechanisms of fainting, and I think they show clearly the essential differences between hysterical and vegetative neurotic symptoms. In the former, the experience is understandable in terms of symbolism; in the latter, in terms of physiologic changes occurring concomitantly with the emotional experience.*

DR. BROSIN. The time is growing short. I would like to call attention to Dr. Alexander's classic essay on organ neurosis.† He distinguishes three categories of anxieties. The first is reality anxiety—the person is threatened, for instance, by a bull or by a cat. The second category is that which you have now heard repeatedly described in terms of conversion hysteria, where the body manifestations of the anxiety have meaningful significance in working out a solution to the person's problem. The third is the organ neurosis (specifically, the ulcers and the hypertension and perhaps even the skin cases we saw yesterday). According to Alexander it is too much to expect that the ulcer as such or the hypertension, which is a system of physical balance, should have a specific psychologic meaning. His point is that a series of forces has been set in operation. In the hypertension it is a thinly subdued hostility; in the ulcer, it is the dependency needs that are denied. As a concomitant to this pattern, certain incidental physical forces are set in operation, such as hypermotility and hypersecretion. Whatever the x, y, and z factors of the etiology of physical gastric ulcer are, however, and whatever the physical manifestations in the organ neurosis, these are only adventitious concomitants to the emotional life pattern.

DR. ROMANO. I think that's very important to stress. I know that medical students and many doctors faced with the proposition that certain psychological experiences eventually end up, let's say, in changes in arteriolar structure think that there are certain gaps or breaks in logic which are very difficult to reconcile. In the organ neuroses there are certain concomitant physiological changes which are part of certain types of emotions, while in the hysterical conversion neuroses there is not that concomitant physiological change; instead, the somatic reaction is sym-

* J. Romano and G. L. Engel. Studies of syncope: III. Differentiation between vasodepressor and hysterical fainting. *Psychosomatic Medicine*, 7:3–15, January 1945.

† F. Alexander. Fundamental concepts of psychosomatic research: psychogenesis, conversion, specificity. *Psychosomatic Medicine*, 5:205–210, July 1943.

bolic and does not follow the traditional pattern of physiological responses in the body.

STUDENT.   When an hysterical patient faints, would he fall just any place or would he pick out a nice, soft place to fall?

DR. ROMANO.   Many hysterical people hurt themselves. I think at times there is danger in exaggerating some of the differences between hysterical fits, for example, and epileptic fits—to think that hysterical persons only have a fit when someone is around, and that they never hurt themselves. Sometimes they do hurt themselves. It all depends on the intensity of the emotional factors at play.

DR. JENSEN.   I wonder, Dr. Romano, if this might fit in here? Gillespie, in his book *Psychological Effects of War on Citizen and Soldier,** says there are three ways in which the emotional states can influence the individual. First, certain emotional states can cause illness. I think the psychiatric conditions under discussion here illustrate that. Second, certain emotional states can precipitate illness. A practical example is that of the individual who is subject to asthmatic attacks suddenly coming into a threatening situation. He gets an asthmatic attack. There are many other factors involved here, but certainly the emotional reaction may precipitate the attack. Third, the emotional states may be sustaining factors. Dr. Brosin's case would be an example—the matter of gastric ulcer and perhaps hypertension. The individual who is under a good deal of pressure over a long period of time may express the disturbed emotional state through somatic complaints. When I read that analysis it helped me to get away from this either-or point of view; that is, in every situation we are called on to deal with, it isn't a question of "either, or" it is "both, and." As I see it, one of our big jobs is to determine the relative importance of each factor and, having done that, to work with each factor in its proper proportion.

* R. D. Gillespie. Psychological Effects of War on Citizen and Soldier. New York, Norton, 1942. (Thomas William Salmon Memorial Lectures.)

Clinical Problems

IV

1. A PATIENT WITH ASTHMA

Complaint. This patient, a married woman forty-seven years old, has had asthma for the last eight years. The trouble started, she said, with a hay fever attack that lasted several months. At that time she was spending much time caring for her only son, ten years old, who was a complete invalid. The son died three years ago.

The patient attributes her asthma attacks to excitement. She has had very thorough checks for allergy but has obtained no relief. Fearing excitement, she has completely withdrawn from her former social life in the church and does not walk even the few blocks downtown without taking some adrenalin. Asthma attacks can also be precipitated by dreams. She has very realistic dreams, usually concerning her son. In a recent dream she saw him in a wheelchair and went up and put her arms around him; when she awoke she had difficulty adjusting herself to the fact that he was not there.

The most recent attack of asthma was precipitated by the unexpected return of her younger brother from war. She had not seen him for several years. He telephoned and said he was arriving to visit her that same day. The patient immediately went into a severe asthmatic attack that lasted throughout his visit. When a young girl she had taken care of this brother as a mother. Her son resembled this brother closely. The asthma attack she had during her brother's visit six months ago was the worst ever; no medication could relieve it and she was confined to her chair throughout his visit. Since then she has had short periods of relief but, in the main, the asthma has persisted.

Personal History. In addition to the facts stated above, it was learned that this woman was the middle one of three children, the one younger than herself being a baby when she was ten or eleven years old. She spent much time with this youngster, who was a great favorite with her. She married a kind, understanding man who has been sympathetic with her troubles, though less disturbed than she has been by their son's death. They have had three children, the son who died and two daughters who are married. That was about all that was learned in this first interview, for the patient said she was always one to keep her troubles to herself.

DR. ROMANO. I think the interesting point in this case is that the on-set of this disorder occurred eight years ago when the patient was in the midst of caring for an invalid son and that the present severe attack was precipitated by an unexpected long-distance telephone call from her loved younger brother whom she had not seen for years. You can speculate about the possible connection even at this point—namely, the relationship between this brother and her son. The question is, what emotions are being experienced in relation to this brother which may be similar to her emotions to this invalid son? There's another similarity; not only was she the mother of the invalid son but she was also the mother—the "little mother"—to this younger brother. There may be a lead there in her feelings about being a mother—her feelings about giving and having others dependent on her. These may be mixed feelings.

The point is one which goes beyond this patient; it is one we have mentioned in previous cases. I think it's important to be aware of the possible mixed feelings that a person has in taking care of an invalid, particularly an invalid person whom he loves. One feeling is that of love, of wanting to help, but another, sometimes not conscious, is that of annoyance and hostility.

In the next interview with this woman, without asking direct questions, I think you might get into the area of what some of her responsibilities were. "It must have been difficult for you," for example, you could say, "it must have been difficult for you to take care of a person like that, knowing he was sick, and loving him very much." At that she may cry. Then you can say, "That's all right, Mrs. X." Then she may begin to talk a bit about some of her problems in caring for this invalid child. In that way you may eventually get an understanding of what some of her feelings were toward her brother also. Remember, she was a teen-age girl taking care of a baby boy. She probably had mixed feelings about that, too, you know. Perhaps you've had experience with that in your own family. Adolescent girls who have responsibilities in respect to younger members of the family often feel that this keeps them away from other enjoyments, much as they may like their younger brothers and sisters.

Why this woman developed asthma instead of migraine, hypertension, or some hysterical disturbance, we don't know. In considering the various determinants of the choice of symptom you may be dealing with, some factors such as breathing disturbances may have a special psychological significance, as in sexual excitation or rage, or you may be dealing with a breathing disturbance which is patterned after the behavior of someone else. However, at this stage we don't know what the determinants were.

STUDENT.   Couldn't there be the possibility—this son was a heart case—he had difficulty in breathing all through those ten years?

DR. ROMANO.   You mean identification? Yes, this is a possibility. Identification is a term which we use to describe something like the unconscious imitation of someone else's behavior, attitudes, or symptoms. It is different from imitation or emulation in that the patient may not be aware of acting like someone else. The possible reasons for identification in this instance may be dependent upon the mixed or ambivalent feelings this patient may have had toward her invalid son.

STUDENT.   I'd like to ask about the relation of asthma to the emotions. This is absolutely new to me; I've never considered asthma as anything but a strictly physiological process.

DR. ROMANO.   We are far from complete understanding of the role of emotional factors in bronchial asthma. It has been known for a long time, and is more or less evident in folklore, that the actual experience of the asthmatic attack may be altered significantly by certain emotions. However, more recently the approach has been from the other side—namely, that emotional factors may play an important part in provoking the attack. With this type of illness—as in many psychosomatic illnesses—the problem of causality is a complex one. We are probably dealing with multiple factors cumulative over a period of time. It is important for all of us to keep this in mind. I think there is a tendency in medicine for us to think of single or unitary cause-and-effect relationships when actually nothing in nature that I know of is as simple as that. Some of the most interesting work which has been done in this field has been done by Felix Deutsch in Boston and by French and Alexander in Chicago. The latter have pointed out that in certain instances the asthmatic attack may be provoked in situations in which the patient is sexually tempted and in conflict which leads to anxiety.

STUDENT. I would like to ask now what to do with this patient who has been described today. My idea would be just to explore further and with great caution these zones of sensitivity and by the patient's own conversation make the connection in her mind without telling her that there is a connection. If this were my case, I would have to have more interviews before even trying to tell her that there is this relationship. My question is: should one, after an interview or two more, say, "Now do you see there is a relationship?" or should you just let that patient see the relationship for herself? My present feeling is that I should let her gain insight purely by her own reasoning power.

DR. ROMANO. I think you've answered your question. The premise that we've tried to give you all the way through this course is never to make an interpretation unless you have fairly good evidence that it is right and that the patient is prepared to accept it. For example, at the present time what benefit would there be for the doctor to say, "Look, Mrs. X, it's very interesting that the beginning of the asthma happened at a time when you were caring for your son, and that the present severe attack occurred when you were talking to your brother whom you took care of in your childhood much as you had cared for your son." What benefit would that be to her at this time? None.

All that the doctor needs to do when he sees her again is to continue as he has been doing. He can take the lead in a few questions. He might go back to the onset and say, "Well, naturally it must have been difficult for you to have a sick son and to know that he might not get well, and to have to care for him all that time." Then she may start to talk about that. It may even be possible for her to talk a little bit about some of her feelings toward the boy. I wouldn't push that too much with respect to negative, hostile feelings or feelings of annoyance, but maybe you could let her know that you know a bit about such things, that you share her feelings, and that it's perfectly normal to have such feelings.

Then perhaps you could take this scene of her brother coming home and discuss that realistically by saying, "That must have been rather exciting, not to know that he was in this country and then to have heard that he was so close to you," and so on. Those are two possible areas, it seems to me, that you could discuss and continue to discuss in the next two interviews. But don't make interpretations as yet.

STUDENT. I was interested in the previous comment. I certainly wouldn't feel capable of opening up anything about the nature of her feelings about her son. What might I do if I get into that?

DR. ROMANO. Let's anticipate that she does have mixed feelings for this son. If you find that is so, I would just remain at this level and say, "Well, Mrs. X, maybe you don't know this, maybe I can help you to understand this, but every doctor knows that when a mother or an older sister or whoever it may be has to take care of someone she loves very much, it is perfectly natural at times to think some of those thoughts and have some of those ideas. That's all right; that doesn't mean that you love the person any less; that means that you still love him. But a person feels guilt because he thinks, 'How can I think such things about a person I love?'" I think you can go that far. Reassure her, if she seems mature enough. If she seems to be disturbed, you can explain the ubiquity of the feeling, the normalness of the feeling, and its value. That's the only point I think I would probably go into. Do you agree, Dr. Hinckley?

DR. HINCKLEY. Yes, there's just one other point. Even at that superficial level of reassurance on a point that you're already sure of, I think it best to use the interrogative form of question, "Isn't it normal for all of us to feel that under those circumstances?" A question rather than a statement, "This is normal."

DR. ROMANO. I think that is a very good suggestion. After all, our primary aim is to help the patient see as clearly as possible what some of his feelings and attitudes have been and to try to help him deal with these feelings at a conscious and mature level. This can only be done through the emotional relationship between the doctor and the patient, so that the patient knows that he can share his feelings and attitudes with the doctor without being scolded or punished, or without losing the doctor's interest and support.

We don't know in which direction further study of this patient will take us. It may be that certain medical factors will appear to be more important; it may be that certain psychological factors which we have not touched on may be of great importance.

2. A PATIENT WITH DIVERTICULA AND
DEPRESSION

DR. BROSIN. Dr. Bauer, Dr. Wolff, and I saw a patient of Dr. P.'s, a woman with massive hypertension. Dr. P., what was your reaction when these doctors said her physical condition had nothing to do with her complaint?

DR. P. (STUDENT). Here is a patient with hypertension, massive destruction in the kidney.

DR. BROSIN. Undoubtedly; but what has that to do with her complaint? What have the diverticula to do with the present disease?

DR. P. They cause her discomfort. Those diverticula can be inflamed.

DR. BROSIN. Did you see the diverticula inflamed? Is this a typical picture of diverticula that are active in current symptomatology? What I am trying to discuss is your feeling about the concepts rather than this case. These men also asked what the relation is between the physical symptoms and current complaints. They (Dr. Bauer and Dr. Wolff) have come to the conclusion that there is none. How can you justify your feeling in the face of your own lack of convincing evidence? What is the evidence?

DR. P. I will grant that she has superimposed upon organic disease these conflicts that she has had for many years. In her history you would find that she had disturbed emotional development as a child. Her father left her mother.

DR. BROSIN. How did you feel when the big men with reputations (not in psychiatry) said that the present complaints could not be caused by physical disease?

DR. P. I became doubtful. I am appalled that they dare say such a thing in the face of such structural changes in this woman.

DR. BROSIN. That is a painful business, because they surely are not foolish. Why do you think a professor of medicine, who is not a psychiatrist, saw no relation? Are you sorry for them?

DR. P. No, but I am confused. I mean, seeing that patient without having had this course I surely would have focused on the organic disease. I accept their opinion but I am confused. I have a conflict there.

DR. BROSIN. I think that is an honest statement. As far as diverticulitis is concerned, I know that an x-ray diagnosis doesn't make a clinical diagnosis. What it amounts to is this: the conflict is very genuine both by training and immediate circumstances. We are trained as organicists and we like to be doctors, in fact we must be doctors, otherwise we are no different from a great many people who are called unkind names, like various healers; but then we come to a person with a good many organic structural changes and we find that perhaps there is no necessary connection between all that pathology and what she came to the hospital for. That causes conflict. I think it is the best kind of teaching not to by-pass it and politely evade the very real issue. What is at stake? It isn't only your personal opinion but the whole philosophy of medicine. Does diverticulitis in the absence of activity cause symptoms? No. You can't treat a Wassermann test, you can't treat a PSP; you treat a clinical condition.

Let us wind up on the treatment.*

A fifty-six-year-old woman, a good hard-working soul; unhappy most of her marriage. Her husband was a truck driver who traveled at the time of their marriage. No evidence of syphilis. After marriage and the birth of the child transferred to stationary job. Pretty consistent drinker. To be retired on a pension of $55 a month. Her immediate problem is curtailment of income. Husband getting more senile, increasing loss of memory. A brother older than he is suffers from senile psychosis of advanced grade, and she sees the real problem: for the rest of an already hard life she must take care of this senile psychotic. He treats her badly. She had had gastric complaints a few years before marriage, periodic exacerbations for years. Now she comes in afraid of dying of cancer.

DR. P.   Had a tumor in her breast removed about seven years ago. Has been coming to the tumor clinic every seven or eight months.

DR. BROSIN.   She has all the marks of depression: facies, tone of voice, tempo, has typical tension (yawning); and yet it wasn't too bad, because with jokes and a little interest she could laugh and responded quite nicely. The problem, then, I think, is for the physician to work in two directions. One, as we outlined it to you—the doctor is the best medicine; she needs a friend; she needs support. She is condemned to live the rest of her life with a senile psychotic, curtailed income, loss of children through marriage. For the depression you can do a very

* This case is presented in greater detail at page 414.

great deal by encouraging her through your good spirit and good will, which takes just so much time. The other area in which the doctor may be useful is through social service. . . .

DR. P.   I see that but my concept of this—and I think it is important —is that if I have a patient who comes to me and says, "I am afraid I have cancer of the stomach," I have to prove to my satisfaction that she doesn't have a cancer before I can tell her so.

DR. BROSIN.   That is the first obligation we always teach, but we are trying to go beyond that. That isn't the point at issue. We give you *carte blanche* in discovering the physical status.

DR. P.   She comes in with fear of cancer. But the x-ray of the colon was taken a year ago.

DR. BROSIN.   All right, you have a note of triumph. If I had known this was bothering you, we would have started one step back.

DR. P.   No, I am not certain in my own mind. Looking at her grossly, she is not emaciated, she does not have pallor, she does not have anything to remind me of cancer.

DR. BROSIN.   If she has a malignancy, then we must handle that. You started out with the fact that she had diverticula. We don't want to retreat into endless examinations while we are waiting for her to develop her fear of cancer.

DR. P.   But she says she has the fear of cancer. By this reassurance you do feel we can make her overcome that fear of cancer?

DR. BROSIN.   What she really fears are her death wishes. She probably could wish her husband dead.

DR. P.   She would like to divorce her husband but she can't. She has tremendous problems but she also has an organic problem. I think she is just bumping her head against the wall.

DR. BROSIN.   Our job is to help her stop bumping her head. Here is more a nonspecific, generalized fear. Those depressions react very well to treatment. Those fears have excellent prognosis. With a little push, social support, you could expect fairly good results.

ANOTHER STUDENT.   Just anatomical proof that she has no cancer won't do any good.

DR. BROSIN.   Correct. We must be very sure that first we are doctors and understand the organic status. Even if she does get into kidney decompensation the psychological problem will remain.

3. DRUGS AND PSYCHOTHERAPY

STUDENT. One of the hardest problems I have had to face is to try to help a woman get along with a premature, artificial menopause. I have never, of course, done anything of a psychologic or psychiatric nature. I have depended a lot on estrogens—replacement therapy—and I have felt that the results have been excellent. I recall one woman of about thirty-five who went away—she hadn't been my patient before— and had a total hysterectomy. She came into the office in a little town where we have office hours a couple of times a week—I had known her very casually before she came in—and she was just wild, just a picture of frustration.

DR. ROMANO. After the operation?

STUDENT. After the operation. I did give her some assurance that perhaps her condition could be changed by giving her estrogen. Whether it was conversation or estrogens I don't know, but she was back to her normal self after a short time and with decreasing injections of estrogen she maintained herself very nicely. I have seen this many, many times.

DR. ROMANO. How would you interpret it?

STUDENT. Well, up to the present point I would interpret it as a good result from estrogens.

DR. ROMANO. Well, I haven't had as much experience—my experience in giving estrogenic hormones is to another group of people, people who are seriously depressed, and in such cases they have been of no value other than to control hot flashes and other vasomotor changes. I think what happened with you is that you did two things: you were a person who gave evidence of your interest in this patient; you reassured her, you corrected some of her misinterpretations, and gave her medication which probably did help to control some of the symptoms of the acute surgical menopause. Now, how much of one, how much of the other, I don't know. My hunch is that the psychological factors are probably important.

ANOTHER STUDENT. Dr. Romano, this brings up an idea I have had with regard to therapy. Given an individual who has been reasonably normal before but who has a stress, if you relieve that stress by tiding him over or lessening the intensity of the disturbance for the time be ing, the patient will make an adjustment of his own accord. In many patients the psychological approach is not necessary.

DR. ROMANO. I may misunderstand you but I would disagree. It all depends on what you mean by "psychological approach." If you mean it's a show of interest and the establishment of confidence and a relationship with you as a doctor, I'd say the psychological approach is the warp and woof of our medical structure.

STUDENT. I agree with you there. But the idea I have had is that if I can make life more tolerable for the patient (I'll grant that there is a psychological implication there), he will probably get well enough to live as before without the kind of interviews we've been talking about.

DR. ROMANO. I think I see more clearly now what you mean. I think I would still challenge that in part. It all depends on how you handle the patient every day and what you actually do. We all know what relationship means to a patient, what the expression of confidence and interest means. You may not say anything but your facial expression, the way you nod, the way you look—all those things may be extremely meaningful in helping a patient. Now whether you give that patient vitamins or whether you give him phenobarbital or use a hypo needle, it depends on how you do it and what your relationship to the patient is.

There is a principle in any type of patient-doctor relationship. Where there are two people who relate themselves as a doctor and a patient do, something happens between them. If the patient met someone on the street and had a talk with him, that would be different from the doctor-patient relationship. The reason is that the patient is sick and in being sick he is anxious, and in being anxious he is more dependent, less mature, and therefore his relationship with the person who is going to help him is not that of an adult to an adult. It is more like that of a child to a parent. That's why it is important to have some knowledge of what the doctor-patient relationship may mean. It is not an intellectual experience alone; it has to be an emotional experience as well. The doctor doesn't have to act emotionally but he has to be aware of the fact that the doctor-patient relationship is determined emotionally.

FIRST STUDENT. Thinking back to that patient I just spoke of, I tried to reassure her, but I think I went a little further than that. I said, "You are missing these substances that you were used to. I can replace them, and I am absolutely certain that if you will take these injections you will feel as you did before."

DR. ROMANO. You reassured her and used suggestion in a good way. Now, however, you are faced with a problem in such a person in that many times patients are given substitutive therapy all the way through and this sometimes delays their need to realize what they are facing. Sometimes the patient has to face the issue and you may delay it too long by using substitutive therapy.

Substitutive therapy can, however, be used to wean the patient, to prepare him to face his problem. There's a similar situation with patients with a sudden attack of polio. "This can't happen to me," they say. "This is a dream, I'll be all right." Are you going to go in that first day and say to them, "Look, this or that is involved; you won't be able to move." No, you don't do that. You reassure, you help. The patient has to get a realistic understanding of what he has—not what he has lost but what he has left and how he can utilize that most efficiently. The timing is important. You did the right thing. This woman was furious because someone had taken away her womanness. You were kind to her, and you told her she was going to be a woman again. That helped tremendously. Personally, I think that was much more important than the estrogens.

The question of when it is wise and when it is unwise to use drugs and other medicinal therapy in conjunction with or as a substitute for psychotherapy brings up a great number of considerations. There is a tendency on the part of some doctors to be either for or against. They say that it's not wise to use any drugs, even as adjuncts, while one is endeavoring to give the person either some insight therapy or reassurance, education, or support. It's been our experience that it is possible to use both, and together, so long as the doctor has a reasonable grasp of what his goals are and what he is doing. Many individuals who are somewhat sleepless, restless, tense, or fatigued can be helped by an internist to find out and face some of their more obvious problems and also be aided by certain drugs. It all depends on how you use the drugs. You can help the patient in taking the drugs by saying, "I'll give you these drugs and they will help you; however, at the same time it's important to find out why you feel this way." In other words, I think it is possible to use drugs wisely, so long as you're honest about it and know what you're doing.

DR. BAUER. Don't you think in most instances you should actually tell the patient why you're giving the medicine? I've always made it a routine practice to say, "This is just to tide you over, to help you, but please don't look upon this as therapeutic. We still have the difficulty to contend with, but we can perhaps handle it better (and you can handle your own day's job better) if you take this medicine. In the meantime, we'll carry on with some further discussion of you as an individual." I'm sure you have to be honest about it; otherwise you're hoodwinking yourself.

STUDENT. My thought was that it might delay the individual in gaining insight, inasmuch as he has the idea the pill is the thing that does the trick.

DR. ROMANO. Well, that's a matter of management again. That's a matter of knowing when to wean a patient from a drug, and knowing, too, that it can't be done abruptly. You can't wean a child, or wean anyone from something he's become dependent on, too abruptly. For example, I've used drugs—principally chemical sedatives—to allay anxiety during the day or night or to help the patient sleep for a while, and then decreased gradually the dosage of the drug. One can do something like that. Then one can use some of the distress that the patient feels in the weaning period to point out his dependence on the drug or his dependence on supportive treatment, and then give him the positive factors in his improvement to help him stand on his own. It is very much as we said the other day about convalescence. Convalescence is essentially weaning a person from the normal regressive experience of illness back to mature living. It usually has to be done gradually. If it's done too abruptly it may provoke further regression and the recurrence of symptoms. The point is—progress, go forward; but the speed and the direction of the progress must be determined by the nature of the illness and who it is who's sick as well as by the nature of the doctor's relationship with the patient. Each is an important determinant.

General Principles of Psychotherapy

JOHN W. MURRAY, M.D., AND
HENRY W. BROSIN, M.D.

WE go on this afternoon with our consideration of the problem of psychotherapy. Our special angle will be the treatment situation—the factors in the emotional relationship involved in it, from both the patient's and the doctor's standpoint. These factors are very important in treatment, for, dynamically speaking, much of the treatment situation depends upon them.

This morning Dr. Romano showed you that a patient with an illness becomes a different person from the one he is when he is a healthy individual living normally in his environment, with normal outlets for his needs in the many varied areas of his life. The neurotic patient is somewhat similar to an ill person, in that he is chronically denied certain outlets in life by the nature of his disorder. He is not able to relate himself to people in the normal way, so that his work and various other aspects of life suffer. As such a person grows older, he is likely to become less and less satisfied with his neurotic compromises and to want more and more, consciously or unconsciously, to do something about it. And ultimately, the sick person seeks help.

It is a fact, as Dr. Romano indicated this morning, that when a sick person comes to your office seeking help, he is a different person from the one he is outside the office. In the relationship that exists between him and the doctor there is an emotional coloration which is different from anything he experiences in life outside this special situation. The adequate utilization of the dynamic forces existing in this situation makes treatment possible, makes effective the ideational interplay which, under ordinary circumstances, would have little influence upon the life of the patient. This is a vital point to understand. The doctor-patient relationship is as important as the catalytic agent in a chemical experiment, or, to put it another way, it is as important as the blacksmith's heating a piece of metal to the proper temperature before working upon it. By and large, what you do with your patient will not be well done if the relationship between the two of you is not the proper one. You may hit the patient with your ideas, just as the blacksmith hits the iron with his hammer, but if the temperature is not right, nothing will happen.

You already are aware of this fact. As you said the other day, when you sit down and talk with a patient, in a very few moments something happens. The patient's attitude changes; he knows or senses that here is someone who understands him, who is plugged in on the same wave length as he is. Therefore, the first thing you need to do in the treatment interview is to give your patient the feeling—by your manner, by your demeanor, by your response, and by the very fact that what you show the patient is true—that you are in a position to tune yourself to his wave length. That is the first thing you need to do.

Dr. Romano has said that ill people have regressed, that they have become, in certain of their attitudes, like children. That's a good way to describe simply the basic attitudes of the patient in the treatment situation. Such persons know that they are somewhat helpless against the forces of illness that have been battering against them day in and day out; they have become tired by that battering, and they are deeply anxious to have some relief from it. But in the situation that gives them relief they're like children, at least in part, and they need support. Your response, as we have often said, should not be to play up to the helplessness of their situation, but, like wise parents, to go along with them, side by side, with your greater experience and your greater capacity for objectivity, guiding, leading, assisting, but not trying to take over the experience which your patient has to go through. The patient, like a child who grows up properly, has to experience certain things himself, has to appreciate their importance, has to develop the capacity to master some things which he could not master before and thereby to control this thing which has overwhelmed him.

We have talked about emotional conflict, about its meaning behind the symptoms of the neurosis; we have talked about the conflict being overwhelming and about anxiety being a reaction to the conflict. Therapy, therefore—psychotherapy—if it is effective, particularly if it is permanently effective, does one thing always: it helps the individual to master previously unmastered conflicts in some or many areas. We have shown you that certain devices may be used to achieve this goal. Dr. Romano has outlined them for you. But the catalytic agent through which such devices can be translated into effective use is the emotional relationship which develops when the patient knows that he is going to be treated by an understanding, kindly, and mature person.

The question properly arises in your minds: What do you mean by that, Dr. Murray; just what are you driving at? How do you bring about this special attitude in the treatment situation, as you handle ideas which up to now have been so painful that the patient has been forced to run away from them, to repress them? What do you mean when you say "handle this person right"? What is the attitude toward these people that will let them feel that you have that proper relationship with them? I am reminded of an experience I had in the Army that may help to answer these questions.

When I first landed at Fort Logan there was a difficult situation out there, a morale problem. The lads had been taught to believe that they were sick and that they therefore were not responsible for their behavior —that they could do anything they wanted, that they could go to town and raise hell, that they could get in fights, that they could kick out windows, and so on. They would do this, that, and the other thing, and they would get away with it; they would be excused because they were in a convalescent hospital for NP cases. So one of the first problems I ran into when I got out there was to straighten this mess out. They said, "What are we going to do about it?" I said, "That is very simple. Whenever these lads go to town and get into trouble, bring them out, and if the offense is serious enough court martial them. After the court martial is over, I will examine each lad individually; I will review the case and I will see Colonel Graham and express verbally and in writing what my idea is and how much the punishment should be modified to meet that individual's needs. In other words, we will let these lads feel that they are being held up to the responsibilities of the adult world but that we are also going to take into consideration the fact that they have been hurt by the war and that this will make a difference in what their punishment will be. They will know that we are people who ask them to be mature and to live with their maturity; but if they are not able to do so, they will find us kindly and understanding. Nevertheless, we won't go off the deep end and let them feel that they can regress to the behavior of infancy. They can't do that because life, being constituted the way it is, doesn't permit it."

Now if we can take that situation and translate it to the usual treatment situation in a doctor's office, this is what we see. The patients there find in us the same thing: they find in us kindly people who understand them but who, being realistic and mature, know that life is not all good and that it has its pains and that many times the surest way to ease the pain is to take a straightforward and steadfast stand in relation to the things that cause the pain, even though this may be difficult at the time. In this way one creates and builds up the morale of the treatment situation. I may tell you that we soon built up an outstanding morale at Fort Logan and that after three weeks we had no cases I had to see in regard to behavior problems downtown.

This effect is never accomplished by discussion or any explicit handling; everything is implicit in your relationship and in your attitude toward your patient. Perhaps this something which the patients sense in us is our own confidence—that we are capable and competent. Just as I said the other day, Bobby Jones has come to know that with an easy attitude and an easy swing the ball goes on the fairway about the way he wants it to. We know that, and you saw the other day in the treatment room how responsive to it patients are. The approach must vary a great deal, of course, with different patients. The dependent person who is close to a depression or close to a schizophrenic breakdown because the forces of life have been hammering and battering against him a long time needs a different type of handling from the less serious psychoneurotic, who is potentially able, or potentially almost able, to stand up and face the thing that has been hurting him. In general, however, quiet understanding is the way to make your first approach to a patient.

As treatment progresses, the patient will more and more assume toward you the attitude of a child toward his parents. The expectancy which the patient will have in relation to you will often become, in a sense, childlike. Much more will be expected of you than you can realistically give. Then, denied what his fantasies have led him to expect, the patient may become somewhat aggressive and hostile toward you. Children, when frustrated—either through having something done to them that they don't like or through having something taken away that they dearly want—become angry and are apt to express their anger toward the parent either directly in terms of action or indirectly in terms of behavior. So likewise in the treatment situation. Because in the beginning the patient has made you out to be an omnipotent person, he may become angry and upset when you are not able to rise to his overhigh expectations of you.

Now the wise doctor does one thing at this time. Either by direct interpretation (which usually is not the best way in this treatment situation) or by indirection and the use of allusions or little stories which bear upon the main point, he shows the patient that he has expected too much of the doctor on the one hand and too little of himself on the other. Dr. Bauer has laid stress on that latter point—on how, in the psychological treatment situation, you call upon the patient to mobilize his own personal resources in order to get well. And so you likewise show the patient that perhaps he has not fulfilled your earlier expectations, that perhaps there is something more he can do now. Thus you turn the aggression which was directed against you into more productive channels.

What I want to tell you is this—that you can come upon a critical situation in your relationship with a patient when he finds that you are not an omnipotent person and can't give him the tremendous help he was hoping for when he walked into your office. There comes an end to that, because we are not God and we can't give that stuff out. So about this time you usually run into a burst of rejection. This is what you need to do in handling the situation: in your quiet way (1) modify this overevaluation and (2) show the patient that the two of you are going down the road of treatment together; you are working as a mature person and expecting him to be mature, and in that kind of journey together you can do something that will help him to attain the goal he is so eager to reach. That is one of the first and most important steps in getting treatment under way.

All of this, again I tell you, is done by indirection and by implication. By and large, the patient senses it by the attitude you express in the situation rather than by any formal speech you make in regard to it. At the same time you find that one very, very important thing is taking place. I am speaking again of identification. When you have set the treatment situation up realistically like this, you have put yourself in the position of the mature, reassuring, and powerful father or mother figure—that person to whom the child looks up and says, "I want to do things his way," or that person about whom the gunner in the tail end of the bomber speaks when he says, "At any cost I'm going to be like my pilot." When that happens, identification has taken place, and from this alone frequently develops a capacity for mastering the conflict. This is a very important factor in the dynamic influences that enter into the sound process of cure. Many times the cure will be a response to this identification and not a response like that of a child who wants to be a good child for you by getting well. I think it was Dr. Kaufman who mentioned the fact that many patients will do the exact opposite of this: they won't get well as long as they're with you but will turn in the other direction and go to another doctor in order to punish you by getting well for the other doctor when they wouldn't get well for you, even though you were the one who has done the essential work on the road to the cure. In the average patient that you work with in your office, however, the factors that I have just stressed are the ones that are of importance dynamically.

Many times, of course, the process goes astray. For instance, in the case of a paranoid person, particularly a paranoid person who is in a therapeutic situation with a therapist of the same sex. You mobilize such deep and powerful desires that the insight you give and the security of the treatment situation aren't powerful enough to set aside the tendency to act out the illness in the treatment situation. As a result, you get deeper and deeper into expressions of hostility until the treatment situation becomes quite impossible. I have never seen more intense situations of this type than those which occurred when I was acting as consultant to young social workers. One of the aggressive, demanding, domineering clients would get the little social worker into a place where she would commit herself to giving some small financial help. Then the client would blow that up to great expectations, far beyond anything the social worker had committed herself to, and begin making demands with great pressure. The poor social worker would try to resist the flood and try to interpret, but she would be just powerless in the wave of those tremendous, infantile hostilities. That reaction on the client's part was predetermined by life experience. It's always so in a case like that—and it is often very difficult to overcome. So it is important, you see, to be aware of the dynamic forces that are at play in the treatment relationship situation.

There is another angle of this problem which we should consider, momentarily at least, and that is the meaning to the doctor of his relationships with patients. This could grow into a very involved discussion, beginning with the question of why the doctor became a doctor in the first place. Many of us had varied reasons for becoming doctors, some good, some not so good. Most of them have been modified into a pretty sound personality development that makes us, on the whole, pretty good people. As pretty good people, we are desirous of doing what we can to help others. But it is important what patients mean to us and also what the power we have over these people means to us, and, too, how we use this power which the patients give us over their destiny. It is very important, as you can see, that we respond as mature people to the tremendous amount of power that the situation gives us over a patient once the treatment situation, properly speaking, is established. We need to understand that—perhaps not in a deep and involved way but deeply enough at least so that we do not express any of our own insecurities, any of our own needs for power, any of our own needs for dominance, or other aspects of the inner life which are perhaps not so healthy and mature as they might be. We need at least to understand the pitfalls inherent there and, by being aware of them, to minimize or exclude their appearance.

Dr. Brosin will discuss this special aspect of the doctor's relationship to his patient.

DR. BROSIN.   Dr. Murray explained the doctor-patient relationship in such excellent detail and with such true feeling for its quality that my exposition may be a little superfluous. Meeting my new group this morning and trying to introduce myself, I offered myself as a subject for study. You *are* the subject for study by your patients. When two people meet, in whatever situation—at breakfast, in a railroad coach, in foxholes or box cars, or even in a classroom—a certain interchange of energy takes place. Most of us don't have a vocabulary with which to describe that exchange of energy; we are not particularly interested in doing so unless we're philosophers or metaphysicists or, perhaps, psychiatrists. But it is worth while to spend five or ten minutes on the very basic proposition that you should become self-observing, self-critical, and, in the narrow sense, self-conscious organisms because you are being observed, more or less critically, more or less expertly, by everyone who comes in to see you. Your patients certainly will study you in great detail, and your success or failure will in some measure be a function of the attitudes you consciously and unconsciously adopt and your expertness in maintaining the role Dr. Murray is outlining for you. So I'll offer you a proposition: I'm new to you, you're new to me. What are the forces acting between us? What do you think? What are the cues by which you study anyone?

Now I have a certain height, shape, color, clothes, and so on, and so have you. We all have certain motilities. Dr. Romano and Dr. Bauer, like myself for instance, are addicted to the use of chalk. As students and teachers you know that the use of chalk at times is a wonderful crutch; it spares you when you are trying to think of the next paragraph. You will detect certain motilities which are the signs of ease and others which are the signs of anxiety, some which represent a desperation to escape being the cynosure of fifty eyes, and some which indicate complete freedom or even histrionic enjoyment. By such means is it possible to study the forces which are at work in the impact of two new personalities.

Dr. Romano gave a valuable exposition this morning when he outlined the stream of regression, and I'll start again with that same scheme with certain additions. We find that the sick person is not the ordinary man with good integration; he is not a normal adult by our standards. We discard the use of a statistical normality in which a person is a hypothetical point in a scale of some sort. We also discard the myth of normality of some medieval or even eighteenth-century conceptions, the myth that normal man has no troubles. All of us were born, all of us grew up, and in one way or another we all had our troubles growing up. To quote Dr. Bauer, whether we look relatively normal depends on our façade. May I also add that it depends on the acuity of the observer? That's one reason psychiatrists are supposedly such disagreeable people; their acuities lead them to have "dirty minds." The chief characteristics of the adult are those of maturity and freedom (freedom from anxiety) or, if you are very mechanically minded, free energy. The best exposition of maturity as a concept is that

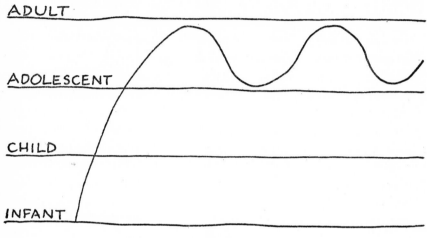

LEVELS OF MATURITY

given by Maurice Levine in the twelfth chapter of his book, *Psychotherapy in Medical Practice*[*]; the best on free energy is Alexander's in *Our Age of Unreason*,[†] which is a remarkably clear statement of the difficulties most of us have suffered.

Now down here we have the helplessness of infancy [points to low point on curve. See diagram], then the development of childhood, then adolescence and its competitive interests, its trials, and its requirement that we prove ourselves. (This competitiveness, if you like, is one of the great diseases or curses of our time.) Only as we develop a healthy freedom, the energy to live productively, can we be good, happy, and creative human beings.

[*] Maurice Levine, M.D. Psychotherapy in Medical Practice. New York, Macmillan, 1942.

[†] Franz Alexander, M.D. Our Age of Unreason. Philadelphia, Lippincott, 1942.

Now in this two-man situation where doctor and patient scrutinize each other with hypersensitive eyes—the doctor because of his training and professional interest (excluding, we hope, certain neurotic curiosities); the patient because he is sensitized, wants help, and wants to know whether the doctor is the fellow who can prevail. You have heard about the patient's side of the story; I'll carry on a little more with the doctor's side. You also are biological organisms subject to the same stresses of life. You also had to learn habits of feeding and toilet training. You also suffered at the hands of authority and encountered more or less oppression and intolerance. Your own ideas about dominance and submission, your needs for prestige, are variable, and these factors, in spite of any façade you may develop, will show themselves in the intensive living which you must be prepared to do in the treatment of a patient. One must pay the price of time, interest, genuine giving of energy in order to do good treatment. One reason why so many physicians are incapacitated is that, raised in the nineteenth-century tradition of medicine in which the cadaver was the ideal patient, as B. D. Lewin says, they don't have the capacity for the understanding of man as a whole. In order to be a good clinician in the best sense, one has to achieve techniques of even greater subtlety than those of the physiology and chemistry laboratory, however good they may be. And these techniques involve a certain self-knowledge. One has to know something about one's self, and not have huge blind spots. If a whole lot of you develop into cynics, which is another curse of our age, or have a pseudo-adolescent type of competitiveness, it will be very difficult for you to sit down and have genuine, mature interest in the lives of the people who are entrusted to your care. Furthermore, unless the physician brings decent free energy into play, he falls victim to certain incapacities. One of you pointed up this concept by asking where the quality which makes for intuition comes from.

The test of the physician is that he must maintain himself as a mature person with free energy though he too is subjected to the strains and stresses of our world. But if he permits himself hurry, fatigue, toxicity, alcoholism, or other neurotic outlets, he cannot function efficiently as a therapist. If you have blind spots, if you react excessively to other people's irritability, you should know what you are doing.

Restraint of oneself may not be enough. Perhaps you are too smooth; you have learned through the years that a doctor never, never becomes angry at a patient who is a nuisance to him. So you can defend yourself expertly *ad nauseum* and *ad infinitum* by series of laboratory work which Dr. Bauer and the rest have told you can become the great weapons against studying the problems of the patient.

Even more, the penalty for lack of the genuine maturity and free energy which are necessary to work is that you yourself become a damaged organ. With free energy one has a certain ability to deal with abstractions. But if you are hurried or fatigued or neurotically involved, you lose the most important asset or tool required in the diagnostic treatment situation.

I am afraid I am cutting this too much. I had a chance to talk about it freely this morning, and now I am trying to reorganize my ideas into a much shorter presentation. You will forgive me for trying to define intelligence briefly. It is the ability to deal with a number of variables, to maintain a superior organization of those variables, to deal with abstractions. Organization, of course, depends upon endowment as well as upon teaching and learning. Those people who are, shall we say, poor in endowment will never be good therapists. But, surely, you can see that as you regress in the scale of free energy you lose the ability to handle the number of variables that God gave you initially the power to deal with, and you also lose the ability for abstractions. If you are too worried or anxious to see too many patients in one day, or if you have an ambition to be the most successful physician in the community, as judged not by what you do for people but by the size of your motor car, then you are going to go down in this scale. You will be a damaged organism; you will impair your ability to deal with the fragile multiple factors which are mental disease.

DR. MURRAY. Now, have you any questions in regard to this treatment relationship, this patient-doctor relationship? If you have, we will try to answer them.

DISCUSSION

STUDENT. I don't know if I can put into words what I want to know —but it has been brought to my attention that in the development of psychosomatic disease there are people who get into their difficulties just because of their independence and others who get into difficulties because of their dependence, and in both these groups of people there are dependency and independency needs. Is it proper to conceive of normalcy as being a balance of such dependency and independency needs?

DR. MURRAY.   Yes, it is a balance, particularly a balance that can be maintained within limits of flexibility, such as Dr. Brosin has outlined, without the production of conflict or, shall we say, crippling conflict. The circumstances of life are such that difficult, complicated situations will arise; that is inevitable in the nature of life. The important thing is that we shall rise to the challenge with an answer—in a minimal space of time—that reduces the conflict to the point where we do not have persistent, nonpurposive, nonadaptive, nonproductive reactions. Being human beings, we have our independence strivings—I want to be like father, who seems to be a big, independent, strong individual. But we also have dependency needs—I also like, at times when I am tired, to be taken care of by mother. Both of those strivings are in the same child and both are normal.

STUDENT.   And both are components of maturity?

DR. MURRAY.   And both are components of maturity, but subject to adjustment in maturity.

STUDENT.   Dr. Brosin, where does the big mass of our population fit in on your developmental scale?

DR. BROSIN.   It seems to me that for the normal, educated professional man there is a seasick undulation somewhere around adolescent competitiveness and pseudo postadolescence and adult maturity. This undulation goes on day by day. You and I are not stable and fixed like the laws of the Medes and the Persians. We are biological organisms subject to the same onslaughts Dr. Romano so clearly told you about. We, too, may suffer severe, acute illness which pushes us down the regression scale in our behavior. Possibly it is a meningococcus or a bullet or a taxicab that is the traumatic agent; possibly it is some loss of affection, a girl turns you down, you lose a good contract, somebody else gets the job that you wanted, you don't get your promotion. Getting a new competitor in your community who happens to take some of your finest patients may be as severe an onslaught as an illness and may push down a reasonably good maturity to a childish level of activity.

DR. ROMANO. About the doctor-patient relationship in some of the areas, the actual clinical areas, there may be generated in the physician certain attitudes of hostility or annoyance toward the patient. I would like to point out that there are three types of patient who present such a problem rather clearly. One is the patient who is more or less of a nuisance to the doctor. Sometimes he is suffering from irreversible organic disease, say hemiplegia; sometimes he is a considerable problem in care to the doctor or the nurse. It is quite easy at times for the doctor and the nurse to become annoyed with the constant attention such patients require. The second type consists of the patients who have organic disease, sometimes hypertensive, cardiovascular disease, diabetes, cardiorenal disease, about which the doctor feels he can do very little. He feels in a dilemma; he has exhausted his armamentarium of therapy; he doesn't know what else to do. All this generates, localizes, a feeling of frustration on the part of the doctor; he doesn't know what to do. In anyone when frustrated, the feeling of not knowing what to do may generate hostility. In the third group are those individuals who have chronic neurotic complaints with no pertinent, demonstrable physical findings, whose neuroses seem to be beyond the skill or understanding of the physician. It seems to me that the common denominator in the latter two groups is that the doctor's anxiety started from his inability to understand and to deal effectively with the patient's problem on the basis of knowledge that his medical education has given him.

DR. MURRAY. I think that, as Dr. Kaufman said in one of his talks, it is very important for the doctor to understand these things, because it is so much easier to refrain from hostility when you understand why a person is hostile to you. It thereby becomes that much more of an impersonal thing. You know it isn't really a hostility to you but is based on the situation we have spoken of today—that a person comes to you with great expectations, the expectations of a small child, something you can't live up to, and that that is at the bottom of his hostility. It's nothing personal against you. Moreover, you know that you can turn and use your insight as a fulcrum to aid the person in his way toward recovery. You can now, by your psychologic manipulation, get the person to see that this tendency toward hostility, which is so clearly evident, shows the feelings that have been hampering him for such a long period of time and that play such an important role in the illness. Here, you see, by continually being the physician and maintaining the physician's role, you are able to utilize your understanding in the right direction toward a cure.

Dr. Bond, would you say a word or two regarding the treatment situation or any special angle you may have in your mind?

DR. BOND. I don't think I really have anything to add. Dr. J. had an interesting experience the other day that points this thing up, and I don't think he'd mind my telling about it. He had a man of twenty-four come in, who was having considerable difficulty with his lower gut; he had a diarrhea that had been going on for at least two years. About three years ago he had been involved in an automobile accident in which his brother had been killed. The second time Dr. J. saw him, the patient blew right up. Dr. J. had asked him something about his brother, and this fellow said he wasn't going to talk about that. "I'm through," he said, and he stormed out of the office. The doctor was quite impressed with all this, and at the time, he said, it made him as sore as the devil. He felt a good deal better when the patient did the same thing to me, and also when he realized how clearly inappropriate the emotion was. The patient did not hate Dr. J. that much; he did not really hold anything against Dr. J. He was pulling his feeling in from somewhere else and was bestowing it gratuitously on Dr. J.

I think that's just an elaboration of what you were saying of how much easier it is to handle these things when you are aloof and a little away from yourself. In psychotherapy such emotions as these are the stock in trade of your daily practice. Anger, fear, and their expressions are grist for the mill of your daily work, and you miss them when you don't accept them as such. It becomes a second part of your nature to handle them as gracefully and as graciously as a good laboratory worker does the excreta which at first were so unpleasant. You get a professional attitude toward the things you deal with in your daily work and they become a matter of interest to you.

Dr. Jensen has a way of putting this that's rather good, I think. I wonder if he would give it to us.

DR. JENSEN. Well, I think it's just another way of saying what has been said, but it is this. In doing your work as doctors you are playing simultaneously two roles. The first role is the one which involves all that has been said today—the intimate personal relationship that springs up between two people. If the doctor is trying to do a good job with his patient, as has been said so well by others, he must be unhurried, must not be distracted by other things that may be pressing in on him; he must devote his entire attention to the situation. In doing this, however, he must also assume the second role, in that he must be very much away from the situation. He must be not only a part of the situation but also apart from it, so that he can critically observe and evaluate all that is going on. And he has to play the two roles simultaneously. Once we can get the idea that we are a part of the situation but that, as we become a part of the situation, we are also apart from it, we can feel comfortable in the two vantage points and then learn to deal with them. I think we are able to be effective in our relationship to our patients because we ourselves don't get snarled up with them.

STUDENT. In the situation that you spoke of the patient places you in the father relationship. How do you finally dissolve that relationship?

DR. MURRAY. In the average treatment situation you will not find too great difficulty in handling the relationship. The only exceptions you are likely to find are those very, very severe cases in which the patient is on the edge of a psychotic breakdown and grasps at this treatment situation as a support for his strong dependency needs. The amount of good judgment which you men have shown here as we have worked along with you will be sufficient to carry you through in handling the usual doctor-patient relationship competently. In the Army, for instance, we found that we never ran into serious transference problems (problems of the patient clinging to the doctor), particularly if we'd helped the men with their anxieties. They took leaving automatically. I think you'll find the same thing except in the deeper type of regressive illness.

You'll learn in your treatment work what brings that type of sticky dependence upon you. (Get that word I used—"sticky" dependence.) Such dependence is quite characteristic of that type of patient—the dependence that is like a little child's. You continually feel that the emotional quality of the situation is always the paramount thing in the attitudes of such patients and that the intellectual interplay that goes on between you is at a minimum. Usually there appears to be a strong positive relationship; nevertheless, the patients use their intellects in it only as an excuse for acting out their inner emotional difficulties. I think you men will learn quickly to recognize that type of patient. They are the ones who are probably on the way to a more severe sickness anyway.

In general, you needn't be afraid of the transference situation in work of the kind you will do when you go back home.

DR. BROSIN. Unless your own curiosity or your own uncontrolled need to do something for the patient encourages him to become unduly attached to you, you won't get into trouble. If you have an overly urgent need to be "good" to children or dependents, or if you must show, in reaction to the deprivations of your own childhood, that you are a generous person, or if you feel best when you have a number of very admiring stooges around, you're probably a bad doctor. There is danger that your humanitarianism is only an expression of your neurotic needs. As long as you maintain conventional behavior and show decent, kindly appreciation for the patient's basic problems without falling into the many traps which are laid for you, you will not get into trouble, for you have something within you—your own conscience, let us say, your own feeling for the fitness of things—which will control the treatment situation.

At every step in the game try to define to yourself in quite ordinary language what your role is, what you are doing, what you are there for—"Am I really being a doctor and not a pawn in the neurotic plans of this patient?" With experience and reading and consultation with professional psychiatrists (usually you can get some help even at a distance these days), or other physicians who can play the role of Dutch uncle, you will get along all right. For unless you work hard to gain deep transference situations, which then need adequate interpretation, it is quite unlikely that the intricate defenses of the patient which have protected him against the onslaughts of a hostile and alien world for many years will be disrupted by you.

Special Therapies

DONALD W. HASTINGS, M.D.

TONIGHT we want to take up a few of the special treatments that have come into being during the last decade or two of psychiatry, treatments that bring drugs or electricity to bear on the patient. The main idea in calling them to your attention is not to tell you that these are treatments that you may find useful in your practice but to emphasize that they are all hospital treatments, not office or home treatments, and, like marriage, are not to be entered into without deep thought. All these treatments have certain dangers. For effective use all of them require precise knowledge of psychiatry and most of them call for knowledge of the psychoses. I don't know what the situation is here, but I think it is well to draw to your attention that in certain localities some of these treatments, particularly electro-shock, are used in rather helter-skelter fashion—in the home, in the office, and so on. In some eastern cities, for instance, electro-shock convulsive therapy is apparently becoming a favorite method of home treatment. We will mention its dangers and its possibilities later.

First I'll tell you about *metrazol* and *electric shock*, which we can consider as one type of treatment. In 1929 a physician in Budapest, a psychiatrist by the name of von Meduna, made an interesting analysis of a large series of patients who had mental disease, and he discovered that they had a much lower incidence of epilepsy than the population as a whole. On that empirical basis he speculated that there might be some antagonism between convulsions and mental illness. Carrying the idea one step further, he set about to produce convulsions in his psychotic patients. He first used camphor and oil. This had the disadvantage that one could never predict when the convulsion was going to come; on his wards some patients convulsed in the middle of the night and some did not have convulsions until two days after he had given the injections. He then cast around for another drug and found it in metrazol, which you know as cardiazol, a heart and respiratory stimulant. He gave about ten times the dosage you would give when you use it as cardiazol. He gave it intravenously in a dosage of about 5 to 8 cc. in a ten per cent solution and produced a convulsion. A little later, around 1934, two Italians, Cerletti and Bini, tried electricity. They simply adopted a method which had long been used in testing anti-convulsive drugs and applied it to human beings to produce a convulsion.

The results of metrazol and electro-shock treatment are about the same. Both are useful mainly in the psychoses and specifically, according to present-day thinking, in involutional melancholia. Without going into its symptomatology, involutional melancholia can be described as an illness which, it is generally agreed, has a poor prognosis for recovery. The statistics of the Pennsylvania Hospital show that fifteen per cent of the patients recover within a period of five years, which is a low recovery rate. With metrazol or electro-shock treatment the recovery rate has jumped to approximately eighty per cent within a period of three to four weeks. Follow-up on these cases at the end of three years, which is the longest the series has run, shows that the recovery rate remains in the vicinity of seventy per cent.

Both metrazol and electro-shock require hospital treatment. The danger of both of them lies mainly in the fractures they produce. It is well worth remembering, if you are tempted to give these convulsive therapies in your office, that the fracture rate with metrazol runs around twenty-two per cent; in other words, you will fracture about a fifth of all your patients. For the most part, the fractures will be compression fractures of the bodies of the thoracic vertebrae, but you may fracture arms and legs. I remember one case in which the patient in the convulsion fractured both hips; you could literally hear the heads of both femurs snap. A rather frightening experience, to say the least. The same thing can happen with electro-shock therapy. A drug known as curare, put out by Squibb as Intocostrin, has been used to reduce the severity of the convulsion. In most series of cases in which this drug was used—Bennett's of Omaha and others—the incidence of fracture has been very low.

These shock therapies, then, constitute dangerous treatment from the point of view of the skeletal system of the patient. Certainly such

treatment should not be entered upon without very serious consideration. It should never be given without psychiatric consultation, and it
should never be used without specific indication. The psychiatrist has
to weigh which is the greater danger—to try shock therapy in the hope
that it will jolt the patient out of his illness or to wait and see what happens without it. My own advice is certainly to follow the latter course
nine out of ten times.

Insulin shock treatment, another shock therapy, was introduced by
Sakel. I'm not too clear about the reasoning behind it, except that
Sakel thought it helped morphine addicts, and so, seeing some changes
in the personality develop out of that, tried it in the psychoses. Insulin
shock therapy is another hospital treatment. It is a treatment that is
expensive and requires much nursing care. Present-day thinking is that
it is useful in dementia praecox or schizophrenia. Referring again to
the Pennsylvania Hospital statistics, we find that if you lump all cases
of dementia praecox together there is about a ten per cent spontaneous
recovery rate, while with shock therapy you can discharge about
twenty-six per cent of your patients as recovered. If you follow those
patients for a period of five years, you will find that the recovery rate
has dropped to around thirteen or fourteen per cent. In other words,
there has been a total gain of three or four per cent over a period of
five years, which may be nonmeaningful from a statistical standpoint.

Sub-shock insulin is a treatment that has had a good deal of popu-
larity. It consists of giving the patient enough insulin so that his blood
sugar will go down to a certain degree but not sufficiently to produce
coma. This treatment was used by Sargent in England quite extensively during the war, and it seemed to have some value in quieting
very anxious patients. It has, of course, the additional advantage of putting a lot of weight on the patient, who may have been run down physically for one reason or another. It is obvious, however, that sub-insulin,
or sub-shock insulin, really does nothing in getting at the patient's
problems unless psychotherapy is carried along with it simultaneously.
It may or may not be a fairly reasonable adjunctive therapy if the
patient is worn out physically, is underweight, and so on.

Lobotomy, a fairly recent venture in treating psychiatric patients,
consists of the heroic measure of opening up the skull with two burr

holes and putting a wire loop down through the frontal cortex. Certain of the frontal pathways are interrupted. There was high hope several years ago that lobotomy might be the answer in dealing with some of the severe psychoses. In general results have shown that lobotomy has use in old cases of psychosis which have not responded to any other means, old cases in which the patients are very agitated and present hard nursing problems. In certain cases lobotomy seems to have the facility of cutting down activity, making the patient easier to handle in the hospital. There are some psychiatrists, however, who would disagree with this very pessimistic statement.

Narcosis therapy consists in the giving of large doses of sodium amytal to patients. In its classical form it consisted of giving such amounts that the patient remained asleep for about twenty-two out of each twenty-four hours and continuing that for a period of ten to fourteen days. This is again a fairly heroic treatment and a difficult one from the nursing standpoint. It has very specific dangers—hypostatic pneumonia, cardiac collapse, and so on. The blood pressure often falls to very low systolic levels and must then be supported. In narcosis therapy the patient is not infrequently fairly close to the pearly gates.

Narcosis treatment is perhaps useful in the psychosis known as manic-depressive disease, when the patient is very manic, so near to wearing himself out that the doctor fears he may literally wear himself to death. The results of narcosis treatment have been very equivocal, much depending on whose reports you believe. At best I think the treatment solves the problem for only a couple of weeks; all too often when narcosis therapy is stopped you find that the patient is still as manic as ever. This kind of treatment does have one advantage, in that during it the patient talks, and so one may learn a good deal about his conflicts and inner turmoil. This, perhaps, will give something to work on with the patient, some hints to follow after he has made enough recovery to be accessible to psychotherapy.

Pentothal or *narcosynthesis*, as it was called during the war, is one treatment I'd like to spend a little bit more time on. With the advent of sodium amytal, the date of which I forget but I think it was around 1930, Lorenz and Bleckwenn tried giving this drug intravenously to psychotic patients and found that they talked. For example, when a patient with a mute type of dementia praecox was given intravenous amytal, he would open up and perhaps for a period of two to three hours seem almost normal. However, he would lapse back into his disease as soon as the drug had been excreted. Sodium amytal has been used for that purpose by a good many workers for many years. A more recent refinement of the treatment is to give the patient five grains of caffeine sodio-benzoate and then in ten minutes follow it by intravenous amytal. This often makes a patient with dementia praecox quite conversant for a few hours, and thus the doctor may get some insight into his difficulties and problems.

During the African campaign Dr. Roy Grinker, who was the psychiatrist for the Twelfth Air Force and was also working with some of the ground force personnel, saw a number of the rather gross reactions which resulted from combat, in which men were markedly tremulous, speechless, sometimes stuporous. Grinker wanted to use sodium amytal to see if it would have the effect of releasing these men and making some of them more accessible to psychotherapy. There wasn't any sodium amytal in Africa, but there was a lot of sodium pentothal for intravenous anesthesia, so Grinker used pentothal instead. He found, interestingly enough, that the soldier who had been through a campaign or through a battle or through a very trying experience would, under the influence of intravenous pentothal, not infrequently act out in the present tense the traumatic experience through which he had gone. One case of Grinker's I remember offhand. He was an infantryman who was in a semistuporous condition when he was brought to the hospital where Grinker was. Grinker gave sodium pentothal to him, and he reenacted the whole affair that he had been in. Under shelling in the Tunisian campaign he had tried to get under cover in a foxhole, found it already filled with two dead soldiers, threw them out of the foxhole, and lay practically covered by their bodies during the remainder of the shelling.

Sodium pentothal is given in either 2.5 or 5 per cent solution, intravenously and very slowly. The usual amount that would be needed is in the neighborhood of 5 to 7 cc. of the 2.5 per cent solution. The technique is simple. As the needle is introduced, the patient is asked to count backwards from a hundred as far as he can. The drug is continued until the patient's speech is very thick and he is pretty groggy. The needle is then withdrawn. This treatment is useful as a short cut to finding material which is buried; it is an uncovering technique to find out what is at the bottom of the patient's illness. It is useful in the war situation, when one suspects that a recent, overwhelming trauma has produced the difficulty. I doubt very much whether pentothal would have any real use in civilian neuroses where the conflicts of the patient may lie many years behind him, in his childhood. It is useful, however, as a short cut to therapy in uncovering what may be at the basis of the patient's difficulties if a recent traumatic episode is thought to have precipitated the neurosis.

Pentothal is given only after the doctor gets to know his patient. It is not given in any hit-or-miss fashion; only after three or four interviews with the patient, in which the general scheme of things is sized up, may pentothal be used. There is no magic in the drug itself. It is useful simply as an adjunct to talking with the patient. I remember going into one airfield at a time when pentothal was becoming quite popular. The doctor who was using pentothal on a rather widespread scale said, "Colonel Hastings, I don't think the damn stuff is any good," and he asked me to come along with him while he gave it to a patient. He stretched out a patient in the dispensary, gave the pentothal, and put the patient to sleep. He waited until the patient woke up and then said, "See, nothing has happened!" Of course nothing had happened.

Let's assume that we have our patient, one of the war cases, under pentothal, that we know something about the man's general setting, what he has been through as far as he can tell it to us, and let's say that we now have him at the point where we have just taken out the needle and the patient is partially anesthetized, still able to talk in a rather thick way. Let's ask him one question; for example, let's ask him what is it he is trying so hard to forget, what is the trouble, and so on. Then just let the patient talk, and at times one will see his experiences relived, experiences for which he has a good deal of guilt, and so on, relived with a great deal of emotion.

Let me tell you about one instance that occurred at the Don Ce Sar Hospital. We had a cook from the Tunisian campaign, a mess sergeant.

He came into the hospital with the chief complaint of depression, felt down in the dumps, blue, felt life wasn't worth going on with, irritable, was having dreams at night in which men were being killed. He was a mess sergeant and, by his own statement, hadn't seen any of the war; all he had been doing was seeing that the meals were cooked, and so on. He had gotten sick in the neighborhood of Bizerte. I saw him perhaps three or four times, in an across-the-table type of interview, and learned almost nothing about his situation except the theater he had been in, what leaves he'd had, and what air raids he had been through. When asked under pentothal, "What is it you are trying to forget?" with a tremendous storm of emotion he replied, "I didn't mean to kill him, I didn't mean to kill him." To make a consecutive story of it, although it didn't come out in that manner, I learned that one night in the campaign around Bizerte he was in the mess hall when they were alerted for a parachute attack and were given arms. They had had air raids every night, and when the air raid sirens went off again he didn't think much of it, went right on working in his kitchen and making the trip down between the kitchen and the storeroom to get some potatoes for the morning. About halfway down the mess hall he looked out of the windows, which were in relief in the moonlight, and saw a body swinging in front of them. He went over and saw that it was the body of a German parachutist who was trying to cut his parachute straps free— his parachute had become fouled in the chimney and he was dangling over the edge of the roof in front of the window. The sergeant pulled out his forty-five and shot the man twice through the belly. Then he ran through the kitchen, out around the side of the building, to see what he'd done. When he got to the edge of the building he saw another German parachutist attempting to cut down the man he had just shot, and so he shot this second German three times, right in the face. He killed both of them. Without going into too many other details— the sergeant had a tremendous amount of guilt because of this killing. Instead of recording that he had killed these two parachutists, for which he might have got a medal, he dragged their bodies off to a ditch and covered them over with brush. Two days later, when the bodies were discovered, the commanding officer held a roll call of all the enlisted personnel, asked them individually if they knew anything about the bodies, and the sergeant denied that he did. From that point on he began to feel irritable and depressed and had dreams of killing the parachutists.

This was an episode that we learned for the first time under pentothal. Now we might ask ourselves whether that material was truly repressed—was it pushed out of conscious memory so that he couldn't talk about it even if he wanted to—or was it something that he remembered but couldn't talk about without feeling too much guilt? I don't know. In any event, pentothal was a short cut to this man's treatment; it certainly speeded up treatment by some weeks. Cases like this are being enumerated almost endlessly. In some cases, however, the pentothal reaction is more or less sterile; you get no more information than you already have from the across-the-table interviews.

There are some civilian cases wherein pentothal might perhaps be used. One such case was brought up for discussion here a few days ago— the twenty-six-year-old girl whose husband was killed. She had had marital difficulties for a long time, and because of them she felt that in a sense she had sent her husband away into the Army. Five or six months after he left she got the Adjutant General's telegram, "Missing in action"; and a few months later the message that her husband had been killed in action. Her depression and difficulty started after she received the first telegram. In that type of situation, a situation in which trauma has occurred within the recent past, one might think of short-cutting treatment by giving pentothal and securing information which would take some time in ordinary psychotherapy.

Pentothal has all the dangers of intravenous anesthesia. Again my belief is that it should not be given except in a hospital, where if you bump into trouble you've got oxygen and other forms of resuscitation available.

Dr. Murray, would you like to add anything to this?

DISCUSSION

DR. MURRAY. In many cases pentothal is extremely useful in having the patient act out his emotions with pristine clarity. It gives one an opportunity in the subsequent interviews to work out the meaning of the patient's traumatic experience and to relate it back to his whole personality and perhaps earlier experiences that may have conditioned him to be especially sensitive to a particular kind of trauma. The working through in subsequent therapeutic interviews is the thing that is important.

STUDENT. What are the dangers of pentothal, other than those of intravenous anesthesia?

DR. HASTINGS. The amount and quantity of the patient's production are particularly difficult to control. You really make some people a lot sicker because they open up too wide; you always have to run with the brakes on and keep the patient from giving you more than he can integrate at the time he gives it. This is particularly true of people who are a little schizoid; you can make them considerably worse. You are often rather seduced by the wonderful mechanisms they display and the clarity of their discussion, but you certainly can do harm with pentothal. It has to be used with a certain degree of caution and judgment.

DR. ROMANO. I would like, for purpose of emphasis, to confirm that. In the very brief experience we had in Europe in studying several combat infantry units and the use of pentothal in evacuation hospitals and in hospitals in the communication zone, we were struck principally by its abuse and misuse. It was used by inexperienced people, and it was used with specious premises: that all one had to do was to introduce this drug, bring about a certain degree of decortication, afford a release of certain withheld and unresolved emotional tensions, and that release in itself would be therapeutic. This is specious and wrong. It seems to me that the techniques and method outlined should be used only by skilled people, for you not only have to know how to use the drug but also have to know how much emotion to release and what to do when it is released. It seems to me that in the hands of other than skilled and experienced people this is a method which may prove quite harmful.

Now, if I may say a word about electric shock and other such treatment, I feel that electric shock is being used indiscriminately and promiscuously throughout the country. I think it is used that way both by psychiatrists and by general practitioners. It seems to me that electric shock and similarly drastic treatments should be administered by skilled people in specialized institutions that are able to take care of psychotic patients. At present electric shock is used indiscriminately in office practice and with a very wide variety of patients. It is true—I think almost everyone will agree with me—that electric shock does something for depressed patients; that is, it relieves them of some of their symptoms, and there is some kind of clinical improvement.

Why this occurs no one knows at the present time. So far as I know, there is no rational, physiologic explanation for any of these therapies. A number of hypotheses have been advanced. It is felt, if I remember correctly, that in schizophrenia particularly there is a type of vegetative imbalance with an exaggeration of parasympathetic or vagal factors, such as bradycardia, skin changes, pupillary abnormalities, and so on. It is believed that the common denominator of all these therapies is that they bring about an increase of sympathetic stimulation. It seems to me that the common denominator is that they bring about a considerable disturbance of cortical metabolism—one kind through a fit, another through depletion of the brain's fuel, carbohydrate, a third through actual penetration of brain structure with an instrument, the fourth through ten days' sleep. Psychologically, the common denominator may be a return to a very primitive, undifferentiated, archaic pattern of behavior, for one of the theories holds that the shock shatters false or erroneous patterns of behavior by bringing the patient back to a primitive level, after which you help him grow up again. Such was one of the conceptual ideas in respect to *Dauerschlaf*.

Interestingly enough, the only psychotic behavior which seems to be consistently helped with electric shock is the depression. It is extremely interesting from the psychological point of view that in the depression the most striking phenomenon is a very exaggerated degree of guilt, a very exaggerated need to punish oneself for this guilt. The question arises, therefore, whether or not the convulsion acts as a punishing medium and thus brings about some expiation of the guilt. Experimentally we have tried electric shock with two or three people who were not depressed but who had repetitive and chronic pains, had been operated on many times, and had a psychological structure essentially the same as a depressed person's; that is, they were unable to handle even normal aggressive feelings and had a tremendous accumulation of guilt concerning these feelings. Electric shock has relieved these people of pain for a period now, in one instance, of six to eight months. I offer that as an experimental contribution to the theory that the benefit of shock therapy in depression may be attributable not to any physiologic medium that we know of but rather to some psychological process.

DR. HASTINGS. There is one other interesting point that comes up with narcosis in relation to convulsive therapy. It has long been noted that if overwhelming doses of sodium amytal are given for fourteen days and then the treatment is abruptly stopped, it is not uncommon for the patient to have a *grand mal* convulsion within the next twenty-four to forty-eight hours. In our series of narcosis patients I don't think any were helped by this convulsion itself. In this connection there is another point to remember. If you are giving barbiturates on an outpatient basis (or any basis that lets that patient have reasonably heavy doses of barbiturates over a fairly long period of time), and if for one reason or another you stop treatment, don't regard the convulsion that the patient may have as necessarily meaning that he has epilepsy.

STUDENT. Can a patient remember what he has said under pentothal?

DR. HASTINGS. This is an interesting point because it is a very consistent one. Given a patient in whom this abreaction occurs and who ventilates material that you are learning for the first time, pentothal has the advantage that it is a fast-acting barbiturate and you can keep discussing the material with the patient right up to the time he becomes fully conscious. The result is that in twenty minutes, say, you have a wide-awake patient who is discussing material with you which at one stage was beyond his memory. Often when the patient finds himself talking about some event or incident or you remind him of it, he'll say, "Who told you that, doc?" He's surprised that he is now talking about something that lay pretty close to his heart. If you stop the discussion under pentothal and let the patient go to sleep, then when he wakes up he often has no memory of what he has told you. The disadvantage of sodium amytal is that it is long-acting, and so the patient almost always goes to sleep on your hands and has no memory of what he was talking about.

STUDENT. In your experience with pentothal in the Army, using that relatively small dose, did you run into any trouble? Complications? Respiratory difficulty?

DR. HASTINGS. There were slight respiratory difficulties at times, but if the drug was well given the patient never went down to an anesthetic level. I think we ran into a few cases of the tongue dropping back in the pharynx, producing obstruction.

DR. MURRAY. There is a tendency for edema of the glottis, but if one is careful not to proceed any time the patient starts to cough, that can be avoided. There should always be an airway around; it may be needed. There should be some metrazol around, too, because sometimes the patient really goes nuts and starts thrashing about.

STUDENT. Do you ever use pentothal in cases of amnesia—to bring back the memory?

DR. HASTINGS. The question is whether pentothal is useful in gaining insight as to what has taken place during a period for which the patient has amnesia. Yes, it can be extremely useful for that. After all, that is about what we were doing in cases such as that of the mess sergeant. A neurologist, Dr. Fabing, in Cincinnati has recently reported that in some cases the events which have followed organic lesions or head injury with structural trauma of the brain can be recovered with pentothal.

STUDENT. Dr. Murray mentioned that pentothal narcosynthesis is of value in a negative sense. I just wondered if material can be repressed so deeply in the unconscious that it can't be brought out under pentothal.

DR. MURRAY. Well, I don't know that we say it is repressed so deeply that it can't be brought out. I wouldn't say that, but I do believe that men can lie under pentothal, and I likewise know that men can hold material back under pentothal if they are not ready to let it come out. I have seen patients do that. If we have established a strong positive transference, if the patient is completely cooperating with us but has no volitional control over the memory of his trauma, by and large we can get out of him the important traumatic facts. Contrariwise, if for one reason or another this person is, let's say, of the psychopathic variety, and he has murders behind him that he doesn't want to bring out under pentothal, he can hold those back. In the average case, however, as Grinker points out in his book, you can tell by the quality of the spontaneity whether or not the patient is bringing out all that is there.

In many cases a negative result from the pentothal interview lets one know that it is best to continue with the routine vis-à-vis interview type of therapy. It indicates that this method will be more productive and that the material one gets there will be sufficient. In such cases, apparently, it is not deeply repressed material that is important. What is probably important is the relationship of the patient's life experience to what one already has at hand; the indication is to work that through and find out why the event was specifically traumatic to him. That's what I mean by the negative value of pentothal.

DR. HASTINGS. I think, too, we have all had the experience of giving pentothal to one of these combat casualties and finding out very little under it, but after you have gotten to know the patient better and vice versa, just as in across-the-table type of interviewing, events come out that are exceedingly traumatic to that individual.

DR. BOND. Dr. Hastings, I had a case in my own experience that illustrates a good many of the criticisms that have been pointed out by Dr. Romano and Dr. Murray. This was a young soldier who persistently kept crawling off his litter or bunk and falling on the floor, giving an excellent demonstration of a combat infantryman crawling without exposing himself. He would make a few whimpering cries and once in a while he would say something about his gun; that was about all the contact we could get with the man. The doctor who was demonstrating the use of pentothal for me got a splendid reaction from the soldier, who told dramatically of his battle experiences. He was a rather immature, emotional, inadequately trained lad. He had been in combat just a matter of minutes when a German bullet smashed his rifle out of his hand and he was so frightened by this that he had lost all contact with his friends. He got up and ran back toward his own line. Apparently somewhere in the course of that he developed an amnesia for the whole affair and probably had a terrific guilt reaction.

We concluded the interview and sent him back to his room. In the course of the next four or five days he seemed to improve—he was getting up, going about to his meals, had no recurrence of the falling on the floor, and so forth. It occurred to me I'd better check up and see whether this man knew what he had told us. I found that he had absolutely no recollection of it. When I told him what he had told us, he developed a terrific anxiety reaction. Apparently all his feelings of guilt recurred, and it took another two weeks for me to get him straightened out.

DR. MURRAY. That illustrates the importance of what we have been saying. Restoring the memory is really only the first step in the therapeutic result. You have to work this through so that the individual really accepts it; you have to work out all the significant emotional relationships to a deep personality structure. That is why Dr. Hastings says an experienced doctor is needed. Fundamentally, pentothal is no more in this treatment situation than ether is in a surgical operation; it prepares the state wherein a good operator can work.

STUDENT. Dr. Hastings, in connection with insulin or metrazol or electro-shock therapy, is it important to start your psychotherapy just as the patient is coming out of sleep, or can you wait a day or two?

DR. HASTINGS. With metrazol and electro-shock, the patient is inaccessible immediately after the treatment, even if he was accessible before. With insulin shock that depends on the severity of the illness. The patient may be immediately accessible to psychotherapy.

DR. ROMANO. We forget the tremendous significance of what has happened in many state hospitals with the introduction of insulin shock. Most state hospital patients are schizophrenics and seniles who have been on back wards for a great number of years. Take them off the back ward and put them on a hospital ward where an insulin unit is operating. There they will find much attention paid to them. Tremendous details are involved in the preparation and management of shock treatment. Nurses, attendants, orderlies, doctors hover over the patients, feed them by mouth and nasal tube, watch them closely, pat them, and are extremely solicitous. Then with recovery, they again get a tremendous amount of attention. It is awfully difficult to regard any of these methods solely on the basis of physiological or chemical factors.

STUDENT. I would like to ask what the brains of people who have been subject to electric shock look like?

DR. HASTINGS. There are a good many experimental reports on the pathology, but not a great many patients have died as a result of electro-shock or metrazol. The brains of patients who have died under convulsive therapy have usually shown a lot of a scattered petechial type of hemorrhage.

A BRIEF DISCUSSION OF DELIRIUM

DR. ROMANO. In my experience as a psychiatrist working in a general hospital for a number of years, I have found that it is important for house officers, interns, and general practitioners, and particularly for internists and surgeons to know something about the diagnosis and basic physiologic and psychologic characteristics of delirium and its management and prevention. The term *delirium* is used in a great number of ways. The French use the term *délire* as a synonym for delusion, but in this country the term is used to denote an acute psychotic episode which occurs in the course of a structural disease or as a result of a metabolic disturbance or intoxication. It is sometimes called symptomatic psychosis, i.e., symptomatic of some underlying chemical, metabolic, or infectious disorder. The term originally came from the Latin *de + lira*, to go off the track in plowing, and the term still has part of that meaning. The patient seems to go off his usual track; his behavior seems erratic and draws the attention of those about him.

Traditionally the delirious person is thought of as a rather excited person with increased motor activity, who is hallucinating or misinterpreting various stimuli, experiencing illusions, and possibly showing great fright. However, when one studies delirious patients in any general hospital, one sees a great number who have as their primary symptom a disturbance of consciousness, a disturbance of attention to the stimuli about them. This may vary from states of fatigue and sleepiness to coma. There may be periods of great motor excitement and thrashing about, dashing about halls of the hospital, jumping through windows, throwing things, and so on—the usual picture of any excited person.

The common denominator from a psychologic point of view seems to be a disturbance of consciousness or awareness. This may not be a constant disturbance; it may be only a fluctuation, very much greater than usual, in the level of awareness and consciousness. Normally, during the waking day, we all have considerable fluctuations in our level of awareness. The normal person's awakening may be very similar to the experiences of delirious patients. A person may awaken and be somewhat confused; the bell of his alarm clock may be involved, somehow or other, in his terminal dream; he may have illusions, may think his shirt, hanging on the bedpost, is a white-robed figure. A great number of such things may happen normally on awakening. Such experiences are very much exaggerated and caricatured in the delirious person. There are great fluctuations, great ebb and flow in his state of awareness; he may be able to be vigilant for a few seconds or longer, and then he will ebb back to a state of relative unawareness or even unconsciousness or stupor. So one sees as a primary disturbance in delirium this increased fluctuation in the level of awareness, with a tendency to be inattentive, unaware, and eventually comatose.

There are other symptoms, too, symptoms which relate to the emotional aspects of the patient. There may be a tremendous increase in anxiety, a tremendous concern that is due to an inability to perceive or apprehend or understand what is going on about one. There may be release of emotional tensions previously well controlled. Similarly, there may be lack of control of the normally well-modulated movements with respect, let's say, to handwriting. Handwriting is an excellent means of testing motor coordination and other things. In delirium it may become quite disrupted, with elisive words and gaps and tremors and off the line and so on. There may be tremulousness, there may be awkward dystonic movements, there may be a great number of other indications of lack of motor control. Then, too, in the intellectual sphere there may be some disturbances, not only in the perception of objects but in the ability to deal with a number of variables. The adult capacity to use abstractions is lost. These symptoms (namely, disturbance of consciousness, lack of control of emotional forces, lack of certain motor actions, and inability to abstract) suggest that delirium is some type of release mechanism. The higher control areas seem to have lost their control, and the behavior becomes less integrated, more archaic, more primitive.

Concerning the physiology of the brain, you know that its respiratory quotient is essentially unity, that the brain burns carbohydrate. One can experimentally produce delirium or disturbances of consciousness very readily by introducing a large dose of insulin parenterally and thus depleting the amount of sugar in the blood which is available for the brain to burn. With this running out of gasoline, so to speak, the brain cannot function adequately. One can make certain tests of basic physiologic factors in this situation. First, when the rate of flow of blood in insulin shock is examined, it is found that there is probably no essential change in the rate of flow. Second, when the amount of oxygen that goes to the brain and comes from the brain is measured by taking blood from the internal jugular vein as it leaves the skull and blood from an artery, one finds that there is a change in the uptake of oxygen, due to the fact that oxygen was not utilized to burn carbohydrate. Third, the electrical potentials which arise from the brain through the intact skull and scalp have been examined to learn what changes, if any, take place in them when certain agents such as insulin are used to alter the metabolism of the brain. Normally in a considerable percentage of adult men and women there is a "brain wave," called the alpha rhythm, which is essentially an 8 to 12 per second rhythm. One can alter this with a number of agents. When insulin is used in a dose large enough to produce a disturbance of consciousness there is a change in this frequency; it is slowed sometimes to 3 or 4 or 2 per second, and there is an increase in voltage and an increase in irregularity. These three methods can be utilized physiologically to indicate, then, that the changes in consciousness, with their coincident release of emotional and motor disturbances and the loss of the capacity to abstract, are correlated with changes in cerebral metabolism. Now so much for the background.

The signs and symptoms of delirium may vary tremendously, as I said; they may run the gamut from sleepiness to fatigue, through tremendous excitement and motor hyperactivity to coma. The neurologic signs may vary according to the primary disturbance, but in all instances there may be increased activity of the knee, ankle jerks, and tremulousness and, at times, reversal of the plantar signs. There are no specific neurologic signs which are correlated with delirium in the broad sense.

Now, in clinical practice what are found to be the most common causes of delirium? That depends on where you live and what type of medical service you have. In some of the larger municipal hospitals, for example, the most common causes of disturbances of consciousness are those of alcohol and trauma. Such is the case in Boston City Hospital. In other hospitals—for example, at the Peter Bent Brigham Hospital—the most common causes of delirium were diabetes, cardiorenal disease, cerebral hemorrhage, and drug intoxications of one kind or the other. In clinical practice it seems to me the most common causes are various infections, pneumonia, infections of other organs of the body; chronic infectious processes of long standing; certain drug intoxications, such as those related to sulfa drugs, bromides, and barbiturate drugs; certain metabolic disturbances, such as Addison's disease, with primary disturbance of carbohydrate metabolism; such cachectic diseases as carcinoma, heart failure, and uremia. These, together with trauma and so on, are the most common causes of disturbance of cerebral metabolism. These are causes which are not primary in the brain. They are causes in which there is either a disturbance of food substance going to the brain, not enough oxygen in the brain to burn the foodstuff, or changes or alterations of certain enzymes in the cells of the brain. There are many, many conditions whose causes are unknown at the present time, and there may be combinations of a number of these agents.

Now with respect to diagnosis—many times patients are called uncooperative or stupid because they don't seem to answer us correctly or quickly enough. We find this the experience of medical students, house officers, nurses, and doctors. Frequently the delirious person is unable to understand or has not heard or is unable to grasp what you are trying to say; much less is he able to execute what you ask him to do. To ask him to do something is equivalent to asking a legless person to walk. The delirious person is unable to understand what is said to him because of disturbance of consciousness and coincidental changes. So it is important to know how to diagnose a delirious person.

Essentially this is very simple. It consists in finding out whether the patient is able to attend to the task that you give him. Questions asked as to where he is, which day it is, the name of the hospital, and so forth test his capacity to orient himself to his environment as to time and place. Then some very simple tests may be used. For many years many clinics used the very simple expedient of giving a person a task such as the serial subtraction of 7 or 3 from 100. This task is a test of vigilance and persistence—one which may show very quickly the person's ability to attend. One isn't interested so much in arithmetical errors as in the way in which the patient errs; namely, whether he has difficulty in bridging the changes at the ten mark, whether his computation is labored, whether he has to repeat, whether he uses his fingers, and makes the situation concrete, so to speak, or whether he insists on doing it with pencil and paper. All these deviations, up to complete inability to do the task, may give you an inkling as to the patient's level of awareness; essentially he is unable to keep to the task, to attend to it correctly, and to follow it through.

Now as to treatment—the treatment of a delirious patient is essentially the treatment of the underlying cause. Whether it be cardiac decompensation, drug intoxication, uremia, trauma, or something else, the primary factor in treatment is the treatment of the underlying disorder. But there are also other aspects of the treatment to be considered. First, one must be careful not to provoke or superimpose on a person already delirious a factor which may increase the delirium; that is, we should use chemical sedation very carefully. A person who is delirious and who for physiologic reasons has some difficulty in excreting certain substances, and whose whole regulatory apparatus is disturbed, tends to become more intoxicated with a drug than another person. Special care should be taken not to use long-acting, cumulative drugs such as phenobarbital. If chemical sedation is to be used, paraldehyde is by far the drug of choice. As you know, it is a polymer of acetaldehyde, has an awful taste, an awful odor, can be disguised only partly in iced grape juice or iced lemon juice, and can be given, as you also know, parenterally, in the muscle and in very small amounts in the vein. It is a drug which has few side effects and when used without other drugs is very safe, has no cumulative action, and is excreted rapidly. It is very valuable in the treatment of the aged and of delirious patients. The ideal quieting agent could be hydrotherapy, the use of the continuous tub. I think the general hospitals of the future will have one or more such tubs adjacent or contiguous to a medical service. Then a delirious patient, whether he be suffering from cardiac failure or intoxicated with a drug, can be put in a neutral tub—called neutral because the temperature is held between 95° F. and 97° F.—and kept there, sometimes, for many hours. However, most hospitals do not have such tubs, and so one has to use chemical sedation. In instances of doubt and when it is necessary to use a drug, paraldehyde is the drug of choice.

The next thing to be remembered is the need to avoid shadows and misinterpretations and extraneous noises. Many times a bedside lamp on the table is much more injurious than allowing the light to remain on in the room all night, for this prevents shadows and misinterpretations.

Third, patient and tactful attendants at the bedside are needed. Many times a relative can be of much more benefit to a delirious patient than a trained person. The sight of a familiar face may be very comforting to a person who is dipping in and out of consciousness and is frightened with each reawakening.

The next principle in the treatment of delirious patients is to avoid any measure which may frighten them. When you are about to do something, explain it simply and repetitively in words of one syllable to the patient. The hypo which is given without any explanation or the oxygen tent in which the patient may awaken in a delirious episode may provoke behavior reminiscent of panic. So explanation, simple reassurance, tactful attendants, avoidance of argument about the validity of the person's sense perceptions (one shouldn't argue whether the person is hallucinating little red men or mice or this, that, or the other)— these are important measures. To reassure the patient you may tell him that he will be all right, that he will go to sleep. In many instances sleep, good sleep, is a tremendous aid in helping the patient to recover.

Now as to special treatment of delirium tremens. Delirium tremens, in a person in a relatively good nutritive state, without the complications of old age or pneumonia or head injury or other factors, can be handled effectively in a period of two or three days with the use of paraldehyde, tactful attendants, and adequate food and fluid. In the past a great deal of attention was paid to dehydrating the brain by spinal drainage or by the use of magnesium sulphate or glucose and sucrose, the theory being that alcoholism was sometimes associated with what was called "wet brain." What "wet brain" is I don't know. If the lumbar puncture is an index at times of a certain type of fluid balance in the subarachnoid space, the incidence of elevated spinal fluid pressures in patients with delirium tremens is very low. However, there may be certain other types of intracellular edema which are not reflected. The special point is that, for the most part, patients with delirium tremens do much better when they are given adequate amounts of fluid and food and adequate sleep is induced.

Finally, in prevention, who are the patients most apt to become delirious? The anxious patient, the person with limited intellectual endowment, the aged, patients who have been receiving drugs for a long period of time, patients in poor nutritive state, patients with inadequate food and fluid intake, and patients who have experienced intractable pain over a long time.

DR. BROSIN. Will you add a word about psychogenic delirium? I have only seen a few such cases and feel uncertain about it.

DR. ROMANO. No more uncertain than I am, probably. I have seen a few instances of psychogenic delirium which resembled panic. I have two patients in mind, two Negro boys, who experienced this panic with many delirious manifestations after a homosexual attack. They were boys in a county jail who actually were subjected—it was confirmed later—to homosexual advances by some older men. Whether one calls a homosexual panic a psychogenic delirium, I don't know.

Another point I didn't mention is that there are some drugs, perhaps mescaline and probably one of the antimalarials, in which the delirium does not consist of this primary disturbance of consciousness but rather of a hypervigilance, a hyperalertness, with a tremendous amount of anxiety.

I also didn't mention that the actual content of the delirium is dependent not on the noxious stimulus but on the previous personality experiences of the patient. There are many, many interesting questions there, the details of which we hope will be worked out in the next few years. In many instances patients have an organic or structural disturbance of a certain part of the brain. For example, a few years ago we saw a little Irish spinster seamstress, aged seventy, who had had both breasts removed because of carcinoma. She came into the hospital very sick and about to die, possibly with some metastatic lesions in the brain. She was experiencing certain scotomata. In these she had figures which went from right to left, at first geometric figures in a sort of buff color against a background; they looked like triangles and circles. Then suddenly she began to see the Knights of the Round Table. She saw them coming from right to left. There were Sir Gawain, Sir Modred, and Sir Lancelot, and the fair Elaine sitting side saddle on a shaggy horse; there were draperies on the horses; and page boys with page-boy bobs were leading the horses, and so on. As she was telling us about these, we tried experimentally to change their size and configuration and color by the use of amyl nitrite in dilating the vessels, by carbon dioxide, and by changing her posture, but we were unable to do it. On learning her story, we found that this little spinster seamstress had lived her life in a very narrow fashion between the church and her sister, that she had read Tennyson and all the variations of the stories of the Round Table and had a very rich fantasy life about them, which was expressed in these scotomata.

After the last war Goldstein in Germany showed that many times in stimulating certain areas of the brain visual experiences were obtained and that these visual experiences were those that the soldiers had had in critical combat situations. So there are many reasons why a patient sees and hears what he does. In one of our morning sections last week I told about a delirious man who at the height of his delirium had described his mother, and it was later confirmed by his sisters and others and by pictures that the person he had described in detail closely resembled his mother when he was an infant. So there are many facts concerning the repositories of memories and reproduction in hallucination and other sense perceptions which are not completely understood. I think we are going to find that they are related to the earlier experiences of the patient, stored somehow or other, and evoked somehow or other by irritants or releasing mechanisms.

DR. WOLFF. I want to make one additional point to demonstrate that there is no specificity about the delirium in relation to a given agent. For example, it is possible to have a patient who has had three or four different delirium episodes, precipitated by entirely different agents, and yet the content and form of the deliria will be so similar that you couldn't tell one from the other. Dr. Romano, in his review of this important psychosis (which, after all, is the most important psychosis the medical man has to deal with), has mentioned four cardinal features: disturbed consciousness; extreme restlessness and tremulousness; emotional disturbances, notably fear; and sensory disturbances, which are chiefly visual. Now it is a grave sign when a person in delirium has auditory hallucinations. Visual hallucinations are common enough and benign enough, but when a patient has auditory hallucinations which are true hallucinations, it is a serious sign. It is, however, often hard to be sure that a person is having auditory hallucinations, for a delirious patient is so easily disturbed that the sound of voices from an adjacent room, sounds in the hall, or sounds of the clock may be misinterpreted. Finally, variability is an outstanding feature of a delirium; the patient is affected by the time of day—notably worse in the evening when shadows are getting longer, and somewhat better after he has had a rest.

STUDENT. Can we go on from here into the subject of dreams?

DR. MURRAY. To discuss dreams is a dangerous sort of thing. When you come to interpret the symbolic meaning of what is going on in a dream, particularly in the analytic situation, you need a lot of background facts and long association with the patient; for you regard the dream as something that is going on in the foreground, against the background of knowledge you have about the patient. When you have that background knowledge the dream begins to make sense; you begin to relate it to a totality. If, instead, you pick a dream out here and there and begin to tell somebody what it means, it may sound a bit bizarre. It seems as if you are spreading it too thin. That is one of the reasons why we are a little bit loath to run a chance of confusing you by discussing dreams. Interesting as they are, important as they are, and although we would like to tell you about this part of psychiatry, we haven't done so because we doubt very much that what we could give you here would be very helpful to you in your daily practice.

STUDENT. When a patient tells you that he has been having dreams that disturb him a great deal, what are you going to tell him?

DR. MURRAY. Well, now what would you say one should tell him?

STUDENT. Well, I'd just try to assure him that it was only a dream.

DR. MURRAY. That's exactly what I'd do. When I am in short psychotherapy with a patient and he asks me about a dream, however good a guess I can make without knowing his background, I devise a euphemistic answer and give it to him. I don't go underneath the surface, I don't do what we call uncovering, because that isn't what I want to accomplish with this particular patient. So I look for some rather obvious meaning for the dream and say, "Well, it looks as though it might be that."

You know, you can't really pull a dream out of the hat and interpret it. Sometimes a dream is very helpful to me in a diagnostic way, but it is very seldom that I use dreams in any short psychotherapy. I think of other things to which I can relate this person's emotional experiences, for it is a pretty obscure thing to do, to pick out the meaning of a dream and throw that at your patient.

DR. ROMANO. What we have told our medical students is that they can use the fact that a patient is having disturbing dreams as an indication that he may have some emotional troubles. I would stop there and then. Usually when a patient has recurrent, disturbing dreams you have other data to corroborate the suspicion of emotional difficulties. I concur completely in Dr. Murray's tenet; namely, that you cannot practice medicine successfully by taking one datum, such as the EKG or the dream, and decide the destiny of a man's life. You would have to have many other data. The manifest content of the dream, that which the patient remembers, may have many meanings, determinable only against the detailed background of the patient's life. The capacity to put a dream in its proper setting is, so far as I know, a special skill.

Common Psychopathology

HENRY W. BROSIN, M.D.

IT is my important obligation this afternoon to discuss in leisurely detail the subject about which you heard this morning. Dr. Romano's extremely neat definitions really get to the heart of psychopathology, and a good many hours should be spent both in formal exposition of those concepts and in demonstration by cases. I'm going to start on conversion hysteria, talk a little about anxiety hysteria or phobic states, then discuss briefly the obsessional states and the depressions. I hope time will then be left for a brief description of the paranoid states. At the end of that time you will be free to ask the faculty questions to clear up difficulties.

To begin with a recapitulation of what you have heard—psychiatrists believe that there is causality in mental disease and emotional disorder. Its symptoms and signs serve a purpose, and it is our job as physicians to discover that purpose. As we grow more expert we recognize characteristic patterns, which are summarized in the formal diagnoses. A footnote should be made here—psychiatric diagnosis is not like physical diagnosis, since it doesn't usually subserve a limited entity but is rather a shorthand notation as to the kind of person you are dealing with. Obviously, diagnoses do injustice to the wealth of possibilities of personalities and situations which you meet; any shorthand notation that this man is a hysteric or phobic or obsessional or paranoic doesn't give the entire picture. Possibly the best total summary one can make, as Dr. Adolf Meyer said, is in the form of the man's name: John Jones —his psychosis. Then would follow a huge biography, which will be in your minds if not on the charts, as to how the man managed to achieve his present state of equilibrium. Whenever you are in doubt—as all of us sometimes are—about what's wrong with a patient, go back to the basic data of the life history. That's where you will find your ultimate security—not by dashing to a book to see if you can find some syndrome which corresponds to the man's complaint, but by sitting down quietly and thinking, "What is the man gaining, what has he done all his life?" Most of the neuroses that you'll meet will have a long, chronic background with only a relatively few acute episodes, perhaps only one. It is the long history, the moving picture, the living biography of activity which will give you a clue to the solution that the patient is trying to arrive at in the present situation. You can find your own place in this picture. If you see how you can manipulate the one, two, three crucial points with which he is most troubled, you will find your job as an intelligent therapist made much easier.

Psychiatrists are also committed to the belief in the economic principle that if a great deal of emotion is being mobilized in relation to guilt, fear, anger, it has to go some place. If you know that a man hates you or his boss or his competitors, and he still acts like the perfect gentleman, then you might well ask yourself, "Where does this hate go?" Which of the behavior forms that Dr. Romano analyzed does the man utilize to get rid of his hate? When he faces frustrations does he kick the door as he enters and leaves the office; does he take it out on his children; does he take it out on his wife; does he, as many physicians including myself are willing to admit, restrain his aggressions as much as he can during the daylight hours and seek the tennis court or the handball court where he may become freely aggressive later? There are hundreds of ways of letting off steam. Most of you in Minnesota hunt and fish; you may well examine those procedures as safety valves, as outlets, not to mention the Saturday night party and the convention. All these are legitimate objects for examination as to how we manage to retain our equilibrium. Mind you, I've said nothing now about maturity, immaturity, normality, abnormality; most of these mechanisms are constantly used by mature individuals in order to maintain equilibrium. There are no moral values attached to any of these descriptions. I hope as I go along and describe some of the perhaps socially less desirable outlets for emotion you won't feel that I am making any esthetic or moral evaluations.

The operation of the economic principle must be sought not only in the field of the psychological activities of thinking or mood but also in the somatic sphere, which you as physicians have primary obligations toward, and in the social sphere. To paraphrase Dr. George Henry, it isn't always clear to the layman whether certain problems should go to the judge or the lawyer because they are social, or to the doctor because they are somatic, or to the priest or his equivalent because they involve a man's behavior. We feel, of course, as physicians that we have a function in all three fields, but it remains to be seen whether we'll retain those functions for the rest of the century.

With that general summary I'll remind you of Dr. Romano's case of the girl with quadriplegia who was sensitized by her ambivalent wishes toward her brother-in-law but on opening the door found only the cat. I'll tell you a similar story. On a Sunday afternoon in the dead of winter, with the temperature about five degrees below zero, a youngster of about nineteen was picked up by the side of the road, far away from the army camp in which he belonged. He said he had fallen down the gully and couldn't move his legs. Careful examination, including x-ray, showed no organic disease, and so after some debate he was sent over to the psycho ward for an examination. There the following story was elicited.

This boy, this nineteen-year-old (I shouldn't call him a child although he looked and acted like one), had a brother about three years older than himself. Both of them had been reared principally in orphanages. The older brother was aggressive, fairly independent, beginning to be alcoholic, and had had much the best of the deal; he had tended to infantilize the patient. The most recent of his demands was that the younger brother play nursemaid to the older's little baby. Now during the period of courtship, the patient and his future sister-in-law had known each other slightly; they had been good friends but there was no great attachment. However, immediately after the marriage, during her pregnancy and the first year of the baby's life, he had come to know his sister-in-law very well and had become erotically attached to her. This was forbidden, of course, and he had quite a time of it, but he repressed his desires fairly well. Then, after the two brothers went into the Army, the older brother had to move on but his wife lived near the patient's camp and continued to use him to help her with the housework and the care of the baby. In effect, then, the patient was supplanting his older brother as husband. The situation was getting very dangerous indeed.

On this particular Sunday afternoon the patient knew that his sister-in-law would be alone, for his older brother was in Florida. Their friendliness was reaching a degree that threatened his sense of right and wrong, and he found it most convenient not to go to see her at all. But how was he to justify this? There wasn't any reason he could give why he shouldn't continue the relation. He was too guilty, too afraid to face the reality of supplanting his brother, and so he used what we call a relatively simple solution—he converted the conflict into somatic disability, paralysis of the legs. With that done (as in the case this morning, and as in most such cases) he was quite cheerful and bland, had a smiling, happy exterior, no troubles, nothing to bother him—everything was just fine. And he *was* pleased, of course, that he no longer had to face the possibility of accepting responsibility for the sister and the baby, that the threat of wrongdoing was no longer active.

I'd like to point out that *conversion hysteria* differs from the obsessional—which I shall talk about in a moment—in having the conflict externalized. The ego submits to a certain rupture; it gives up a certain part of its function. In this case I think the process is clear; the principal difficulty was the sexual threat. The patient knew he shouldn't try to kiss his sister-in-law; he had to repress that evil thought. But repression wasn't strong enough; his ego defenses weren't good enough to tolerate it. He couldn't sublimate; he couldn't do anything that was socially acceptable. This ego-alien, hateful, painful threat was getting the better of him. This caused anxiety. Anxiety escaped the repression, and there appeared what is known as the return of the repressed. He achieved a solution which was acceptable to his conscience and to society at large. He incurred our pity and helpfulness rather than our punishment.

*

We may now consider the *phobic* or *anxiety hysteria*. Dr. Romano gave us the case of a young lady who couldn't walk on the street without protection, a classic example. He stressed the instinctual needs that were threatening this girl and causing anxiety. Unless she invented some way of protecting herself, she was unhappy. Protection depended upon the mechanism of isolation. She could narrow down her general nonspecific fears to the street, symbolizing the street as the outer world.

Strangers are perhaps hostile, strangers are also sometimes seductive, so she needed the protection of some socially acceptable figure. There was also some condensation in this substitution mechanism. If you want to ask more about the phobic type we'll take it up later, as there are some special technical problems in treatment, particularly those which prevent the patient's dependence from becoming fixed.

*

A great group, perhaps the most important group, of neuroses in the more educated portion of our population is the *obsessional* or the *obsessive-compulsive*, what the Meyerians call the "obsessive-compulsive-ruminative states." It used to be said (I don't know if it is still true) that by and large one found frank conversion hysterias only in the more primitive parts of the population. I mention this because of the suggestion that the form of neurosis may be closely allied to the culture in which we live. In most private hospitals we see few conversion hysterias of the "Charcot type"; I saw more conversion hysterias among uneducated men in the Army in one month than I see in one year in my own hospital. Most of our private practice is in the field of the obsessional neuroses. Now you may well ask why should this be true. The suspicion is that the repressing forces and the social demands are more stringent to begin with, are more subtle and are more all-pervasive because educated parents demand a great deal more of their children early in life. Then, too, the defenses of educated people are more highly developed in accordance with their greater abilities.

In the obsessional neurosis the ego is usually intact and there is a great deal of regulated interplay between the instinctual forces and the anti-instinctual forces. That's what makes them a fascinating group to study. In an example or two I'll try to describe some of the characteristics you ordinarily find in obsessional people.

The classic type is the hand-washing phobia. The person with such a phobia was perhaps trained too early or too severely to regard dirt as reprehensible, trained at a time when playing with dirt and feces and interest in body functions was especially enjoyable, and so he had to defend himself through the use of this mechanism. (To reiterate what we said earlier this morning—mechanisms as they are defined singly are artificial creations for ease of thinking; actually most of them occur in combination, and it is in obsessional people that the combination becomes most involved.) Now in this hand-washing phobia the failure of the repression of prohibited instinctual forces causes again a return of the repressed. Characteristically, two ends are served by it: first, gratification to the person; and, second, punishment, which is also a kind of gratification to the conscience. The next item to be noted is that hand-washing is a denial that there is interest in the instinctually pleasurable activity.

Another example, cited by Dr. O. Fenichel, will show the hostility which is characteristic of obsessionals, though it may not be easy to see clinically at first. This patient was a young man who was engaged to a lovely young woman who used to ride each morning in Central Park. Whenever he went out to meet her, he'd have an overwhelming need to place a little pebble in her path as she came down the road. Shortly before she came up, he'd have to take the pebble out of the road. The explanation uncovered in interviews with the patient was that placing the stone there represented a wish that his fiancée would fall and break her neck; taking the stone back was a retraction—a denial, a reversal—of this desire, to salve his conscience.

One of the things about obsessionals that makes them pass, by and large, for very healthy people is that their affect is blocked. It is not easy to detect the turmoil behind the firm façade (which doesn't vary a great deal with the passing current), and therefore it is hard to realize that the person actually is suffering a good deal. Many of them look healthier, more staid, better adjusted than truly well-adjusted people, who have the freedom to be dependent, independent, to love and to hate. Obsessional people often make a fetish of this implacable stability because of their own insecurity.

A prominent character trait is their orderliness, which can be traced back to their need for obedience. As children they grew up in a rather strict environment, and there was great need to be obedient in order to maintain the love which they feared they might lose. To go back to what was told you earlier, the big needs of childhood are love and the avoidance of punishment. In the obsessional you see this in clear-cut fashion. To be orderly not only subserves the purpose of obedience—

the avoidance of punishment by a strict father or mother or both—but is also a great protection against the "dangerous" temptation, the pleasure that is found in dealing with body function. As an extension of this orderliness we find meticulousness, which can be called a displacement on to small detail. If you work as hard as can be at some little piddling things around the office or around your house, you can avoid doing the big things that you really ought to do. I think that is a fairly common experience for most of us. Orderliness as expressed in a fixed routine is also a good defense, not only for ordinary, healthy people but for those with organic cerebral injury. As I said yesterday, it sometimes is an absolute necessity, in order to avoid overpowering fear reactions and also as a protection against the dreaded instincts of hostility and sexuality.

One of the best examples of the value of a rigid work routine (although this gets me into the controversial sphere) is the so-called Sunday neurosis. There are a good number of people who have no symptoms at all on six days of the week but find Sunday a most trying day. Restlessness, tension, headache, ennui—not in a passive sense but in an active sense—what to do, and so on. Now, the first item of the differential diagnosis in such a case is, of course, what the person did on Saturday night! If this is not the explanation of the person's unrest, then there is the fact that the work pattern of the week suddenly suffers rupture, the equilibrium of the individual—not only his social patterns but his physiologic pattern—actually suffers change over the week-end. Dr. Ferenczi, one of the most brilliant of Dr. Freud's pupils, postulated that this phenomenon is widespread over Europe. It is a function, Ferenczi felt, of the strictness of the society. The greater the repressing forces are, the less people are able to handle a free period when it is given. His feeling was that it is principally the threat of the instinctual forces during the free period, when the person is not reinforced by his routine, that enables the anxiety to arise.*

Another characteristic of typical obsessional neurotics is a great pre-

* At the end of the session Dr. Wolff, at Dr. Brosin's invitation, described the "Sunday neurosis" more fully as follows:

People with compulsive features—that is, tense, driving, meticulous, perfectionistic, inelastic persons—are apt to have trouble with week-ends, Sundays, holi-

occupation with time. They have a magical interest in time. They want to know what time it is, must account for all the minutes of the day, must know what they are doing at all periods of the day. If you ask an obsessional where he was at seven-thirty on the nineteenth of January, he can almost always give you some kind of answer. Many of us, of course, need to know where we are in time and space, to have purpose, goal, and direction. If we are thrown off that track, we may become somewhat unhappy; but the obsessional has this trait to a marked degree.

Another aspect of the obsessional is just the opposite of obedience and orderliness; the sado-masochistic patterns make this more interesting. The little child who wants the love of his parents and does everything in the world to avoid punishment occasionally fails—he is punished, he loses love. Then he finds to his surprise that perhaps he doesn't mind the punishment as much as the involvements of the childhood situation, that he actually enjoys it. He then develops a mirror image of all the traits I have been talking about and finds that there

days, birthdays, and vacations. I have given the slang name of "stress addiction" to this illness because in many ways it resembles the withdrawal phenomenon experienced by a person who has been taking a sedative. It seems to be the outgrowth of need to have the work life full of things to do. The stress seems to be necessary for the individual's comfort. Given a Sunday, which he has learned from others and perhaps from his own experience is a good day to relax, this individual becomes sick in a number of ways but certain features are outstanding.

Striking is the change that occurs on Saturday night. At that time the individual may feel unusually hungry, and this isn't necessarily associated with drinking. He may eat an unusual amount of salted peanuts; and indeed such people often enough eat chocolate, and then you get the story of the chocolate allergy that shows itself on Sunday. He sleeps badly Saturday night, and then perhaps at six or even earlier, perhaps a little before the usual waking time, has a heady sensation or actual headache—and I'll discuss that further in a minute—associated with distention, flatulence, anorexia, and constipation (Sunday constipation is extremely common). The headache (the heady sensation often enough turns into a headache in the middle of the morning) persists usually until the setting of the sun or toward the end of the day. Sunday night is usually a good one from the point of view of sleep, and on Monday morning the illness is over.

Sunday is a common time for patients with migraine headaches to have migraine. Probably more migraine attacks occur then than on any other day of the week. Akin

is fun in rebellion. He may become obstinate and aggressive. The very persons who are passive and submissive in many aspects of life may at times act very differently indeed—may be sadistic, punishing, cruel, hardheaded as can be. If you think over your own experience, you can probably dig up a few people like that.

Because of this love for security, orderliness, submission, and so on, many obsessionals attach themselves to institutions, and may themselves determine the climate of the institution. Many people in the government services and in the Army and Navy are of this kind. They find the comfort which they want there; they get enjoyment out of submission to superiors, which satisfies one half of their mirror image, and they get enjoyment out of being mean to those below them. Consequently, for a reasonably well-adjusted obsessional, there is a very real economy in the institutional hierarchy. Their orderliness, of course, their routine, time sense, meticulousness, their bland affect—all these traits are socially valuable in the institutional field, have high market value. That they lose initiative, imagination, creativity is their great

to this is the situation that occurs on the planned-party occasion. Someone is going to have a party. The first characteristic is for the person with migraine to get his headache on that occasion.

Let's say the first days of a holiday are very hard to manage. After three or four days or a week the situation may be better. My notion about it—and after all it is only a notion—is that the individual is called upon to make a vigorous biological adjustment at a time when he is least able to do it. That is, given a week of energy-consuming activity, a good deal of stress and tension, on Sunday he is called upon to fill the role of a father, parent, husband, the innumerable adjustments of being in a home with a child or children with whom he would like to be in contact, with a wife with whom he would like to have good relations, perhaps in a community that demands from him certain calls or visits, a family luncheon or dinner at which various personality problems are brought together—an entirely different day from the relatively predictable day of a man's work life in which he can pretty much outline what is going to happen to him and what he can avoid. He is better at handling situations during the week than he is on Sunday. Now, at a biological disadvantage and with relatively little energy, he tries to face them and I believe does it at a high cost to himself.

My suggestion from a therapeutic point of view is that such individuals should slow down toward the end of the week so that the adjustment isn't quite such a tough one—that slowing down means all sorts of biological rearrangements as well as psychological rearrangements and the transition isn't so great.

loss. Psychiatrists could write a chapter in the development of institutions because of the influence of the obsessional character.

The obsessional person has characteristics which are the results of the mechanisms that you heard about this morning. Because he finds release through intellectualization, he places a high value on thinking in general. This thinking is not necessarily the logical, orderly, Euclidean type we admire in textbooks. It begins with magical thinking and the superior values assigned to it. Most people, you'll find, have at some time in their lives had the habit of touching. It is generally agreed that this touching, or stepping on cracks, or similar behavior, is like the child's game of "I've killed my grandmother, I haven't killed my grandmother," depending on whether you touch the post or not. I recall to you Samuel Johnson's biography. In Boswell's book you will find one of the richest descriptions of truly magnificent obsessions. The value of such behavior to the individual is that he gets rid of his anxiety (he'd like to kill grandma but he can't) symbolically by touching; that is, by behavior that he can undo and therefore say, "Well, it isn't so after all. I didn't really kill her, so I don't have to suffer."

Another characteristic of obsessionals, especially as they become of clinical grade, is the practice of rituals. I'll give you an example. A boy, twenty years old, in his second year in college, became severely incapacitated with an obsessional idea. He had a brother two years older, a mother who died early, and a father who had been going to a doctor for many years. I'd like to point out that there was no demonstrable genetic relation between the patient's symptoms and his father's symptoms, although as you go over his psychopathology you may see a real or fancied resemblance. The father was clearly an obsessional. His means of protecting himself throughout life was to go about once a month, sometimes once in two months, to a proctologist, who did a massage and a colonic irrigation. The youngster's troubles were in the field of bedroom and bathroom ritual. (If you see severe obsessionals with these symptoms, you will recognize their picturesque quality. They may comb their hair by counting as many as five hundred, eight hundred, nine hundred times. They may sit for hours at hand-washing. They may sit on the stool for hours, meanwhile having "magical" thoughts.) The boy's bedroom ritual was something like this. He would open the windows by the bed, then take four steps at a right angle and fix the rug at the end of the bed. Then he would take four more steps and arrange the pillows exactly in position; then four steps back (his brother slept on this side) and he would get into bed. Analysis showed that his hostilities toward his brother probably caused a great deal of this; he had to protect himself against the idea that he wanted to kill his brother.

*

Earlier I mentioned magical thinking. At its best the thinking and over-intellectualization of the obsessional result in great interest in abstractions and generalizations. There is economic value to this interest. Thinking is often, not always, preparation for action. Many obsessionals behave as if they want to anticipate everything; they are afraid to face the events of life without much preparation. They'll spend a good deal of time and effort, perhaps make a whole life career of preparing for something; it becomes a question whether they ever do what they prepare for. There are people with the most magnificent intellectual endowment who spend a whole half century preparing for something that they'll probably never be able to do. Characteristically these people are attracted by things like symbolic logic, semantics, theology, psychology, philosophy, tests like the Rorschach, etc.; they have a tremendous libidinal investment in abstract thinking and the whole field of generalization. This behavior serves a further economic purpose: the substance of life is removed into the field of ideas; the less one has to do with people, the more one is protected from their onslaught.

An interesting characteristic of obsessionals is their social rituals. I won't mention many of these; enough to say that if a person is very insecure, because his own fears and hostilities are great, he walks into every situation with people with the feeling that he is very likely to be angry at them. However, if he isn't angry to start with, he can avoid difficulties by maintaining formal patterns of behavior. His dependence upon others for prestige and self-esteem is very great indeed, and he has to take great pains to maintain that. Characteristically, also, the meticulosity which I have mentioned carries over into dress; in attention to details, orderliness, these people are very often caricatures of the well dressed. From the top of the patent-leather "hair comb," every hair minutely in place, sometimes fixed there by special devices, the elegant shave, the absolutely correct linen, the matched necktie, the impeccable pressing, down to the marvelously clean and polished shoes, he presents a model appearance. Now in the sick (not in the well-adjusted) obsessional ambivalence characteristically shows up in dress; for while the patient's external clothes may be the last word in style and correctness, his underwear may be very dirty.

I have mentioned the sleeping ceremonials of one youngster, and incidentally mentioned his father's colonic irrigations, to show you that psychotherapy is done at many levels. While on this topic, I might add a footnote on the chance that it will be of interest. A very real fear of falling asleep may be a part of this ritualistic behavior. Now if a patient comes to you complaining of insomnia, it may be many a long hour before your questions come down to the bedroom rituals and ceremonials which prevent him from sleeping. I am throwing this in gratuitously to show you how very difficult it sometimes is to arrive at a good psychiatric judgment. Only by recognizing the character pattern (the stubbornness, the penury, the extreme orderliness, and the sado-masochism) can you quickly make the inference that this fellow's insomnia isn't due to hay fever or indigestion and you may have to think about emotional factors. This is true of other situations as well. I have mentioned various pathological aspects of extreme adherence to work or devotion to duty or great interest in reading and so on, all of which may have clinical significance in the proper setting. I have also mentioned perversity. Impotence is common in this group. Dr. Romano has said that some people cannot equate in one life, at one time, the tender, giving emotions with frank sexuality toward one woman. That's also a characteristic trait of obsessionals. Many of them are patrons of houses of prostitution, which, in Berlin, London, Paris, furnish means whereby perverse infantile needs can be gratified for money.

*

So much for the obsessional. The next group of neuroses I want to discuss is the *depressions*. Depressions come in many types; they are not all equivalent. Just like reality anxieties, there are reality depressions. Depressions may be caused by loss of something in which one is deeply interested—a friend, a job, prestige, intimates—and we don't consider these of clinical importance. Where the loss of a person has tremendous emotional significance (a mother, a father, a loved one), we have the period of mourning when what is called "grief work" must be done. The attachments built up intensively through the years are not easily cast aside, but must be slowly worked out during this period. That involves, among other things, getting rid of the hidden hostilities toward the person for whom there had been so much affection.

Dr. Bond will talk, I trust, about the three main types of non-neurotic depression: mourning proper, the acute reactive depressions, and the manic-depressives; so I won't cover them. Depression is the concomitant of the great bulk of all the clinical entities we see. You really ought to look for it in every individual and then rule it out rather than rule it in, so to speak. The key mechanism of depression is usually described as the introjection of the object toward which we have great hostility. (Introjection is one of the few mechanisms that weren't mentioned in the morning's lecture.) If we have a great deal of hatred as well as affection toward papa, if we can't beat him in some other way, one solution is to incorporate him symbolically into our own system and punish ourselves—that is, punish him through his image. This hostility does not fit into our common conception of a depressed person. Most of the time the depressive gives the impression of a poor, meek soul, like the woman we saw yesterday who is fifty-six, her husband past seventy and rapidly losing his memory; he has always been a punitive alcoholic, now he is becoming more cranky and more punitive and is on his way to what she recognizes as senile psychosis, like his older brother. She's willing to get a divorce, sees no future ahead. It's hard to tell her (and I wouldn't) that a good deal of her present depression is due to her hostility toward her husband. One can only manipulate the situation to help her avoid as much of that feeling as possible. When you study depressions, actually spend day in and day out with depressed persons, you will learn to see the hostility that is there.

*

The last of the groups that I am going to speak about is the paranoid state, the *paranoid character*. I won't speak of all the clinical concomitants; I take for granted you know those—loss of weight, lack of eating, sleeplessness, difficulty with the bowels and various organ systems, and sense organ disturbance. I am talking just about dynamics. These groups are characterized principally by the mechanism of projection. Dr. Romano defined it this morning. We all use it; we all project. Many rationalizations involve projection. The story of the King of Denmark is an excellent example in reverse of projection, the projection in that case having to do with unacceptable impulses toward the father.

In everyday life you meet the attenuations of the paranoid psychosis. People of this sort are characteristically and chronically suspicious; we all know them. No matter what goes on around them they wonder why should this be, who is doing this, who is doing that, why should he be doing it. They interpret. I think that is the other primary characteristic. Everything has meaning; even the leaves which fall from the tree must be given a meaning. They are uncomfortable unless they can find some way to explain everything that happens. They are ideal participants in rumor-mongering and intrigues. And I might add that one of the big areas of difficulty in psychiatric diagnosis is that between paranoid characters and severe obsessionals who take on paranoid coloring. As you can see, the magical thinking of the paranoid and the obsessional may have great similarity.

Now it is getting late; so feel free to ask any questions, and the faculty will try to answer them.

DISCUSSION

STUDENT. A good many patients express the fear that they may do something in the way of acting out their hostilities. Is it possible to reassure them? Are they likely to act on their hostilities?

DR. BOND. Well, people apparently do kill other people. Very frequently, if you know anything about a murderer, you can see where the impulse came from. It doesn't come out of the blue as much as you might suppose. Generally speaking, I think, an obsessional person is too involved in his obsessions to accomplish his act; that is a general rule. But an obsessional can break loose and does so occasionally. Certainly a schizophrenic person can commit murder.

Generally speaking, I think, murderers who are psychotic are schizophrenics of a certain type. Very frequently there are other forms of murderers as well: people who have involutional depressions, people with tremendous feelings of guilt, who feel they are passing on their feelings of guilt to their children. Epileptics with certain kinds of character may murder in the sudden bursts of irritability and aggression which occur frequently in epileptic furor.

DR. BROSIN. I think that is right. Catatonics, epileptics, encephalitics, schizophrenics generally, paranoids are the groups which may employ violence. A true obsessional who can commit murder is by definition extremely hard to find. I don't think I've ever really seen one; I don't know that I've ever heard of one. Dr. Murray, does the true obsessional with strong ambivalence ever kill anybody?

DR. MURRAY. No; you see, by definition, the obsessional has a very severe and strict conscience. Though he is engaged in tremendous quantities of hostile fantasy, that's all in the magical realm of thought; he can't translate his thoughts into action, for his conscience is too strong. It's quite different with the paranoid with simple fantasies; he will follow through on his fantasies, will simply say, "That guy is doing this to me, therefore I have a right to retaliate." It may be that an obsessional will regress to a schizophrenic level and on that level will act out his hostile impulses; by this time the corrective value of his conscience is lost.

*

STUDENT. I don't quite understand the concept of depression. Is hostility the moving force behind depression? Does that result in punitive feelings, so that by your own reaction you will punish others?

DR. BROSIN. Yes, that's true, I think. The attitude of that fifty-six-year-old woman toward her husband, in the case I mentioned, was clearly one of hate. By incorporating his figure into herself and punishing that part of him which is within her (turning the hostility inward instead of outward) she became depressed. Maybe that needs more elaboration. Dr. Murray, go ahead.

DR. MURRAY. I think to understand depression you first have to understand grief and what goes on in grief. You remember that early in our lectures I spoke of the child who loved the watch because it was bright and shiny and ticked. At that level of his development his way of relating himself to the watch was to stick it into his mouth, showing a tendency toward oral incorporation, as we call it. Now, an individual can maintain that device for a long period of time, 'way up into adult life. It is a mechanism, a device, that is sometimes used by human beings who lose someone they love.

We saw an example of it in the clinic the other day. A patient told how close her mother still was, in terms of dreams and of daily being around the house, in spite of the fact that she had died six years ago and before that had lived five hundred miles away. It came out very, very clearly in our discussion with the patient that, in a sense, the spirit of her mother is closer now than before—because she cannot tolerate this loss.

To illustrate again—there is an old fable of a Japanese girl who got the news that her father and five brothers had been killed in battle. She came from a family with a history of bravery, and so she went into the house and set the table for all of them and had her meal—psychologically denying the fact that they were gone. The next day she took off one plate. She went along for a few days and then took off another plate. So little by little, by this symbolic act, she let go these persons whose loss she could not tolerate all at once. It seems that by the psychologic mechanism of introjection we give up the object we have lost—a loss we cannot tolerate—little by little, gradually replacing it with other objects. This is a sound physiological procedure as long as it is effective. Normal grief is a physiological procedure.

Depression is an abnormal expression of this physiological procedure. There is something else in it than the loss of a loved object. Because we are such narcissistic or infantile personalities, when our feelings are injured by the behavior of another person, we psychologically deny ourselves any positive relationship with him. But the introjection of this person goes on. I rage against him, I blame him, I say it is his fault, he does not love me as I should be loved; I have a right to be loved the way I want to be loved and I haven't been loved that way; therefore, I am a poor person, left all alone, and unloved. So with all this hostility and this ambivalence we rage against that introjected object within ourselves, placed there originally in order to taper off a big loss little by little.

Introjection is a very interesting concept to have, for you see it in all variations of depression, from the depressive reaction of the hysteric to the reactive depression of the melancholic down to the depression of manic-depressive insanity. Another way you can conceive of it is as being like the actions of the little girl who hasn't been loved as much by the family as she thought she ought to be. So she says, "I'm going to go away and I'm never going to come back, and then they'll be sorry they didn't love me as they should." You see, she thinks that by running away she is going to hurt them. She runs down the street, but she hasn't gone far before she changes her mind. The same mechanism operates in the depressed person. He estranges himself from the people from whom he wanted love but for whom he has a hell of a lot of hate because they haven't loved him enough; in a sense, he runs down the street via the mechanisms of his psychotic illness and then he carries on his hostility in his depression.

STUDENT. I think that answers a considerable number of questions. Depression then really can be a variable factor?

DR. BROSIN. Yes. It is very frequently present. Almost all illness has some element of depression, almost all illnesses including organic ones like paresis. We used to talk about the elated, expansive paretic. That was true in the days when we treated lumberjacks, cowboys, rugged, outdoor individualists. I haven't seen many of this kind in Chicago; by and large, there we get simple depressed paretics, sometimes with a little agitation.

STUDENT. Is there still an expression of hostility, for instance, if a person develops cancer and he gets a definite depression after that? What is the explanation of that?

DR. MURRAY. Yes, there can be a serious depression. If the person has had normal gratifications, normal, healthy affective relationships with people, he can accept his fate. But if he hasn't, and if he has developed an overdependent need for love, security, and what-not throughout his life and tends to use this withdrawing or depressive response as an answer to a threatening situation, then when he gets cancer, he will act in the same way. It is almost as if he thought the cancer was something that people could have prevented if they had loved him enough. Such a person will go into a depression. With such persons the incidence of the cancer is simply a trigger situation which sets off an old mechanism that has been there for a long, long time. Similarly the involutional period may be a trigger mechanism for lighting up the rapid case of involutional melancholia. By and large, the person who develops this depression at the time he has cancer has been a depressive personality throughout life and has been using this mechanism in difficult situations; now, in this most difficult situation, he uses it more than he ever did before.

*

STUDENT. There is a process of hysteria that is rather confused in my mind. I wonder if you would elaborate on it. On the one hand, you have paralyses in which the person seems to be indifferent to his condition; on the other hand, what we call, in ordinary speech, an hysterical episode with thrashing about and crying.

DR. BROSIN. The lay conception of hysterical—a person, usually a woman, thrashing about, crying wildly, and so on—has no correspondence at all to the technical word "hysteria," as far as I know. Most writers make a point of differentiating between them sharply. It may be that a person with an hysterical character, as we call it, may become extremely upset, with motor restlessness, but ordinarily this doesn't happen. The hysterical character has nothing to do with the concept of an hysterical episode as you have described it.

*

STUDENT. Will you elaborate on the family background of the obsessive-compulsive? I gather that there would be a very strict father and mother.

DR. BROSIN. The characteristic picture is one of at least a strict father, sometimes also a strict mother; or a strict mother alone. Incidentally, a very good diagram of the typical obsessional is the husband in the movie *Ecstasy*, which some of you may have seen many years ago.

STUDENT. Say the mother dies and the child has to assume the burden of cooking and that sort of thing, is there any factor there that plays a part in the development of a rigid personality?

DR. BROSIN. What is more characteristic of very sick obsessionals is that during a period of great hostility the father actually dies. Then the child is committed to the belief of the omnipotence of his own magical powers, and he becomes a chronically ill patient, unless helped out.

DR. MURRAY. I think there is one other aspect here that we need to consider. One of the impetuses for the obsessive is that which Dr. Brosin has outlined. But you also might get parents of the doting kind who urge the child ahead. They want their child to be trained in the habits of cleanliness before other children are. Each time the child goes to the stool they make a big fuss over his excellent performance, so that he becomes deeply concerned with his bowel functions and attaches a tremendous, exaggerated importance to them. He begins to relate himself to the world in terms of his attitude toward the stool and all the positive relationships he can achieve through the parent. Now, sometime later, if that child is frustrated, he may reverse the field and start using the stool to force his parents to do what he wants them to. You then have a child who is overdetermined in this particular zone, in the anal zone, and who later on may well become a compulsive neurotic, with a fixation on an early emotional era of his life because of the excessive attention applied to it.

The same effect can be secured by the opposite behavior on the parents' part. You see, this thing we call fixation, which goes back to an early period in the child's life, can result either from excessive denial, excessive frustration, or anxiety, or from the exact opposite. Either kind of behavior on the parents' part may do it; either extreme may do it. It is the middle-of-the-road course that you need to take in bringing up children.

DR. WOLFF. I think another word might be said about it. Children who are insecure in early life, for whatever reason, discover the pattern that brings them approval and that becomes the arch or keystone of their lives—namely, "I shall do it better and longer than anyone else and thus gain approval." This system, which works reasonably well early in life, operates at a higher and higher cost during middle life and it always brings with it symptoms in those areas we have talked about.

Common Psychopathology

DOUGLAS D. BOND, M.D.

THIS morning we are going to talk a little about a lot of heterogeneous matters that have been left dangling—some of the psychoses and some practical hints for identifying them and handling them, a bit about suicide and a bit about some of the troubles that you can encounter there if you are not on guard: grief and the mechanisms of grief and what grief means. We'll take that last topic first.

When you love someone you endow him with a lot of affection and emotion, and, in a way, he becomes part of you. When that person dies it is very much like a physical injury to your personality, and you go through a period of mourning or grief or sadness. Your mind is filled with thoughts of the loved person. You are likely to ruminate about all the things you wish you had done with him. You are likely to have a nasty persistence of the feeling that the person isn't dead, that he is still living, that he is still going on. You may even have rather spiritualist-like experiences in which the person seems to appear again in the flesh. That is part of the refusal to recognize that the person is really gone, to cushion yourself from accepting it all at once.

Now that's a very normal reaction and one which everyone has. It is a very simple reaction, not a complicated one. How distressed you feel depends in part on the amount of time you have had to prepare yourself for the loss. If the person was ill for a long time and you recognized that sooner or later you were going to lose him, you built up your own defenses and in a sense weaned yourself away from him, so that when he finally went you were very much more comfortable or very much less shocked than if the death had been sudden. This is the kind of reaction that takes place when a person has a rather whole-hearted and pure kind of love. There is very little ambivalence, very little criticism of the dead person, but a very pure, kindly feeling toward him.

You have all seen a lot of grief; you have all probably had a lot of grief. One of the most important things to remember in such situations is that recovery takes a little time. Time alone is very helpful in the pure grief reaction, for we have a great tendency to heal ourselves. While grieving, a man retreats and regresses; he becomes interested only in himself, and he is likely to feel that he won't dare reach out and love again, because by loving he can also be hurt again. As time goes on, healing usually takes place; the person begins to reach out beyond himself again and to live on in much the same way as he did before.

When a person in grief comes to you as a patient, one of the most important things to realize is that what that patient needs more than anything else is consolation. So console with him. Let him give vent to his feelings. Encourage him to do this, but don't force him. It's much better not to have that action delayed. If a person has been shocked, he may not feel anything; he'll hold all his emotion within himself, and very frequently he will not be aware of feeling anything. The delay of the grief reaction is often terminated by some incidental little event or some new trial that comes up; then, all of a sudden, the person experiences a real flood of grief. Such a delay very seldom helps a patient. So don't be too quick to tell the patient to pull himself together. Let him cry a bit. Don't let him hold his grief back too much. Let it come. Expression of grief is helpful, and time makes all the difference between health and illness.

Two or three months is a very common length of mourning; the grief usually attenuates toward the end of that time. By five or six months there ought to be a real change for the better. There is a natural healing process within us that is strong enough to heal within that time, if it is only grief that is being dealt with. Recovery commences when the patient stops withdrawing into his own preoccupation and sadness and begins gradually to reach out again. This recovery is helped if the patient has some substitutes for the lost one; for instance, has children whom he can keep on loving and on whom he can pour the love he had for his wife.

*

So much for grief. Now I would like to talk about prepsychotic and early psychotic reactions which are characterized particularly by the fact that the individual's psychological defenses are down and the ego pretty much overwhelmed. Mechanisms usually unconscious and covered are now too much in the open. This situation is a field day for you if you are interested in dynamics, but it is very important for you to realize that further breakdown of defenses is what the person cannot stand. What the person in such a situation needs is a strengthening of his defenses. You will have to help such a person to recognize reality, for the part of him that knows reality and recognizes how he should fit into his daily living is gone. He is overwhelmed by the unreasonable part of himself; his unconscious is in full sway and it meets the outside world directly.

It is going to be hard for you to stand for reality, for when a person is wide open it is very tempting to become lost in the fascinating workings of the unconscious with its own peculiar system of logic. But it is not a good thing to do. In such a patient you have a damaged person; you have to give him a splint, you have to be the splint of what sense of reality remains.

In such cases, there is not the usual doctor-patient relationship. You can sense that the patient's relationship to you means very much less than usual. If you are not aware of it, you can easily get into a one-way relationship in which you find suddenly that you are doing all the giving. The psychotic person as a rule has retired to his own inner life, and this inner life has become his reality. People outside it and events outside it have very much less influence than usual. After a little experience you can sense very quickly how different such a person is. He will come right into your office and begin to tell you, without that bridge of friendship, things that ordinarily don't come until after the doctor-patient relationship is firmly established.

One of the easiest ways of telling when a patient is in this condition is from your first interview with him. If a patient suddenly begins to flood you with a lot of sexual detail (particularly sexual feelings toward his parents) and gives you many detailed examples of the sort of psychological mechanisms that usually come to light only after a great deal of trial and turmoil on the part of the patient, then you must be careful. When emotional problems and their connections become too evident, then you know you have a patient who has too few defenses.

The other big thing about such patients is that generally you have the feeling that there is something inappropriate in the way they are—the way they sit with you, the way they talk with you. Things you say are met inappropriately. Often this is rather subtle, or seems rather subtle to you at first, but it becomes evident very soon. Perhaps they are depressed beyond reason. They are flat; they don't make much response at all. Things that ordinarily get a big rise out of others leave them cold. They are perhaps too quick in their change in moods, too sudden or too violent. There is something very inappropriate and a little unreal about this; you often have the feeling that a psychotic person has a tremendous force within him to which he is paying attention. You feel how that power has engulfed him and how he has withdrawn into himself, how he doesn't stretch out his hand to people any more. Psychotic persons often have lost the ability to have thoughts that they keep to themselves. They are likely to put their thoughts too easily and too quickly into some kind of action. It is in a way a loss of social sense. Consequently, perhaps your main job is a social one—that is, to decide whether the patient has enough left to remain in society or in his own particular environment or whether he should get out. Very frequently your decision will be that he should be hospitalized.

*

I'll turn now to a brief description of some of the *manic-depressive reactions* that you will see in your practice—psychotic depression, morbid grief. Morbid grief is differentiated from normal grief by simply one thing: in morbid grief there is guilt. The patient is always saying, "I'm wrong, I deserve it, I'm the worst person in the world." (There is a tremendous amount of personal devaluation.) Or "I'm Hitler's mother," or "I've caused the war." Morbid guilt is conscience gone haywire. Conscience has the upper hand, and is dominating the scene. As a matter of fact, conscience (super-ego) and the unconscious (the id) have joined forces and fight their battle on the overwhelmed ego or social part of the patient. The conscience is a very punishing thing; it keeps reiterating and perseverating, and saying, "You're bad."

I think we have talked about guilt enough to have a pretty good idea of why guilt appears. It is not hard for you to see, I think, that it is based on hostility and other unpleasant feelings toward someone you love. Otherwise the guilt wouldn't be there. If you feel rather hostile toward someone and then become depressed and begin to blame your-

self very badly, you beat yourself as if the person toward whom you
have the feelings were inside you. It is as if the feelings that you should
turn out toward him were turned inside yourself.

Now it's often not so hard to see the aggressive aspects of a depression, in that a depressed person is a helpless, hopeless person who de-
fies any action on anyone's part to help him. "Oh, you can't do anything for me. Don't worry about me. Leave me alone. I can't be helped.
No, no; well, just don't worry, I'm not worth it. I'm not worth your
trouble." The relatives of such a person may take a pretty good beat-
ing, for the person is saying, "I don't care enough about you to have it
make any difference to me. You haven't any power over me. I have
within me things you don't know about that are so strong and so overpowering that they leave anything you may do useless; you are powerless to do me good." The people who live with depressed people contend with this. It is a very difficult thing.

In a psychotic depression there are several signs that are of help to
you. First of all is the way the patient looks—very depressed, sad, unhappy, withdrawn. He talks with great difficulty. He is slowed up in
everything—his actions, his talking, his walking. And he is without
hope. Very frequently he will stop eating and will lose a lot of weight;
very frequently he will lose all interest in sex. These are wonderful
indicators of the beginning of this type of psychosis. It is very helpful,
too, to get from somebody else the patient's history of previous attacks.
Also, in all these cases in which the patient's judgment of his social
person and his social life are gone, it is very helpful to get a description
of his behavior from his family or someone else who has his social sense
intact. This informant can tell you how much the patient usually shows
of what you see in him, to what extent he acts at home as he does with
you. There can be a good deal of variation in such patients' behavior.

Now people with depressions of this type are sick people, and they
are very suicidal people. A skilled person can handle a suicidal depression with a good deal of assurance, but even he will have many qualms
and anxieties. In general this is a serious illness with a real suicidal
danger in it.

How do you find out about suicide? I think one of the best ways is
to ask the patient nicely. You often find out a lot more than you would

expect. It is not bad to introduce your question by saying, "Well, now, everybody who feels this way has a few suicidal thoughts. Can you tell me about yours?" Then it is a very good idea to pursue that just a bit further, if the patient isn't too sick, and find out how he is going to commit suicide and why he is going to do it. The person who is afraid he is going to commit suicide is often not nearly so much the problem to you as the person who longs for suicide, who longs for death, who looks upon death as a release. A release from what? It is really a release from his own conscience and from his own hostility.

The depth of the person's hostility toward someone is a very important assay to make in determining whether or not there is a real likelihood of suicide, how serious a suicidal danger the person is to himself, for he sits as judge and jury and hangman, too. If he feels his crimes are great, then there is only one way out for him. You can do a lot about preventing suicide in very depressed people by hospitalization. It is best not to take the sole responsibility for a seriously depressed patient. If you can't get a person to a hospital or to a psychiatrist, get another doctor to see him, for you should share the responsibility of a possible accident.

Frequently one of the most dangerous times for a person with a depression is when he is swinging out of it. Before that, in the depths of his depression, he is so retarded that he does not have enough motor activity or agility to commit suicide, for he is almost paralyzed. Hence it is good not to stop your observation of a person with a serious depression too soon. The intensity of the delusions of guilt and the intensity of physiological signs are also very important as indicators of the quantity of his suicidal interest—but to mention this is to say the same thing over again. What does the patient think he has done? How deluded is he? How much of the world's guilt does he take on his own shoulders? Guilt beyond himself? If that guilt is great, the suicidal risk is great.

*

The same kind of guilt occurs in the *involutional depression*. It, too, is morbid grief—melancholia. This reaction is a little different from the manic-depressive in that, to begin with, it occurs in a different kind of person. Although the manic-depressive swings up and down in his normal life, he is quite well between attacks. The person who develops involutional melancholia is likely to be the obsessive type, a rigid person, one who has a very high code, who has lived the life of denial, who has formed himself into a tight little pattern, who doesn't live at ease with himself. That type of person is often the leading citizen of the community. When an involutional melancholia hits, it is rather likely to hit hard; in the more serious form it's a major illness. There are all sorts of gradations in it, however; this is a most difficult field in which to draw lines.

There is the same kind of guilty sadness in involutional melancholia as in the depressions, but here it is mixed with agitation. The manic-depressive sits quietly and is so retarded that he can hardly move at times; the involutional melancholic paces, wrings his hands, reiterates over and over again, ruminates about the things that are wrong with him. He has delusions that are of a special sort, that are very charac-teristic of this kind of illness—delusions that part of his body is gone. The part that is lost is almost always the gastrointestinal tract, but it may be the brain. "I have no bowels," he will say, and will go over and over this, pacing and wringing his hands.

There are a great number of involutionals, too, who at first appear to be paranoid, and there is a lot of paranoid coloring in the involutional picture at times. There is a paranoid aspect to all psychoses, but I think that in the involutional it is a bit more marked. Now, in a rigid person, in an obsessive person who has a guilty depression, you can gather that the biggest trouble lies in his hostility—and his defenses against it. A severe involutional depression is the greatest suicide risk of all, for such a patient is not so retarded as the manic-depressive and the guilt that he is under is enormous.

The finer involutional pictures that you see should be treated with respect. Let's go back to our earlier statement and recall that a psy-chotic is a wide-open person, a person with no social self, for whom you will have to be a sort of social self; a person whom you will have diffi-culty in reaching, whom you will have very great difficulty in joining to you. You'll have to be a lot more patient, you'll have to expect a lot less response on the patient's part to you or to your efforts to help. It is very important to realize, too, that the patient broke because his defenses against his hostility broke. He has no defenses; his hostility and his other conflicts are too strong for him. If they are, then don't point them out to him. It is so easy to see the difficulty that it is tempting to do so. But it is very important to stay away—to follow the patient at some distance. You can let *him* tell you—but don't *you* tell him. And you can let him tell you only up to a point. You have to be the support; you have to be reality; you have to be that part of himself that is gone; you have to hold him back and be his defense.

And then there are a lot of reality factors to consider. A person who has led a very rigid, denying life comes to later life mournful over the things that he has never had, realizing that his chances of getting those things are now past. Very frequently at this time in life people don't have very much to look forward to. Very frequently they have made a poor marriage or a half-poor marriage. Not infrequently they have very severe economic problems that are not going to get better and in reality can't be handled. There is really only one thing to try to do— accent the positive. Try to help them see what they can do. Try to help them get as much pleasure as they can out of the things they can do.

*

Let's go on to early *schizophrenias*. The early schizophrenias are a lot more common than you realize at first; you always have the feeling that all the schizophrenics are in hospitals. Well, they are not.

The chief characteristic of the schizophrenic as he comes in and sits with you is his queerness. You don't mean much to him. The fact that you are a doctor doesn't mean much to him. You are talking to him across a great river. You feel, too, the frequent inappropriateness of his response to your questions.

There is another thing which I think is quite striking and which is not very well recognized, and that is the impulsiveness of a person with schizophrenia. You may make an incidental remark or casual comment or in the physical examination you may look at some part or other, and all of a sudden the patient explodes as though he had brought dynamite with him.

Dr. J.'s case was a good example. This man, after an automobile accident in which his brother had been killed, developed diarrhea. In the course of the medical examination, the physician decided upon a duodenal drainage. When the tube came, the patient wept and said he was going to have none of that. It would kill him, and he was going to leave the hospital. Then, with elaborate precaution, he was kept in the hospital by the device of getting his mother to come and live with him. His reaction to having a nasal tube used was much stronger than you would anticipate, and it is easy to see that this tube had a very special meaning for him. The advisability of using the nasal tube in the first place is, of course, another matter.

Schizophrenia is a retreat into fantasy, to the point where fantasy becomes reality. It is as if you were dreaming while you were still awake; as if you had made your choice and said, "What's inside me is far beyond, in interest and in worth, anything outside me." Schizophrenia is a retreat and a regression to the very earliest levels of development. A striking characteristic is the elaborate use of symbol: everything is a symbol for something else, every gesture that is made means something more. Certainly with the patient mentioned, the tube was no longer a duodenal tube that was being passed; it represented lots of other things —things that were well beyond any reality. For him reality had little meaning in comparison to his inner thoughts.

The fact that such a boy will talk to you, will give his name, will discuss baseball, raising chickens on the farm, and so forth, is often disarming to the physician who thinks that if a patient has islands of reality he is not schizophrenic. But you immediately sense in such a person a remarkable degree of flatness; he doesn't give anything to you when he is talking. He'll talk if you want him to but he'll certainly keep quiet if you don't. And then he gets cut off and he explodes. Dr. J. tried to get this patient to talk about his brother who had been killed in an automobile accident, and up he went and out. In a rage for a moment, but the next moment as flat as before, carrying over very little—that's a schizophrenic patient. You can go and talk to him now; he's glad enough to see you, he's glad enough when you go—it makes no difference. You aren't much to him; you are a little piece of reality he has discarded.

Now, of course, in schizophrenia as in other psychoses, you see the mental mechanisms that we talked about yesterday thrown up in enormous relief. The reservations and inhibitions that we have normally are stripped back in the schizophrenic patient and you see underlying unconscious processes.

There are a lot of little things that a schizophrenic who is hallucinating will do that are easy for you to detect. They are very important and surprisingly often missed. Let the schizoid alone when he is talking to you; give him a moment of silence, give him a chance to listen and to answer. That's often all you need to make the diagnosis. When you're talking to him, always be judging how much of the pressure to which he is responding is yours, and how much is his. Very frequently you will confuse the two. A schizophrenic who sits silent and quiet and unperturbed will have little feeling of discomfort, though you may be uncomfortable yourself. Such actions are very important in your judgment of him. The impulsiveness and the quick change are also very important—quick change in mood, from apathy to resentment to apathy within thirty seconds; quick resentments that quickly die. All these actions are inappropriate to what is going on between you and him. He has far more important things to be concerned about; he is loaded with something else.

A history of the patient secured from somebody else is often another important bit of evidence for you to have. A patient who is withdrawn in the psychotic sense has usually begun his withdrawal in adolescence. Another bit of evidence of a developing schizophrenia is hypochondriasis—flashes, pains, malfunctions of all sorts and in all parts of the body but different from those neurotic disorders you see pretty regularly in the clinic. For these are bizarre symptoms. First the patient's chest is burning, then the soles of his feet; then his belly is aching; then his head is different. The symptoms are divorced from anatomical and physiological systems, but the patient often connects them in a delusionary way. These symptoms are elaborate, and very frequently you find out from the patient that he attributes them to an influence outside his body. They can be very confusing, and you can spend much time and money in tracing each one of these symptoms down. As is the case in most confusing problems in medicine, a good deal of time spent in careful examination before you make half-hearted decisions or embark upon frantic physical search will save much time later. In general, when you are satisfied that you are dealing with a schizophrenic patient, refer him to a psychiatrist.

Of course, there are a lot of schizoid people who by living on a farm, or in some other simple environment, can control their environment and make it part of themselves, can have their fantasy with all its freedom and interfere with no one else. They may be pretty harmless people and pretty happy people, even though they are a little queer.

I want to go back a minute and say that with the schizophrenic there is danger of suicide—of homicide too, at times, particularly if he is a paranoid, for the intensity of a paranoid is often very great. There are a lot of people who are semiparanoid, who go through life with chips on their shoulders and their chins out, and it is very tempting to knock those chips off and knock those chins in. In general, if you have a feeling that here is a paranoid person who feels with great intensity that others are persecuting him, there is one important thing not to do—that is, not to argue with him. He may be able to go a little further than you in an argument. It is very important to know, too, that you should avoid all homosexual topics when you are speaking with a paranoid, for paranoia is a defense against homosexuality.

*

I'd like to talk briefly about just one other topic—a character neurosis or a *psychopathic personality*. Much that applies to your handling of a psychotic applies to your handling of that type of trouble too. People ask what bad character is. It's a little like asking what Betty Grable has that other people don't have. The answer is nothing; she just groups it better. Character is the pattern of the ego's action in handling inner drives in relation to reality.

Now strong character is really a fiber which has been built through a multitude of identifications, and it determines how readily the person's unconscious drives are expressed without proper concern for reality. If this fiber is lacking, the patient cannot assimilate and mold and make firm what insight you may be able to give him. You are going to have to learn this the hard way, I fear, for it is almost impossible to tell you about handling psychiatrically people of poor character. Some of them can be helped by very deep analytic therapy over a long period of time, often in a controlled environment. There is nothing else that is going to help any of them. So you can be led down a very tearful path if you take one on and don't recognize the nature of the difficulty. You are safe if you know what you are dealing with, but you are not very safe if you don't.

Many psychopaths are very attractive, and this makes a lot of difference. Many psychopaths will immediately give you histories of horrible things that have really happened, overt incestuous relations, brutal drunken parents. By the time they get to you they have often married other psychopaths, and so added to their worries. If you get very close to such a patient immediately, you can become too much involved, appreciate too much the tremendous trouble, the tremendous reality difficulty that he or she has had, and live in anxiousness with him. Very frequently what happens next is that the psychopath uses you as part of his symptomatology.

The chief characteristics of this type of person are that he acts out everything; in that way he is somewhat like a psychotic. He puts into action every primitive desire he may have—and he has a lot of them. Another characteristic of these people is that they demand immediate gratification. They can't wait. They want it now. They take it now; then they want to take it again, and again, and it has always got to be immediate. They don't have the capacity to plan how to wait, or to deny themselves now and to get more later. Coupled with this is the inability to learn from experience. They will do the same thing over and over again. This has a lot of deep psychologic meaning which we can explain, but the fact is that they don't learn, they don't learn from punishment, they don't learn from their own troubles.

You won't have so much trouble with psychopaths who are men or psychopaths who are elderly. You may have a little trouble with psychopaths who are feminine, young, and very pretty. Frequently it is easier for a doctor to bring forth his sympathy for such a patient. Such a psychopath will defer to you to engage your sympathy and will tell you her very disturbing thoughts or difficult experiences, so that it is very easy for you to take her under your wing for a short time, but soon you will find that she is playing you.

You can often tell this type of person by the way she dresses and acts.

She is the kind who is very much aware of the way she looks at you, bats her eyes a little bit and is very understanding, perhaps a little tolerant; takes the attitude, "You and I know these things, doctor; others are less fortunate." She dresses rather flamboyantly; does not dress to cover up what nature has endowed her with but rather to emphasize it.

Now one of the characteristics of the complaints of people in this category is that their reactions are those of an immediate frustration. They may be a little depressed and may sit very quietly while talking to you, but you can usually see that they are depressed because they can't get everything they want right now. They will often describe to you how bad they feel, how retarded they are, how much they hate to talk, how they want to be by themselves, but you'll have a difficult time getting them out of your office, for they want to talk and talk.

These are people who threaten suicide, who use suicide as a club, an aggressive act against someone else, saying in a petulant way, "I can't do this, you won't give me that, so I'll end my life." They are the people who make suicidal attempts with an evident purpose, plan the time, plan the place. It is hardly a planning in the conscious sense, however; it is an impulsive act. More than that, they usually don't get the impulse unless the person they want to put under their control is near by. Now I don't mean to say that these people won't commit suicide; they may. For one thing, anybody who is toying with a suicidal attempt may make a mistake. Also, in a fit of desperation and frustrated anger one of them may commit suicide.

People with psychopathic personalities aren't very numerous and since this is a category that you can throw people into, be careful about putting too many into it. People like this do exist, but they aren't just the people that you can't help—though that is very often the basis on which a doctor makes the classification.

*

In closing this lecture I'd like to say one word about the danger of suicide in one other mental disorder—that is, in delirium. In delirium, suicide is a little different in that it isn't a planned death; very often it is an accidental, confused death. Delirious patients, however, certainly form one of the largest groups in which suicide occurs. Such suicide is, of course, more frequent on the surgical and medical services than on the psychiatric. As such, it may be of special interest to you.

DISCUSSION

STUDENT.   I would like to ask if there is any set of criteria that will help us to decide between psychosis and neurosis. I'll tell you why. Our main job in that line is the insanity thing that goes on in the county courthouse. We're called in and supposed to be experts to decide whether a person should be institutionalized or not, and most of us are badly equipped. Now, is there any short-cut series of criteria which can be used?

DR. ROMANO.   I think the most valuable criterion is the social one: namely, is this person able to relate himself to society and the social group with which he lives; is he able to adapt to it successfully? It seems to me that is a much more satisfactory means of deciding whether a person is psychotic or not than any I know of. As you know, "insanity" is a legal term; it is not a medical term. And insanity means essentially that a person is certifiable or committable to a mental institution, that he is no longer able to care for himself or to adapt to his society. I think the first decision to make, then, is a social judgment. You as a doctor must collect the data from those about you to find out whether the man is able to take care of himself in his social order. When one studies the reasons why a person is unable to adjust to society (in other words, the medical distinction between neurotic and psychotic behavior) he finds that many of them are quantitative differences. There is the essential difference that the person's capacity to test reality—that is, to face realistic problems and to deal with them effectively—is broken and, as Dr. Bond told you, there is a greater utilization of fantasy than of reality.

Among the psychotic people whom you will see are those with organic brain disease. Whether these are the dementias associated with brain tumor or chronic infection or degenerative vascular disease or due to senility and so on, the problem is essentially the same. There are many aged people who are able to adjust to their society, especially if that society is a rural farm community. They may have memory loss, they may wander about, they may reminisce, and so on, but they are perfectly all right in a rural community. Now, if such a person were moved to an urban area and had to live in a two-room apartment with a son and daughter-in-law, many times psychotic reactions would be provoked—that is, the person would not be able to adjust to that society. I think the answer is essentially your awareness of a social distinction, whether the patient is able to adjust to society.

STUDENT. Is the psychotic amenable to the same kind of therapy as the neurotic?

DR. ROMANO. The answer is no in most instances. In treating a neurotic person you work with his ego, don't you? You work with his ego, so that he can understand more clearly what the opposing forces of the id and the super-ego may be. Through his relationship to you, you help him to see his inner conflicts, view them more dispassionately, and try to handle them in a more efficient and mature manner. That is the essence of psychotherapy.

Now, in the psychotic the ego is shattered. It is more damaged than it is in the neurotic, so that you don't have it to work with. In other words you can't help the person to see what his conflicts are because he is not prepared to look at them. In fact, they have broken through and are revealed in the symptoms and signs of the psychosis, such as the mania or the depression or the paranoid state. In such persons you don't have an integrated ego to work with, you see.

With the neurotic the method is analytic and synthetic. You help the person to see certain things so that he can put them together. With the psychotic, however, the purpose of treatment is to keep the person intact, and so the method must be one that helps him to integrate immediately. The methods used in handling psychotic patients vary. In many state hospitals, for example, the patients are given no treatment except that they are taken out of society and placed in a protected environment which minimizes the stresses and strains they were previously subjected to. Through being in a kindly atmosphere and being given occupational therapy, recreational therapy, and the like, some patients recover. Lately insulin shock, electro-therapy, and *Dauerschlaf*—prolonged sleep—and other methods have been used to bring patients to a very primitive, immature level with the loss of consciousness. Then they are helped to build up new, more mature attitudes.

You see that much. Then, too, a few very skilled psychoanalysts are using adaptations of psychoanalytic procedures with selected patients. Even here the method differs from that used with neurotic patients.

*

STUDENT. Will you discuss a little bit what is meant by the term "reactive depression"?

DR. MURRAY.   A reactive depression is that type which comes to a person when some life event has overwhelmed him to the point where he uses the depressive mechanism in an effort to find an adaptation to this event, which seems greater than he can tolerate. The precipitating event may be the loss of a loved person, as Dr. Bond told you this morning, or it may be the loss of some of the world's goods. Usually you will find in taking a careful history that this person has been a somewhat overtense person, sometimes even an anxiety-ridden person, that he has had minor neurotic upsets, anxiety reactions, prior to this more serious breakdown. You sometimes get the feeling that he has been only two or three jumps ahead of the breakdown prior to this trigger situation which sets the depression off.

The reactive depression is different from the so-called psychotic depression, usually in depth and in the character of the symptoms. There are usually no hallucinations or frank delusions. The patient's ideas may border on frank delusions, yet you can usually see that these are delusions that have a great purposiveness in solving the individual's reality problem rather than delusions that come because the individual has given himself over to the inner world of which Dr. Bond spoke this morning.

You also usually find in the reactive depressions that the patient's previous anxiety is still present. Many times in the frank psychotic depression the anxiety, the affective reaction, is glossed over. This is not always so, of course, for there are agitated depressions in which anxiety persists. In reactive depressions there is much less departure from, or breach in, the normal course of a man's life than in a psychosis, which is almost an attempt to cut oneself off from external reality.

The reactive depression is much more available to you as a therapist. In your efforts to restore the patient via the treatment situation, you experience a much greater feeling of rapport, of being closer to the disease process than with a psychotic patient. Your capacity to help him in the therapy situation is greater; he is apt to be much more responsive.

STUDENT. Will time take care of this kind of depression even if it is not treated, as happens in ordinary grief?

DR. MURRAY. By and large, yes. It depends though, of course, on the patient. If the reactive depression occurs in the middle fifties and the person has been of the compulsive, rigid type (the type that ordinarily gets involutional melancholia) and the life ahead of him is pretty grim, and if he hasn't got enough normal personality to rise above it, the depression may turn into the mid-life or late-life type, with agitation and a more serious outcome. In the earlier years of life, however, ordinarily you are safe.

*

DR. BOND. I wonder if Dr. Brosin will say a word about the use of vacations. That is one of the commonest decisions you doctors have to make—whom to send away for a rest; who will get a rest from a vacation and who won't?

DR. BROSIN. The doctor's problem of a vacation prescription as part of treatment is one that involves his own judgment and social-psychological orientation as well as the patient. We come back to that very good thesis that very often the prescription of sedation for a patient in a hospital is for the purpose of giving the doctors and nurses a rest. It's the same thing with sending a patient on a nice long sea voyage or out to Colorado Springs.

That point I think is important. Is it your own need to get rid of this patient? What devices are you defending yourself with? Are you doing more and more x-rays, are you using more and more vitamins or essential amino acids, and so on? If you think in those terms, the problem will straighten itself out. I took several voyages in the Caribbean on banana boats in prewar days, and I will tell you that they were floating hospitals. Now you have heard enough of the dynamics of mental illness to know that the patient carries his problems with him; he is his problem—John Smith, his psychosis. The history of his illness is the equivalent of his own biography. In certain cases, however, the reaction situation can be changed by going on a vacation. You must estimate what is the real problem. Prescribe vacations only when situational factors, not intrinsic personality factors, are involved.

*

STUDENT. Has the psychotic ever been a normal child? How can we as practitioners recognize the so-called prepsychotic and what can we do in preventive therapy?

DR. BOND. Well, I think one can say categorically, first of all, that as far as you are concerned the answer is yes; it is possible for psychotics and neurotics to have been normal children. Often one's looking back is very much better than one's looking forward. It is very difficult to make predictions. I think, however, that the introverted child, the child who lives alone in his fantasy more than other children do, is one of the most important early problems. Perhaps Dr. Jensen would say something about that.

DR. JENSEN. I was just thinking back and was struck with the real paucity of material that we have to answer that question. Certainly as one goes back into life histories one does find many times, in fact almost every time, that the situations that the individual found difficult to face early in life made a very real difference in his behavior as he got older. In the last eight years here at the university, since we have been paying attention to some of these personality factors, we have found many disturbed children who might have been overlooked in the past. We have encountered a number of very real depressions in children; in fact, right now we are watching with great interest a young lad, ten years old, who has been depressed for two years to the point where he is unable to function adequately—cannot go to school, cannot go out of the house. We have encountered, I suspect, just offhand, a dozen or so children who would fall into that category. I think, too, we have had a number of children who have exhibited the classic signs of schizophrenia; they have recovered rather spontaneously in a surprising manner. We've encountered a good many severe anxiety states, many more than we would have ordinarily suspected. We have also encountered a good many children (children as young as eight years) who would fall into the category, if one were to classify them, of psychopathic personality.

Now in every instance, as far as I can recall offhand, there have been factors in the children's situation which have been important in the production of those kinds of behavior. We have found an unusually large number of disturbed homes, homes broken by death or divorce, or homes that ought to be broken by divorce. We have found in many instances that there is very intense sibling rivalry, intense to the point that you rather marvel that things go along as well as they do. I remember, for instance, one youngster who threw an ax at his sister because he was so angry at her. We are also finding a good deal of disability arising out of the threat of failure in school. I think we have underestimated the tremendous threat that failing in school is for a good many youngsters. Many of the problems that are brought to us day after day—the tummy aches, the headaches, the vague, ill-defined muscle pains and joint pains—often stem directly from failure in school. Threat of failure may be due to inadequate capacity; a good many times it is related to lack of understanding on the part of the school authorities and the teachers; it is quite often related to such things as unrecognized reading difficulties. Summing it all up, I do think that as we become better acquainted with the force of circumstances in childhood, maybe 'way back in early infancy, we shall find a good many answers to questions that still remain unanswered.

STUDENT. How often can you trace a psychoneurosis to a child's being pushed by his parents at an early school age, skipped in grades, urged to do better work, rivalries worked up, and then finding out he can't carry on in the way the parents expect of him?

DR. BOND. It is very common to find in people who have disturbances in later life that their parents have used them in one way or another, that they have not respected them as individuals but have used them to fulfill their own ends. You yourself can elaborate the thousand different ways in which parents approach a child and use that child for things they haven't been, things they always wished they were. That plays a very definite role in many people's later problems. It is very rarely that you see a very ill neurotic or psychotic patient or a psychopathic patient who has had a well-balanced, happy, stable home.

Clinical Problems

V*

1. A PATIENT WITH ASTHMA AND PSYCHOSIS

Complaint. This man, aged fifty, has been employed in a prison for fifteen years. He has been visiting the outpatient clinic for one month for complaints of asthma, characterized by cough with shortness of breath, wheezing, and difficulty in the expiratory phase of respiration. He claims that for the past six months this disability has prevented him from working at his job. All the work-up on the chart centers around this asthma. Apparently at no time has he been allowed to tell the entire story, which seems to be the main thing troubling him—that is, that the prison officials have it in for him.

To elaborate on the medical history of asthma—the man says that for five years he has had a chronic cold. Two years ago he first began to have asthmatic attacks. These attacks were rather short-lived, characterized by intense wheezing. No one was able to prescribe medicine that gave relief until some friend told him about a mouth spray that apparently has adrenalin in it; he gets relief by oral spraying. For the last six months the attacks have been almost continuous. The work-up in the hospital revealed some emphysema, rather coarse musical râles. Chest plate shows an old t.b. in the right upper lobe and some fibrosis. He has an eosinophilia 9 per cent; sedimentation rate 20 mm. in two hours; gives a history of sensitivity to beans, peas, and one other food. He was diagnosed as having bronchial asthma and was referred to the nose and throat clinic because of the history of nasal surgery two years ago, at which time some polyps were removed. The nose and throat clinic tagged him with chronic hypertrophic rhinitis with polyps. During the course of the last month there was some nasal surgery with removal of polyps.

Personal History. This man told me specifically the day, month, and year that his trouble began. He pulled out a little notebook and gave me the dates of the exact occurrence of things that happened to him and quoted things

---

* Excerpts from discussion in section meetings April 3, 8, 11, and 12. The first case is used here rather than in its proper chronological place because of its obvious connection with the two foregoing lectures.

that were said to him. It was a very circumstantial story he gave. The trouble began when he was called into the office and accused of talking to members of the legislature and giving them information about two inmates of the prison. Because of that, he said he was changed from day duty to night duty. Some time after that there was a murder in town, and the murdered man seemed to be tied up with releasing information about these same inmates in the prison. While on night duty, on about ten occasions the patient noticed that a van came up the road, drove along, and then stopped behind a wall. One night, when he was trying to find a comfortable place to lean against the prison wall, a bullet came whizzing by. Then he found a note in his box which said, "Keep your face shut; just remember." He assumed a prison official was responsible for taking the pot shot at him, for on one occasion while he was on night duty he noticed a couple of men out on the road, one of whom he thought was this official, who had previously called him in and said to him, "Do you know what happened to a couple of fellows around here for doing too much talking? You don't want to quit, do you? Keep your face shut and you will get a rapid promotion." No promotions have followed, however. He has felt very depressed about these episodes and says he has lost a good deal of weight. When I asked him why he didn't change his job, he said he wanted to see this thing through; it was no time to drop out of a job.

Prior to employment at the prison this man had tried to raise stock but lost money at it. He then bought his father's homestead but wasn't able to make a go of that either and had to turn it back to his father. He hated his father because he had kept pressing him to give the farm back. Further troubles were the death of a child and his wife and loss of considerable money through bank failure.

When Dr. Rennie asked him if he was discouraged about this thing, he broke down and started to cry. When asked if he cried very much, he said no, but he was under a lot of tension, which was evident. I had the impression that probably one of the main factors in his not going to work in the last three months was accumulated tension. I was impressed with the fact that he sat across from me breathing very comfortably, like an asthmatic free of an attack, and did not appear to be particularly depressed. I wasn't too much impressed with his being disabled by asthma, at least at the moment. The way that all these dates tied together and the way in which he corrected me if I made a mistake in a date indicated to me that he had a story that was quite well tied together. When I asked him if the officials had it in for him, he said very definitely so.

DR. RENNIE.   Recapitulate the emotional factors in his life when the asthma began. Certainly we would like to substantiate this story if we could, but, on the other hand, if he even thought he was shot at it is important.

DR. M. (STUDENT).   There was much I couldn't assess. He spoke of many senators and political individuals.

DR. RENNIE.   There can be little question that when the asthma began, he was carrying a heavy charge of anxiety and outright fear in view of all these things he says have happened. We are entitled to ask ourselves whether the asthma is really the thing the man is sick about. Has he ever been put to bed because of asthma? Has he had to stop work because of asthma? It has never been an overwhelming thing that needed heroic therapy to relieve.

The more important question is what is really disabling this man at present. If he was free of anxiety, do you think this asthma would keep him out of work?

You have given a pretty good picture of what he looked like but I would like to supplement it. Here was a man who looked rather furtive. I would catch him watching me; he was distrustful of me. He had a notebook packed with incredible facts. It was imperative for his inner needs that the story be precise and organized; the story flowed logically through a long history of terrifying things that had been happening to him. In spite of that there was really little show of emotion until toward the end, when I said to him, "Well, I imagine this thing must discourage you at times." Then came the flood of tears. His voice disappeared. Then we got a history that he was indeed an emotionally very disturbed person.

I tried briefly to evaluate the depth of the depression that might be present. Depression is a very common medical disease, is much more common than most doctors realize. They miss the fact that depression is present. It can be fatal to miss it. It becomes at once a medical emergency as well as a set of emotions that can play into somatic disease. So we had to know whether this man was enough depressed to be at the point of desperation or suicide. We had to fish around. He is a man with a purpose in life, a fixed purpose. Why does he stay on in a situation where he believes himself threatened? Obviously because he has to vindicate himself, because he has so much emotion wrapped in this necessity to prove and vindicate himself to the world that this has become a central and fixed preoccupation throughout his life in the past years. We don't know whether this is reality, is true or not.

Clinically we have a pretty good hunch what is wrong with him from the manner in which he told the story. We hadn't enough time to make a thoroughgoing psychiatric evaluation as to whether this is genuinely psychotic or not. On a quick clinical impression he is psychotic, however, largely for these reasons: first, the unreasonableness of his insistence on hanging on in that situation; second, the incredible circumstantiality of the story, which is common in paranoid people; and, third, the nursing of his grievance for these long years. You were the first doctor to whom he had spilled this.

Let us leave the psychosomatic issue aside. How depressed was he? Did you inquire about sleep?

DR. M. He says the asthma has interfered with his sleep but apparently has not kept him awake all night. I don't recall that I inquired about appetite. His general nutrition looked pretty good.

DR. RENNIE. He is at the age period where one might expect paranoid development. One would want to know whether he is fundamentally paranoid with incidental depression. I doubt if he is a suicidal risk, but one fine day if this situation becomes intolerable he may take a pot shot at someone. His story makes me think some things have happened that have badly frightened him.

Paranoid individuals are extremely difficult to handle. I would say categorically that they are outside the realm of a general practitioner's competence to deal with. When you find a man like this, he should have competent psychiatric care immediately. His real disability is not asthma; it is psychosis.

DR. BAUER. That is an extremely important point. It is missed time after time. It is much more important to treat what he is talking about than asthma.

DR. RENNIE. Time after time what the patient presents initially as the complaint is what he is hanging things on for the moment. The real disability is something of greater magnitude. This is frequently also true of psychoneurotics.

This man needs expert psychiatric care. Such people often do very much better outside a hospital, if you can keep them outside with safety to themselves and to others. A psychiatrist can do that almost in direct relation to the feeling the patient has for him. He must see him frequently and watch for changes in the picture. In a psychiatric hospital one has certain modern methods—electric shock, insulin therapy, or a sensitive type of psychotherapy which might get a clearer picture of the problems in the person. We owe it to this man to get him over to the psychiatric outpatient department service. We will ask the social worker to go to the psychiatric department, so that they can sensitively receive the man when he comes. Your responsibility as a general practitioner stops at this point.

2. A PATIENT WITH CONVULSIONS

Complaint. This patient is a twenty-year-old girl. Recently, following experiences which I shall describe to you, she has had a great many convulsions, during which she thrashes around. A previous examination indicates that there is nothing of an epileptic nature about the seizures. There was EEG corroboration of the reading taken at that time.

Personal History. This girl is the only child in her family and has a stern, restrictive father who seems to be jealous of his pretty daughter. As she says, she "has to punch a time clock when she goes out on dates," and has to give a play-by-play account of everything that happens. She wants emancipation.

Under the pressure of war conditions this stern father allowed her to go to Milwaukee to work in a war plant as a mechanic. She loved that job, but now, she says unhappily, there is no place for lady mechanics. In Milwaukee she lived with a relative, in whose house there also lived a middle-aged man and his wife. She became acquainted with the couple, and though she blandly denies any kind of liaison between herself and the man, she betrayed a very real tenderness for him when telling us the story. She explained to us that he was nagged by his awful wife.

One morning, about nine months ago, while she was in bed, this man came into her room and spoke to her. (She apparently does not recognize that this was a sexually threatening situation.) The man then went downstairs and called to her, but she paid no attention to him. He called again, this time much more desperately, and so she went downstairs to see what he wanted and there he was on the floor with his tongue out and a bottle of poison half-drained. She gave him milk and other things and called the police. They took him to a hospital, and his life was saved. She and the nagging wife spent the whole of the following night at his bedside in the hospital. The next day our patient had a convulsion in which she thrashed around, and since then she has had many of them.

DR. BROSIN.   I talked with this patient along with Dr. P. It seems clear that this is a problem of a pretty young lady of typically hysterical appearance who gives a typically hysterical story. There is nothing to show really that she has an epileptic type of illness. There is evidence of a neurosis—conversion hysteria as manifested by convulsions. What do you suppose the treatment should be?

STUDENT.   Is it possible that liking a mechanic's job is a manifestation of aggression that she wasn't able to release against her father?

DR. BROSIN.   Masculine striving? Sure! Male rivalry.

STUDENT.   Has she left home?

DR. BROSIN.   She has been home and the family poured abuse on her. She has a boy friend, considerably older than she is, apparently a fairly prosperous storekeeper. It looks as if she might settle for him. She spoke of him not with the real alacrity of youthful love but with resigned acceptance.

A number of things could be done. If you got such a girl in your own practice, you could say, "This is too tough. Send her to a place where there are psychiatrists." On the other hand, you could do a good deal in supportive therapy, personal and social manipulation. No uncovering therapy (this is an area for the professional psychiatrist). The case would be a beautiful study for any psychiatrist, but I don't think this girl's therapy necessarily depends on a good uncovering technique. I think the evidence for a diagnosis of conversion hysteria is good enough. The possibilities for therapy by a general practitioner are good, if he knows what he is going to do.

STUDENT.   I don't grasp her relationship to the man who tried suicide.

DR. BROSIN.   That is a question. I worked by inference and I may be wrong that she had erotic tendencies toward him. That is not too significant, however. She identified with him. She is a twenty-year-old learning to be a woman. Her harsh father does not permit her normal experimentation such as necking, going out on dates, etc. This fellow is, as it were, an "accident."

STUDENT. This suicide attempt. Are you justified in inquiring into guilt?

DR. BROSIN. I feel there is a lot of guilt but we will try to map a campaign without getting down deep. Let's say she feels guilty. If we can get her into a situation where a reasonable adult male can meet her needs, emancipate her from her family, she may be all right, that is, symptom-free. If she gets into more trouble with life, then she will require more care.

DR. P. We do have a bit more personal history. One of her episodes occurred when she went out with a fellow and on the way home he stopped the car and approached her. Then she had a blank spell and remembers nothing until the car stopped in front of her home.

DR. BROSIN. Amnesia is an hysterical symptom and supports the diagnosis. The nature of a neurosis is highly conditioned by the culture in which one grows up. If she were not guilty about her sexual feelings, she would not need to deny them through amnesia.

STUDENT. I think you have to get her out of her home and get her a job.

DR. BROSIN. Yes. In the meantime we must see where social service can help her. She is blackballed in her part of the country because all the employment agencies have her marked as an epileptic.

STUDENT. What is the real significance of her convulsions?

DR. BROSIN. I think the thrashing around is real hostility—release of tension. Another thing it may indicate is rejection of the whole world. Another—like amnesia with unconsciousness—"I don't have to tolerate this." Another angle, which is, I think, also significant, is that through this symptom she can say, "I greatly desire affection in all its forms; if it is not given to me I won't be responsible. If I am unconscious I cannot defend myself against sexual advances." It is an invitation. Her conscience at this time is too strong, she can't operate with it. There may be other meanings for the convulsion, but at least there are these four.

VISITOR. There is perhaps another question that comes up. When available, I presume the question of differentiation of the pattern of attack becomes a problem for the physician. Will you comment on that?

DR. BROSIN.   It is part of our teaching that whenever in a history one isolates a series of events, one must try to connect them in a meaningful way into a pattern. First, the conditions under which they occurred are highly important. What is the very first time, the first setting in which the symptoms occurred? In this case this factor becomes doubly significant. Her first and subsequent attacks occur in emotionally significant situations. She responds with a common hysterical defense against her own ego-alien impulses. Many physicians have examined this girl and gone into the business quite carefully as to whether this is a typical attack with aura, etc. What is the aftermath? She becomes quite maniacal after an attack, which isn't the usual aftermath of epilepsy. I think this is a primitive reaction in a very little girl. She is fighting these people who are keeping her from being a grown-up lady.

I have read the patient's record with a good deal of interest. The failure to elicit significant history does not indicate that there isn't any worth-while history. Just as the apparent lack of positive physical findings doesn't indicate there aren't positive findings. Because you can't get a positive history, especially in hysterical people, it doesn't mean that there isn't a good deal of significance in the patient's story. Inability to get a history means one of two things. Here are two people, two sets of forces operating. Either one set, the patient's forces, is too defensive or the other set, the physician's, is inefficient in its operation. That is true for all of us.

3. A PATIENT WITH DISABLING PAIN

Complaint. The chief complaint of this thirty-one-year-old farmer is that he aches all over, has a burning sensation and inward nervousness. The pain began when he was sixteen or seventeen years old, at which time he noticed some pain in his ankle joints when he walked. He had sore throat occasionally. The joints were never red or swollen, but a doctor told him he thought he had some rheumatism. The only thing he has noticed about the ankle joints since that time has been some sensation in them whenever cold is applied. At about sixteen, too, he had what might have been a mild joint involvement, and at about the same time he began to experience a burning sensation all over his body. These symptoms are so bad at present that he is unable to carry on his work.

Personal History. The father of this man is living and is a chronic alcoholic. His mother is quite nervous. There are two brothers older than he is. They drink moderately.

The past history of the man is interesting. He told us quite a bit about how his father drank up all of the money that they had or that he and his brothers as children earned. As a result, this boy went to school in patched clothes, was not properly fed, and certainly did not get the care and attention he was entitled to. He was not even given adequate physical care when injured. He finished the eighth grade and at sixteen ran away from home to stay with his brothers, who were in a mining town. He worked around the mines and then got a job on a farm. All this time he was having the burning pains and aches. He married a farmer's daughter and had some conflict with her father. He continued to work around the mines and managed to save about $1,000. His father-in-law was quite persistent about his becoming a farmer, and so he finally moved to a farm near his parental home.

On the farm he has had successive failures. His horses developed swamp fever and died. The crops did not turn out well. In 1942 an event occurred which he says really made his symptoms worse, and he has been worse ever since. That was when he was working in the garden and the horses or cows broke in and tramped it down. He didn't get very angry at the time, but now says he was inwardly very mad. In 1942 he developed brucellosis, with its usual symptoms. He also had operations on his nose and appendix. He has not been able to support his family on what he makes and has been on relief for several years, getting $68 a month. What he likes best is to tinker around with machinery and to make toys for his children.

DR. HASTINGS. What was this man's attitude toward his illness?

DR. F. (STUDENT). He wasn't much disturbed. He sat there tense, with his hands clenched, during the first interview, but he was easier, more relaxed, during the second one.

DR. HASTINGS. Well, now this is a rather unfair question, but what would you say this patient has got?

DR. F. I wonder whether he is starting to withdraw, to become introverted.

DR. HASTINGS. I asked that question to trick you. I haven't heard you say much about a physical examination or laboratory work.

DR. F. I don't recall that anything stood out. The patient has had x-ray examinations.

DR. HASTINGS. Well, let us assume that the physical findings are within normal range, would you want to make any further examinations?

DR. F. No.

DR. HASTINGS. If this man were a patient in your office, what would you be thinking about him? A young man, father of four children, panic-stricken, on relief even though times have been good and other farmers have made money, not much concerned about this situation. I am trying to hitch these things up. Why should he be this way? Why is there this discrepancy between the way he feels and the way you would feel? What kind of a fellow is he?

DR. F. He was rather pleasant. I thought he was a little tense. He talked freely and was not evasive.

STUDENT. It strikes me that he is pretty unaggressive.

DR. F. He isn't aggressive now but he may have been when he was out west. He saved money then.

DR. HASTINGS. He feels he has to get things done. He is very meticulous about paying his bills. What does that suggest?

STUDENT. An obsessive, overconscientious type that develops anxiety when he fails.

STUDENT. His symptoms are a ritual to deal with his anxiety.

DR. HASTINGS. Do you see any of that in yourselves?

STUDENT. Aren't we all that way in our practice? One doctor says he washes his hands three times whenever he sees a patient.

DR. HASTINGS. May I use you as a specimen? Are you aggressive?

STUDENT. Not on the surface. I keep it bottled up.

DR. HASTINGS. This is a common mechanism. On the surface this man seems unaggressive. The surface may break down under stress or with alcohol.

DR. COTTRELL. How bright is this man?

DR. F. He went through the eighth grade and seems to have normal intelligence.

DR. HASTINGS. Let's go back and look at his childhood. What factors have laid down his personality?

DR. F. Neglect, and the success his brothers have made. Conflict in his childhood about his poor clothing and so forth, which made him feel very inferior at school.

DR. HASTINGS. A child's normal needs include clothing, food, shelter, and security.

DR. F. He was also deprived of security because of his father's drinking.

DR. HASTINGS. Did you ask about his relations with his mother?

DR. F. We didn't get to that in the interviews but he probably had more affection for his mother than for his father.

DR. HASTINGS. The father was a hard man to identify with, and a child's maturation depends on his identifying with those who are close to him. We don't know about this man's childhood relation with his father, but assuming he was a deprived child, could his mother have given him the proper security?

DR. F. Because of her nervousness she probably could not.

STUDENT. She too had conflicts.

DR. HASTINGS. Here was a youngster, then, deprived of clothing, shelter, affection. What happened?

STUDENT. Hostility, resentment, regression, and fantasy.

DR. HASTINGS. Most commonly in such cases you get feelings of anger and hatred and a feeling that everything in the outside world is unfriendly. This makes it hard for the individual to feel close to anybody. What, then, would he be searching for in his adult life?

DR. F. Security. He would want what he has been deprived of.

DR. HASTINGS. He is after a will-o'-the-wisp. Why might he have developed obsessive trends? Was there anything in his early training?

STUDENT. He might have wanted to keep relations with others so they would like him.

DR. F. It looks to me as if he wants to be everything he wasn't as a child.

DR. HASTINGS. Still we have no picture to show why he developed these symptoms. Unfortunately the data about his earlier physical history are unavailable. What do you think about his sore ankle?

STUDENT. He wants to escape.

DR. F. He has had four operations in the past four years—tonsillectomy, appendectomy, and a couple of others.

DR. HASTINGS. What about the symptoms becoming worse when he left home?

STUDENT. In leaving home he may have expressed resentment against his family.

DR. HASTINGS. He chose departure from home as the lesser of two evils. The pain in his ankles might be a string holding him back. I don't know the bridge between psychogenic factors and a symptom like this, arthritis in the ankle, although we can see why the symptom localized there. What about secondary gains here? What is he getting in return for the pain of his illness?

DR. F. He is getting financial support. I don't know about the affection of his family.

DR. HASTINGS. Let's guess. What difference does this produce in the family?

STUDENT. The patient may be getting a lot of attention and may fear loss of attention if he gets well.

DR. F. That would be losing a crutch.

DR. HASTINGS. Well, what are you planning to do next with this man?

DR. F. We expect to go into some more things about his family and about his convalescence and his operations, and some way or other I want to find out if he thinks he has had a fair deal.

DR. HASTINGS. What about medication?

DR. F. I expect to tell him that pains like his are often due to worry. He has not asked for medicine.

DR. HASTINGS. With this approach patients often do not try to force your hand.

VISITOR. Any comment on what you have accomplished with him?

DR. F. The only thing I can notice is that he was less tense the second time. He does come a long way for each visit.

DR. HASTINGS. You can help such a patient with medication if you let the patient know that it won't cure him.

DR. F. Office practice in general is a fast brush-off. You have got to give them medicine if you don't give them psychotherapy.

STUDENT. How is he going to see the relationship between symptoms and underlying factors?

DR. F. Repetition.

STUDENT. A little suggestion along with repetition. Without that, will he ever make the association?

DR. HASTINGS. Summing up, then, here is a man with chronic disease of early origin. Even psychiatrists couldn't set their therapeutic sights too high. Some patterns are too firmly fixed to be relieved. You can help this man a lot and probably you can give him symptomatic relief. You won't do him any harm, and you may keep him away from quacks. In any event, you can help him work through his underlying hostility.

PROGRESS REPORT (FOUR DAYS LATER)

DR. F. We have had two more interviews with this patient. In the third interview we began to discuss his marital relationships and discovered that there was quite a bit of friction at home. He found fault with his wife in that she wasn't quite as meticulous as she should be. He said that, as a result, many things happened around home that were costly to him and quite annoying. On the other hand, his wife was rather critical of some of his habits. She didn't want him to drink beer. She didn't like to go out to dances. She was quite jealous, and they would have days of not speaking to each other. His wife was also very afraid of becoming pregnant. They have four children. With the first pregnancy she developed asthma that wasn't recognized at first. With each of the subsequent pregnancies she had asthma. When not pregnant, she has asthma only when they have intercourse. They have tried contraceptives and they have tried to practice rhythm but this only creates more anxiety.

In the third interview, also, we suggested that probably a change in his occupation might be desirable and said that help could be obtained through the vocational rehabilitation of the state. He seemed quite interested in this. Our social worker had talked with him about it, but it was a little difficult for him to decide just what he would like to do and how.

At the last interview he came in feeling really very good. It was very easy for Dr. Hastings to draw out his recognition of the relationship of his feelings to the burning sensations. He and his wife had been talking it over, too, he said. He stated that he has been able to sleep all night long and has had almost no burning since the second interview. Dr. Hastings reiterated that the burning feeling was due to nervousness. By talking with the man about what happened whenever he visited his parents, Dr. Hastings was also able to elicit his feelings of anger against his father for his drunkenness. In his own words, whenever he went to visit his father and found him drunk he felt "burning up."

He talked about these matters very freely. All one had to do was to start him, and he was completely relaxed and let loose everything. He told us that he couldn't take a glass of beer and couldn't smoke because those always produced a burning feeling. Dr. Hastings told him that would gradually pass away. Early in the interview Dr. Hastings offered us cigarettes and both of us refused them. Toward the end of the interview, Dr. Hastings offered him a cigarette again, and he grabbed one saying, "I guess I'll try it."

I think there will have to be follow-up; there will have to be work by social service to get this man in a new occupation so that he will have a chance to gain some financial independence. I also think his wife will have to be called in and interviews held with her to explain this situation and to get her cooperation.

DR. COTTRELL. In summary we might outline just what happened in each interview.

In the first interview the man's history of his life events, given spontaneously, showed no correlation with symptoms, and so you evidenced interest in other things.

In the second interview some of the inner conflicts became clear and an elaboration of life events was secured.

In the third interview we began to tie up the emotional factors and the symptoms and gave reassurance as to the future, including in this plans for rehabilitation.

In the final interview the patient gained some insight into the reason for his difficulty, gave expression to some of his hostility, and began to feel some self-confidence.

Care of Veterans

DONALD W. HASTINGS, M.D.

THIS afternoon we want to take up the broad problem of the effects of war on soldiers, the so-called war neuroses. First of all I'd like to say—just to make it clear to any of you who perhaps have to talk with the parents of combat returnees—in view of all the statements that have been made in the press, that all the men who come back from combat are not insane nor are they going to be insane. As a matter of fact, the incidence of insanity among combat men is much lower than in the population as a whole. The rumor has gotten around, perhaps by confusion in psychiatric terminology, that great numbers of combat returnees are mentally unbalanced. I'd like to show you as we go along that that is not true. Even under the extreme hazards of actual combat in the Eighth Air Force over a period of a year and a half, dealing with perhaps sixty-five thousand men who were actively flying combat missions, we saw only two cases of insanity. That is a negligible number compared to the psychoses that might have developed in sixty-five thousand men of that age back home who weren't in uniform. So much then for the bald statement that the effects of war are not those of insanity. Some men do develop psychoses and insanity overseas just as they do back here in this country, but the incidence of insanity in the Army as a whole was lower than in a comparable civilian group. The Army in combat does not directly produce insanity or psychosis.

Now this afternoon I'd like to talk mainly about what happens to men as they come back home from war. First of all, we start with the proposition that a man who is capable of reaching an adult level of adjustment stays pretty close to that level as he conducts his civilian life. Well, what about this individual when he enters the Army? A good many of you have been in the Army, and so what I am going to say is no news to you, for you have experienced it personally. What is the Army? It is a group of men gathered together in units, such as squadrons, platoons, battalions, etc. These groups are gathered together for a purpose, held closely together not only in combat but also during train-ing for a definite purpose. If an individual is to feel happy and well ad-justed in the Army structure, he must drop down to an earlier level of adaptation, that of the gang or the group. His loyalties, his devotions to other men are of that type. Our first premise, then, is that adaptation to the Army requires a retreat on the part of the individual from his normal, adult method of doing business to a previous level of adapta-tion, the one that roughly corresponds to the high school level. Those of you who were in the service will remember in yourselves certain forms of behavior which would fit very conveniently in high school but might not fit in your home town as you practice medicine.

There is one point in this that is extremely important as one con-siders later developments, and that is the group loyalties that come to exist between the men in the unit. Take, for example, the ten men on a B-17 heavy bomber. In that group are three officers and seven enlisted men, all bound closely by group loyalty and dependence one upon the other, literally and figuratively. In combat they are dependent upon one another for their very lives; emotional ties are welded in the heat of combat. Men in combat are able to go through terrifying experi-ences, experiences productive of large amounts of anxiety, if they are supported by the other members of the group. In common language, it is much easier to go through a bad situation with ten people all in the same boat than it is to do it all alone. That, of course, is exactly what took place in the group of men we are considering—ten men in a heavy bomber. Let's imagine for the moment that the tail gunner on this bomber, for one reason or another, is carrying a heavy load of anxiety but is able to tolerate it and defend himself against it by the support of the other nine men in that ship. What is likely to happen to that tail gunner if he gets wounded and is sent to the hospital as a lone person without his nine companions? It is quite apparent that the man may be overwhelmed with anxiety which previously had been held in check by the support of the group. That's a point we shall come back to in a few minutes when we consider the effects of coming back home. Another point that should be mentioned is the men's total dependence on their immediate leaders. In our example the leader would be the flight offi-cer or the pilot.

To recapitulate in a sentence then—the setting of the Army demands of each individual that he regress to a level of adaptation in which he develops group loyalty and group dependence. Most loyalties in wartime do not extend beyond the small group. The individual does not usually extend his loyalties beyond the squadron, the twelve airplanes, seldom to the group, almost never to the wing, certainly never to bomber command or such flights of fantasy as air force or headquarters of air force in Washington. These terms he will never think of in his loyalties except in some very abstract way, as in "democracy," the "Four Freedoms," and so on. His main loyalties are concerned with the individuals who are immediately around him.

With this adaptation a formerly mature individual, or one who had the ability to be mature, goes through certain other experiences which show up in clear light as he comes home. First, he wishes he were not in the situation he is in, he wishes he were out of the Army; and, secondly, he overidealizes the former civilian life he had. Specifically, he overidealizes his home and the people in it—his wife, his children, the drug store on Main Street, his plans for the future when he gets back home. As time passes, he will carry this overidealization to a point far beyond the ability of the people at home to live up to. As he returns home he has in his mind's eye a picture of the ideal situation to which he is returning.

Now let's go back to our example again. The bomber crew are united by close interpersonal relations; their anxieties have been held in check by the support of the group, and so on. In addition, they have an overidealization of home. Now at one time in the Eighth Air Force the men flew twenty-five heavy-bomber missions and then they were started on their way home within twenty-four hours. What happened, then, when a plane landed at the end of this twenty-fifth mission? The men who up to this time, perhaps for six months, were bolstered by all these loyalties suddenly and abruptly found them broken. They were no longer members of a certain plane in a certain squadron but were now individuals standing alone without the support of anyone, awaiting shipment home. One might expect that in their anxiety to stay alive and not be hurt or wounded the men would have a great sense of relief. Quite the contrary happened. As a general rule, men were not elated at finishing the last mission. Not that they wanted to fly any more—they simply didn't feel that inward sense of happiness that all of them had expected. I think now we begin to see the reason.

Now let's cross this line with these men and see symptomatically what we find in them. In the Air Force all of the men followed the same routine. Within twenty-four hours after landing at the point of debarkation they were given orders for a thirty-day leave to their homes. If a man came back by air, say from England, it is conceivable that he might be in his own home within seventy-two hours after he had finished his last combat mission. At the end of the thirty days he went to a redistribution station, where he was looked at from both physical and emotional points of view to see if he had suffered damage as a result of his overseas experience. Depending on the result of this examination, he was either hospitalized or given further leave or sent for reassignment to a new unit. At one point (these figures are no longer secret) at the height of the European campaign, approximately twenty-two per cent of Air Force returnees were being hospitalized for emotional reasons. That is, roughly a fifth of these men were found to be suffering from anxiety states—not insanity but anxiety states—and to be in need of definitive care. Something like eight per cent more were missed in that examining line but were found to be unable to fly after they arrived at their next station. That gives us the figure, then, of approximately one third as the proportion of Air Force returnees who needed treatment for their emotional difficulties.

The types of emotional illness these men brought home with them can be put in four large groups. One was the somatic group, wherein the man's anxiety was reflected in physical symptoms. The organ system most commonly affected was the gastrointestinal; to a lesser extent the cardio-respiratory was affected; and there were a good many vasomotor symptoms. The second large group consisted of men who were depressed. The third was the hostile, aggressive group, the men who had large chips on both shoulders—a very difficult group to manage. They were aggressive in their attitudes toward civilians, they resented any hospitalization, they weren't sick, nothing was the matter with them, all that was wrong was the Army, civilians, their homes, and so on. Fourth, an almost opposite group, the passive, dependent group, the men who seemed completely licked, ready to crawl back to mother, doctor, nurse, and so on.

Let's go back momentarily to the situation the men found on their thirty-day leave, for within that lies the focus of the accentuating of symptoms. Remember now that men came home insecure because of leaving the security of their former groups and with rather extreme notions in mind of what home meant. As one sits in an overseas theater of war, one's wife tends to become a very beautiful girl, one's children are little angels, and so on. The reality of the matter—that your wife is no younger than the day you left, that your children get in your hair, that you have to go to the grocery store, that you have to do this and that—such things often come with quite a shock. On the other side of the picture we have to remember, too, that wives and families did not have an easy time during the war—what with the loss of security that the husband's going meant, the living with in-laws, which might literally represent to a girl going back to the bosom of her family and adjusting herself to her relatives all over again. I think all of you are acquainted with wives who became alcoholic or were untrue to their husbands under the strain. Consider, too, that the family of the man who has been gone for two or three years has had to make adjustments which have left him out of consideration.

The point I want to make is that just as one cannot adjust overnight to the Army structure, neither can one come back overnight to the full measure of maturity and re-create the same situation that he left. The result is that the individual returning from the war (I can't give you any adequate picture of the wife's end of it) became a rather confused, upset, insecure individual and often considered trying to go back to his combat unit in a vain attempt to recapture the relative security that he knew there. The Personnel Division of the Air Forces received many requests from men who had just returned, or who had just finished their overseas leave, for another stretch of combat duty. I think most of those requests were made because the men wanted to recapture the feeling of well-being that they believed they had had.

The combat returnee, then, usually belonged to one of the four groups I have mentioned. All combat returnees perhaps showed some hostile-aggressive symptoms, passive-dependence symptoms, and depressive symptoms, and certainly some somatic symptoms. There is an overshading in these groups. I suppose almost every returnee had some deep-seated objection to civilians, feeling that they had not done their part, that he had given so much and they had given so little. Superficially, he meant that people were not showing him the affection he thought he should have.

The hostility and the aggression shown toward civilians often became quite severe in the hostile-aggressive group. Two psychiatrists in the Navy told me that at one of their stations they had constant difficulty with little groups of returnees standing around on the main corner of the small town which lay near their convalescent hospital. A man in civilian clothes would walk by and the group would yell "4-F" at him until he got mad. Then a fight would ensue, the Shore Patrol would be called, and instead of operational fatigue the men now had concussion and brain injury!

I might say a bit more about the depressive group, for it is a very interesting group and one that illustrates some of the factors we have been talking about during the last few days. The depressive group had a fairly characteristic combination of symptoms. The men were depressed, had terror dreams, dreams that were repetitive within each night, dreams in which they would perhaps reexperience actual events, such as the crashing of planes on fire. They would wake up in a sweat, panicky, and finally get back to sleep, only to have the same dream reappear and be reawakened. Loss of appetite was very frequent and, consequently, loss of weight. Gross or fine tremor, vasomotor symptoms, easy sweating, and so on, were found. As one got to the bottom of the reactions of this depressive group in the course of psychotherapy, the difficulty was found not infrequently to be related to the death of a friend, particularly the death of one of the men in the patient's tight little unit or a death for which he felt responsible. In passing I might mention that the chance of doing damage to your friends in wartime is exceedingly great. The pilot who has his hydraulic system shot out over the target comes back and makes a landing, not knowing that his brakes are gone; when he suddenly finds his bomber rolling down the runway with its speed unchecked, he ground loops and kills his navigator and bombardier in the crash, and then with truth says to himself, "I killed those men because I failed to order them out of the nose for the landing." Then there are the overanxious sentry who shoots a friend; the lead navigator who loses his squadron, half of whom run out of gas and go down in the North Sea; the Operations Officer who has part in planning a disastrous mission, and so on almost *ad infinitum*.

Now a word about the management of such cases, management by the general practitioner—the first question you doctors must decide when such a veteran comes to your office is whether active psychiatric treatment is needed or certain manipulations of the environment or simple psychotherapy will do the trick. Is the man sick? Does he have the symptoms that spell emotional difficulty as you have come to know emotional difficulty during these past days? Or does the trouble that he is presenting seem to lie in a simple situational affair? If you regard the man as really sick, apparently influenced by war experiences, and if he is in need of definitive psychiatric help, you may want to refer him to care by the Veterans Administration facilities. If the man is not so sick as that and you think you can handle the case yourself, the treatment principles to apply are exactly the same as those you have learned here in the last week or ten days in dealing with civilian difficulties. Fundamentally the veteran's neurosis doesn't differ from the civilian's.

At this point, Dr. Murray, I wonder if I could call on you for a description of the care planned by the Veterans Administration?

DR. MURRAY. When General Bradley and General Hawley came in and took over, they linked up the Veterans Administration facilities with the various universities and formed deans' committees in various centers to be sure that the personnel they were going to train for work with veterans had a competent background and medical experience. Captain Dan Blain went in from the Public Health Service as chief psychiatrist under General Hawley and tackled the job with the idea in mind that his first task was one of training, that he had to build and develop his personnel, so that liaison work with the teaching facilities in various centers is the cornerstone of the program.

Now you might say there is a four-pronged attack on the question of neuropsychiatric care. First are the hospitals for those requiring inpatient care—the psychotics or the severe psychoneurotics who offer little hope of rehabilitation outside a hospital. The second point is the organization of what are called neurosis centers. These will be in-patient units for the short-term treatment of acute psychoneurotic anxi-ety states that, the doctors feel, will recover with a short-term period of definitive care and treatment. These centers will of course be in-cluded in the teaching-training program. Residents and men like your-selves, practitioners in the outlying areas, will be given the benefit of courses such as you have been given here. The third point of attack is the organization of mental hygiene clinics located in strategic areas to which veterans may be referred, and the utilization of established clinics acceptable to the Veterans Administration for the care of similar cases. Patients are sent to these clinics, and then the clinics bill the Vet-erans Administration for their care. The fourth is the use of general practitioners in outlying communities. I believe that the institution of short-term training courses such as this, plus circuit-riding consultants who can come out and help men with difficult cases, also furthering their psychiatric education, will permit a far better job to be done in the home communities than was possible after the last war. It's a big under-taking and it's gathering momentum slowly.

DISCUSSION

DR. BOND. I would like to say something about the psychology of separation, the kind of thing that hits everybody who separates from somebody he loves. It is really another little study in grief. When this fellow who is going to be a soldier is here with his friends in the United States, he endows them with a lot of emotion, and he gets back from them a great deal of gratification and satisfaction. When he leaves, his body leaves, but a part of him remains right here. In every free mo-ment his mind goes back to his family, goes through a little period of mourning for them; he feels that life is hardly worth living. In a sense, he has left part of himself behind. Our emotions and our attach-ments move slowly and reluctantly.

Now after this fellow gets over to Australia he begins to find it a little tiresome to be in love with somebody six thousand miles away. He can keep that up for a certain length of time, but then it becomes a very painful process to have part of himself so far away. You don't get much gratification or immediate satisfaction from loving somebody so far off. So he begins to withdraw a little of that feeling in order to protect himself, to make it a little less painful, and as he withdraws he is likely to regress. Perhaps he can't get satisfaction in a fully adult way, and so he is more or less forced to go back to those satisfactions that he knew at an earlier time. He begins to plant his affection and feeling upon things that are at hand—the griping he does, the debauches he goes on, the people he meets. He may bestow a considerable amount of feeling on these objects and get a good deal of gratification and satisfaction back from them.

Now when he first comes home he goes through the same little process of mourning all over again. Now his attachments are over there. In his regression he had a tremendous amount of personal freedom. That was pretty good fun. Everybody enjoys thinking of himself as pretty much alone. His body comes home, but a part of him stays behind and it is very evident when this fellow comes home that he is only half a man at home. What does he do? What are his thoughts filled with? What is his conversation filled with? He can talk and think of nothing but the people he left and of his attachments to them. That's where his interests are; that's the only thing that can light him up. He isn't here. Just the body is here.

But the people he knew, and the things he knew and enjoyed are now far away. Gradually he has to pull back the feeling he attached to them, again because it is too painful to let his feelings stay over there. He reassigns his feeling to the people he left at home and the things he did here, and then, in a very short time, he has to grow up again from the age of fifteen or sixteen to being the responsible head of a family.

This process is universal, I think, and will vary in degree with all sorts of things, with how fond you originally were of your family, how satisfactory your relations were with your family, and how much you overidealized them while you were away. One of the big troubles is not that people change through separation but that they don't change in the right way or in the way you hope they will. In a sense, they don't change at all; and that is a disillusionment when you return to your family. The family has pictured you as having changed in the way they wished you would; and usually all you have become is an exaggeration of yourself.

I think this kind of thing takes care of itself with time. There is a real time factor in withdrawing feeling, and usually two or three months are needed for it. There's likely to be quite a lot of friction and difficulty in those two or three months, because this fellow who comes back has a wife who has been waiting for him and who wants to throw herself at him too much; he's not quite all here to receive her and sort of backs off and she's hurt. "Don't you love me any more?" she asks. "Oh hell, of course I love you," he says, "what do you think I came home for?"—and they're off. That takes care of itself in time, if the marriage was originally a good one. Two or three months ought to do it; otherwise look for a lot of trouble.

Or it may be that while the man is away, the woman has grown up, and that also presents a very difficult problem. When the husband was away the wife suddenly found within herself all sorts of resources that she never had been allowed to use before. Now when this fellow comes back from overseas he wants to be the dominant fellow all over again. Perhaps she has found certain little things that she can do a lot better than he can. He resents very much the fact that she is so independent, and she will retreat only reluctantly from the new satisfactions she has found. But those things work out, too, particularly if the original ties were very strong.

DR. HASTINGS. One hears a good deal about the boy who went to war and came back a mature man. Would you care to comment on that, Dr. Romano?

DR. ROMANO. Many times, I think, we probably overstress the negative aspects of war and the deprivations and the loneliness, and the tremendous frustrations, socially and sexually, that the soldier had. There were certain positive values as well, which relate to the breaking of chauvinism, bringing about an admixture of peoples from the four corners of the country and from prep school to gutter, accepting the heterogeneity of people who then became more homogeneous. Some individuals did receive training, and certain opportunities, certain types of promotion may have given some value. Some individuals because of their heroic action received acclaim and prestige they never had received before. Many of these things have large value, positive value. For many boys the experience of having met the horrible stresses of this war and remained reasonably healthy was a positive, productive experience.

Deep down I think this whole problem of the returning veteran is much more than a psychiatric problem and that psychiatry must not be messianic in its role or its ambitions. In dealing with citizens returning to a national scene, economic factors, housing, employment, and the meaningfulness of citizenship in a community are probably more important than any specific medical procedure. Where emotional illness reaches certain proportions, then certain skills may be necessary and certain special provisions may help.

DR. MURRAY. I think we also need to take into consideration that psychiatric social work has had experience in dealing with this special problem. We hope it can be brought to focus upon it. We ought to utilize all that we have, both definitive psychiatric care and medical care, plus psychiatric social work, to meet the total problem in a total way.

DR. ROMANO. It is very important to remember that by and large most of these patients will be ambulatory, won't require hospitalization. By taking courses like this you will become more aware of the problem, and you can lessen the load on men who have to face it.

Life Situation, Emotions, and Disease

HAROLD G. WOLFF, M.D.

DURING this work together we have been discussing the effects on the organism of anything that interferes with or threatens the life or love of the individual or the proper use of his faculties. Obviously when the organism reacts to any of these threats he is reacting as a unit. Since this unit includes a body, such a reaction involves changes in his smooth muscle, skeletal muscle, his glands. Awareness that the body takes part in the reaction certainly is not new. Our language is a treasury of our thought. And even though toward the latter part of the nineteenth century we developed a very elaborate concept of the spiritual man as contrasted with the physical man, the Renaissance, the plays of Shakespeare, are full of awareness of bowels and guts in relation to feeling. The important addition that our time can bring to this awareness is to show that these phenomena have some demonstrable relation to symptoms and illness and tissue change. It is about these matters that I would like to spend the next hour.

Let us consider some of the evidence in our language that men have been aware of these combinations. Applied to the vasomotor system we have such phrases as "red in the face," "hot under the collar," "pale with rage," "the pink of condition"; applied to respiration—"takes one's breath away," "sighed heavily with passion," "his nostrils dilated with rage"; applied to sweat—"went into a cold sweat," "cold hands, warm heart," "he has cold feet," "dripping with suspense"; applied to the gut—"nauseating experience," "it makes me sick," "it turns my stomach," "had a lump in his throat"; in *Henry VIII* Shakespeare refers to Wolsey as "a man of an unbounded stomach." We say, too, "his hair stood on end," "it made his flesh creep," "he's a pain in the neck," "it's a gripe," "he trembled with fear," "he shook with rage," "he had the jitters," "stiff-necked fellow," "he became weak with laughter," "keep a stiff upper lip," "faint heart never won fair lady," and, in current popular slang, "it was a headache." These matters are known to engineers; for example, if a thousand people go to a moving picture theater they sweat approximately a hundred pounds of moisture in one hour under ordinary conditions, and that is taken care of by ventilation engineering; but under the emotionally charged circumstances of a thriller, the moisture rises to a hundred and fifty pounds, that is from a hundred to a hundred and fifty pounds. Kleitman has shown that as a man listens to a rather dull or formal lecture in mathematics, viewed coolly and with detachment, his body temperature may drop a degree, but if he's viewing an impassioned dramatic episode on the screen or on the stage it may go up a degree or a degree and a half.

What I propose to do this morning is to point out certain indications that these interrelations are of much more than passing significance to us as doctors, for if tissue changes, like the blush of an embarrassed girl, persist too long in certain parts of the body, and are associated with other changes there may be irreversible changes which carry us frankly into the category of structural alterations.

Let's start with changes in temperature of the skin (1).* Put a lively, interested, energetic young woman, who likes to do problems, into a constant-temperature room and give her a problem as to where two trains starting from different cities and approaching each other at variable speeds will pass. Charge her to solve the problem in a certain number of minutes. While she is doing this, the operators in the room carry on a cross-conversation in voices just strong enough to interfere with concentration and yet not strong enough to allow her to hear all of what they are saying. Under this conflict situation, with the subject doing as well as she can in a category in which she wishes to do well, there will be a gradual drop in the finger temperature from 34° C. to 24°, or about 2° or 3° below room temperature, which obviously represents the sweat reaction in addition to the vasomotor reaction. At this point she is told that the problem is insoluble, to let it go, and the temperature of the finger returns to its initial level within

* Data drawn from experimental observations in the laboratories of Cornell University Medical College were presented on the screen throughout this lecture. Space limitations make it impossible to report and illustrate this material fully here, but a brief bibliography will be found at the end of the chapter for the convenience of readers who wish to pursue the subject further.

twenty minutes. Under the same physical circumstances she can rest in this room without any change in skin temperature; she is adequately covered so that she maintains a balance as regards the temperature of her hands. If you take another woman, who puts no value upon doing well with problems about railroad trains that are approaching each other at a given speed, there will be no such reaction. To carry this a step further, we experimented with the first subject on different days with the same stimulus situation, under the same circumstances of temperature, in the same room, and in the presence of the same people. The problem was to repeat six digits forward and backward. On one occasion she did this task with a finger temperature drop of $7+^\circ$ and on another with a finger temperature drop of about 3°. That looks as though the reaction were entirely unpredictable. But when we looked into the situation we found that this able young woman, who likes to do well at this kind of digit procedure, or likes to use her wits, lives at home with an aunt who is entering or is in the early phase of a senile mental disorganization. This aunt, with whom the subject has lived for many years, is an extremely irritable, moderately depressed, and impulsive woman. There are certain days when this difficult person is able to injure our subject, by word of mouth or implication, so that she approaches the laboratory in a rather tense mood, already on the defensive; whereas, on other occasions, when everything is going smoothly at home, we have an entirely different reaction.

Now here is a very significant observation in relation to the ordinary patient-physician problem. We have studied finger temperature changes in the same woman sitting first in the presence of Dr. A and then in the presence of Dr. B. Dr. A engenders in her a feeling of security; she is not jeopardized. On the other hand, Dr. B may at any moment ask her questions that are embarrassing and that touch on topics that she doesn't wish to discuss. During an hour with Dr. B she sits with cold, sweaty hands, but with Dr. A she has warm hands. This type of reaction we are all familiar with in relation to blood pressure. One doctor will take a patient's blood pressure and find it within average limits; the same day another physician will find it elevated. Three months later, when our subject has come to know Dr. B and feels that he is not quite as hazardous as she thought at first, she is able to sit in his presence for almost an hour with a relatively secure feeling, as evidenced by the temperature of her fingers, which remain warm. But as soon as Dr. B starts to ask the woman questions the temperature of her fingers falls, just as it did at first, when she merely sat in his company. She is only partly desensitized to the implied threat of Dr. B. In other experiments we chose what we considered bland reading matter to allow the individual to maintain a controlled, relaxed condition. Then we chose reading matter that we thought was highly charged and would disturb anyone; this had to do with accidents on the highway, descriptions of bloody decapitations, steering wheels driven through livers, heads smashed through windshields, and so on. The woman we were observing read this material without any reaction that we could detect, saying that she read this sort of thing every day and that it didn't matter to her at all. Then we gave her the bland reading matter—which happened to be an address by President Roosevelt made on the occasion of the dedication of a hospital in Jersey City (it would seem to be as benign as anything could be)—and the woman had a sharp drop in finger temperature. Behind that reaction was the story of two brothers living at home, laborers on some kind of work ration that was being given out at the time. The patient felt that the brothers were not appreciative of the gift that society, and the President more especially, had given them, whereas they felt resentful that they were obliged to be doing something that wasn't acceptable, and that they couldn't be employed at what they considered proper work. So the words of President Roosevelt, indeed the very name of President Roosevelt, were charged topics in that household.

Now we jump from people who have no obvious disease to a woman who comes in complaining of the fact that under certain circumstances her hand gets blue and painful. Indeed her hands are painful a good deal of the time and the nails are beginning to look abnormal. She has Raynaud's syndrome. We put her in a constant-temperature room, at 20°, and allowed her to lie quietly on the table. She maintains a finger temperature as high as that of any healthy person. Then a physician enters the room and discusses basic problems of her life with her, very much as you have done in the clinic during the last few days. She has had several husbands; she has children by some of them; her financial state is very uncertain; her days are spent in going to court to get allotments from this or that husband; there is always too little coal to heat the apartment; she is lonely; her children are doing badly; and in general she gives one the impression of a timid rabbit swimming wildly in a stream that it cannot manage. She is a frightened, insecure creature. Under the circumstances of this interview the finger temperature dropped to the temperature level of the room or slightly below and she had an attack of blueness of the fingers and pain that brought her to the hospital. Then, because of her discomfort, the interview was terminated; she was reassured, and again she was able to warm her hands.

I'd like to show you how this situation is dependent in part on the physical environment in which the organism finds itself at the time. When this same person rested in a room temperature of not 20° to 24°, but 26°, there was again a drop in temperature at the beginning of the interview, but because she was then in what we might call Florida weather, she went down only to a point which was not particularly low and had no symptoms. She had some vasoconstriction, but not enough to produce her symptoms. In summer or in a warm climate she would manage her problems a little better than in winter or when in a cold place. Two entirely different sets of factors, therefore, join to produce a symptom which ultimately brings on her clinical problem.

I think perhaps there are a few simple points that we can carry over from these skin studies to a discussion of another organ, namely, the stomach. The simplest relation of feeling and bodily function in regard to the stomach and the duodenum is seen in the blood flow and contractions. We have a complicated way of recording blood flow to the duodenum but this is a difficult and indirect technical procedure, and all of us like to do things directly if we can (2). Direct observations were made possible by our finding a man with a large abdominal stoma (3, 4). The story is that this man, now fifty-nine years old, came home one night when he was a child aged nine, thirsty and hot after playing on the streets. Finding on the back of the stove a large beer can filled with what he thought was cold beer, he grasped the beer can and took a large mouthful of what he hoped would be cool, frothy stuff; but instead he had to swallow a large mouthful of scalding-hot clam chowder. During the next few months and years many attempts were made to expand his partially occluded esophagus, but with the passage of time it became apparent that this was not going to be possible. He was brought to the hospital malnourished and scared. The surgeon planned to make a small stoma and feed the child for a while through this opening and then ultimately to close the stoma after suitable arrangements had been made in the esophagus. For various reasons, however, the child did badly at the operating table, and the operation had to be hastily concluded. So instead of getting a small stoma, this child was left with a large opening and a generous collar of mucous membrane on the outside. This man grew up, worked, got married, had children, and conducted himself as a responsible citizen for the next half century. He is a shy, sensitive, lively little man, quick to anger, quick to forgive, unschooled, responsible, overly conscientious. He became a *Diener* in our laboratory and the plan was that he'd come in every morning without having breakfasted, put himself on a table, and allow us to look in the stoma. After preliminary observations we'd discuss with him the important events of the last twenty-four hours, his attitudes about them, whether things were going well at home at night, what his feelings were.

Tom is a man of few words, but he is nevertheless articulate in the sense that sooner or later you know exactly what Tom feels. He has the ability to communicate. I can mention only a few of the observations we have made with his help. On one occasion, when he was resting on the table in a relatively relaxed state, with a redder stomach than usual—which we have learned to associate with some anxiety on his part—one of my associates entered the laboratory, saying, "Where is that protocol? It's important. I put it here last night and I can't find it anywhere." He went through the laboratory rummaging, opening one cupboard after another, muttering imprecations. Our subject, who was responsible for the care of protocols and other material in the laboratory, became frightened and got paler and paler in the stomach and in the face. Then my associate opened a drawer, found the protocol, and said, "There it is," slammed the drawer, left the laboratory—and our subject began to look pinker in the face and his stomach resumed its former state (Fig. 1). That's typical of fear reaction—abject, uncompli-

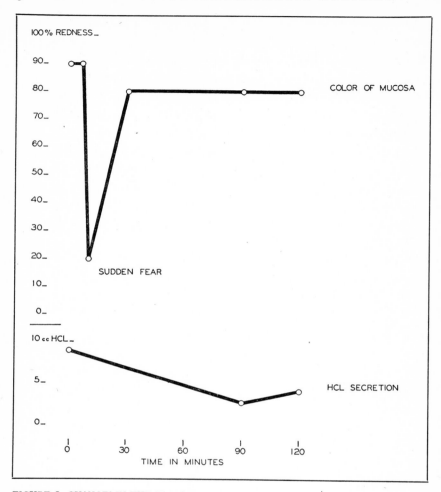

FIGURE I. CHANGES IN THE STOMACH ASSOCIATED WITH FEAR*

cated, without conflict. He said, "I thought I had lost my job," which meant to him a great deal more than the loss of money, although that too was important.

The picture is different under circumstances of resentment and rage. To round out a rather small salary, this man was cleaning the apartment of a member of the medical school staff. Tom did not know much about

* From Stewart G. Wolf and Harold G. Wolff. Human Gastric Function. New York, Oxford University Press, 2nd ed., 1947.

cleaning apartments and he was slow, ineffective, and costly in terms of
the help available at the time. So my associate was going to fire him.
This was done under laboratory circumstances. When he fired him, he
told Tom about his deficiencies. Tom got red in the face, saying, "Yes,
sir," "No, sir," not expressing his anger in words, but exhibiting it by
the color changes. Yet when my associate left, Tom was boiling with
anger and said, "I could choke that man," as a final comment on the
subject. The gastric mucosa got red, the hydrochloric acid secretion
increased, motility increased (Fig. 2). Here you have then a response
of hyperfunctioning, with anger, conflict, resentment, which may last a
matter of minutes or days, weeks, or months. Usually Tom quickly
blows his top, and then his anger is ended. The situation may be sustained, however, and the stomach function disorder may be sustained.

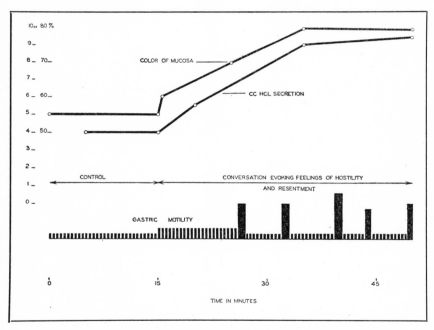

FIGURE 2. CHANGES IN THE STOMACH ASSOCIATED WITH HOSTILITY AND RESENT-
MENT*

* From Stewart G. Wolf and Harold G. Wolff. Human Gastric Function. New
York, Oxford University Press, 2nd ed., 1947.

Tom has a benefactor who gives him a certain amount of money to round out his small income. Tom resents this benefactor because, like many benefactors, this one feels free to meddle in his personal affairs and tell him how to spend his money. He is not being deprived of love or security but he is being deprived of exercising his right to function in the way that he wants to. Following a visit from his benefactor, the stomach has a high color which persists for two weeks.

When there is a high color in the exposed mucosa, the tissue bleeds easily. Whether that's due to the fragility of the walls of the distended minute vessels we're not quite certain, but this seems quite probable. After sustained resentment one can see many small hemorrhages, scattered everywhere over a wet, hot-looking, shiny, engorged mucosa. If the situation is left to itself the hemorrhagic spots spontaneously disappear. If you interfere in any way with the protective action of the mucus, say by putting a little wall of petrolatum about such a spot and allowing the gastric juice, hydrochloric acid, and pepsin to act on it, you can easily produce an ulceration (4). However, when you again allow the mucus to flow over that area, within three days there is no sign of such a lesion on the surface. Unfortunately during the period of noxious stimulation of the mucosa by the action of the acid and juice there is a vicious cycle started in which both increased color and increased acid production result. So once the lesion is started, a self-perpetuating cycle due to the presence of the lesion is established.

What has been observed in Tom is relevant to others. In a patient studied by conventional methods we have seen three levels of gastric acidity at three different times; one associated with a period of relative security, one with relative insecurity, one with extreme insecurity in which he was being pursued by the police (5). He is a professional beggar, and his begging is part of a pattern of getting even with society for supposed injuries that he sustained as a child and as an adult. He insisted on coming into the hospital via the private entrance and then coming up in the private patients' elevator. The doorman knew of our work with him and never interfered. However, on one particular day he found a stranger at the door, a substitute doorman who, not knowing our subject, sent him to the back entrance, so to speak, and up by the outpatient elevator. The man entered the laboratory in a humiliated, resentful state, and with a small amount of fresh blood in his stomach which was greatly increased during the interview. When the topic was rediscussed, bleeding was renewed. Whether this was bleeding around the already existing ulcer or the breaking up of a small blood vessel in the now engorged mucosa, we don't know, but it seems clear that this man's reaction, like Tom's, includes the stomach. One man will use his stomach more than another; this man, under circumstances of insecurity or conflict, has the kind of mucosa that behaves in this way. I wish to emphasize that it is not his emotion *per se* but his situation that does this; his reaction includes feeling and changes in the stomach.

Let's turn to something akin to this, to the symptom of halitosis. A woman we studied produces, under relatively optimal circumstances, about 30 cc. of saliva in a two-hour period. In Tom's esophagus we have a closed tube, so that we can easily collect the saliva produced simply by pouring it into a bucket. The normal production runs about 50 to 70 cc. under optimal circumstances. Under these circumstances our patient is relatively relaxed and the halitosis, though present, is very slight. When our female subject comes to the laboratory feeling slightly anxious, and inarticulate about it, the saliva is much reduced, the halitosis moderately severe. On one such occasion we gave her amytal intravenously. She then told us a good story of her bitterness and resentment about a situation at home and her chances in life; this interview actually cut down the amount of saliva and there was greatly increased halitosis. I can't say whether halitosis is strictly a function of the mouth, but certainly there is a close relationship between the quantity of saliva, the degree of halitosis, and changes in life situation and emotional state in this particular woman.

The nose is an organ that is easy to study; by means of the colorimeter and by criteria of secretion, swelling, and obstruction you can follow changes in the nasal mucosa. In the case of the nose, as elsewhere, some people react more than others, but we'll postpone deciding why some are nose reactors and some stomach reactors. I think anybody who knows anything about human beings at all will agree that the nose is associated with strong feelings. I have a few indications of some of these connections (6).*

* Several cases presented diagrammatically are omitted here.

Daily observations on nasal function and structure, including changes in circulation, size of the turbinates, secretion, and evidences of obstruction and pain, were made on healthy and on diseased persons. Daily records were also made of the subjects' life situations, attitudes, dominant emotional reactions, effectiveness, energy, fantasies, and dreams. Chronologic relationships of the two sets of observations were then formulated. The subjects could be classified as reactors and nonreactors in the sense that the changes in the nose in relation to life situations were far greater and more frequent in some persons than in others.

Although swelling of the turbinates and mucosal vasodilatation often paralleled each other, there was also observed a dissociation of function, in that swollen turbinates were noted in one side of the nose with mucosal vasoconstriction in the other. Mucosal edema and pallor sometimes followed prolonged mucosal vasodilatation.

Chilling of the body surface (remote from the nose) was associated with initial mucosal vasoconstriction (pallor), swelling of the turbinates and increased secretion, followed by mucosal vasodilatation, prolonged swelling, increased secretion and obstruction, until the chilling was removed.

Abject fear, dejection, and disgust were likewise associated with vasoconstriction, or pallor, of the nasal mucosa, decreased secretion and shrunken turbinates. On the other hand, conflict with anxiety, resentment, frustration, anger, and rage were associated with vasodilatation, or redness, of the mucosa, swelling of the turbinates, increased secretion and obstruction. When the latter emotional states were sustained, the associated nasal changes, which were at first usually predominantly unilateral, became bilateral. Also, when swelling and obstruction persisted, pain and tenderness sometimes occurred, spreading over the zygoma and into the temporal region.

Frank weeping, as well as the feeling of being on the verge of tears, associated with frustration and resentment, was accompanied by pallor and extreme swelling of the nasal mucosa, profuse secretion and obstruction, with complaints of difficulty in breathing. These observations indicate the relation of such sustained swelling, vasodilatation, increased secretion, and obstruction with pain, to disease of the nose and the paranasal spaces.

Even in Tom, if you look at the stomach and the nose at the same time, you'll find that when he is disgusted a simple reaction of nausea is associated with pallor in the stomach and pallor in the nose; when he is very angry—as he was one day because someone on the street car was reading a newspaper in which he was described, and was laughing about it—he has a red nose and a red stomach and a nose bleed. If you read any of the old textbooks in medicine you will see it mentioned that nose troubles are probably a cause of peptic ulceration. I suggest that they may both be manifestations of the individual's troubles.

In the case of the stomach a bad situation associated with anxiety and conflict may lead to mucous changes and possibly ulceration; in the case of the nose a situation of insecurity, loneliness, or rejection, often associated with weeping, may lead to occlusion, symptoms from occlusion, and perhaps secondary infection due to the closed ostia. The latter pattern results in a kind of closing out.

Faulkner demonstrated by looking in the bronchoscope that in the average person in the average optimal state of relaxation or relative security, the bronchus will appear full-rounded, with a slight movement of the wall with respiratory movement; whereas if, with the instrument in place in an elderly, insecure man, he suggested a situation of insecurity, the bronchus became small, immobile, and appeared wet. Then if he could reassure the old man that nothing much would happen to threaten him, he got a dilatation and opening up of the airways. It looks as if the individual, with weeping and insecurity, with edema in the nose, is shutting out a noxious environment as much as he can. As we have seen in these weeks, we pluck from our past various patterns or reactions that have helped us in one way or another. Usually they are inappropriate, and we are left with a closed nose, for example, and not much change in the environment or improvement in the situation.

We are so put together as organisms that we are capable of reacting to symbols as though they were in themselves significant biological events. Hence all we need in later life is a symbol that is associated with an earlier trauma to set us off. It may be very trifling. As we learn more about people and how they use symbols, and what the important dynamic factors in early life are, we will attach an entirely different significance to what now seem to be superficial stimuli.

Now I'd like to change the line of investigation completely and describe to you some studies on the heart and the vascular apparatus (7). The method used is as follows. A group of individuals living their workaday lives were brought into the laboratory daily at the same time. A basic reading was made of the pulse, the blood pressure, the minute volume of the heart, stroke volume, and the ventilatory efficiency (that is to say the volume of air that had to be breathed in order to get the necessary oxygen out of it). A variety of other tests were done from time to time. Our notion was (and it was soon confirmed) that the average individual, working under the daily stress of home and the job, would probably not show many variations in his basal level. That is to say, if he came into the room at the same time, and apparatus and circumstances were the same, there wouldn't be much change. But if you put a slight additional burden on that man—the simpler and the more reproducible the better—namely, a simple physiological burden, perhaps you could bring out day-to-day variations. The simple task that we put on these subjects was that of walking up steps a standard number of times— the simplest uniform burden that we could imagine. We recorded the pulse and blood pressure just before exercising, one minute after exercising, two minutes after, three minutes after, and ten minutes after. We computed ventilatory efficiency, the cardiac output, and the stroke volume (using the ballistograph). Remember that these men and women were all doing their work. They would have said, "I'm fine," in answer to a casual question. There was no difference from day to day that anyone would notice. But when the person had appraised his mood—how he slept the night before, whether there were any dreams, whether he was aware of any anxiety or any insecurities or tensions—when the matter was carried beyond the superficial "How are you?" and when the situation each individual was living in was brought out by an interview which followed the standard test, it was perfectly apparent that there was enormous variation in these healthy, average men and women at work.

Figure 3 shows a rather typical situation. The individual has been asked to give an address. He happens to be a teacher, talking is his job, and so the basic situation is that he is simply given a special task to do, one to which he is accustomed. But he is uncertain first of all as to the

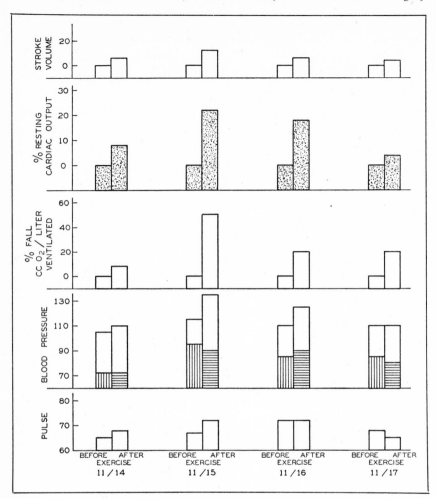

FIGURE 3. CARDIOVASCULAR CHANGES (AFTER EXERCISE) ASSOCIATED WITH ANXI-
ETY, FRUSTRATION, AND ANGER RELATED TO THE GIVING OF A LECTURE ON NO-
VEMBER 15. THE PER CENT FALL OF OXYGEN UTILIZED PER LITER OF AIR VEN-
TILATED (THIRD LINE OF CHART) REFLECTS A DECREASE IN VENTILATORY EFFI-
CIENCY*

kind of audience that he is going to address. He is in doubt, first, because
the audience is a lay audience; secondly, he is not sure whether the

* From George A. Wolf, Jr., and Harold G. Wolff. Studies on the nature of
certain symptoms associated with cardiovascular disorders. *Psychosomatic Medicine*,
8: 293–319, September–October 1946.

thing is being done under the proper auspices, at any rate whether what he is going to say will be understood or badly utilized or publicized, or whether he is being exploited. He is in conflict about whether the whole thing is worth while. November 15 is the day the address is to be given. You see he is under tension, his blood pressure responses are now different, his cardiac output is different, stroke volume is different. Then the address was given and it was a flop. The arrangements were poor, the audience in no way was the sort that would be capable of receiving the information that he was able to impart. He felt humiliated, angry, let down; the whole thing had been a waste of time and his energy had been misspent. The next day he was extremely bitter and sarcastic about the whole thing, he had a hang-over; but he was still operating, doing the same task at a much higher output in energy; then at the end of three or four days he began to see the humor of the situation, let go his tension, and got back to work on a normal basis. During this time this individual was doing everything in his daily life at a greater cost as regards his cardiovascular system.

Take another instance—that of a woman who gains her personal security largely through a conviction of overwhelming and superior health and her loyalty to her friends. She has to be conspicuously loyal to people and expect the same of others or her whole system totters. That's obviously a caricature, but for purposes of discussion those are the two matters that I wish to bring into focus. She has an alcoholic friend. This alcoholic friend asked if she might live in the home of the subject. At first the subject said yes; but when she realized the difficulties of managing a chronic alcoholic in an ordinary household, she wrote her friend, after many hours of conflict, saying that she was sorry but there wasn't any opportunity, no room available at the time, and so on. Feeling very guilty about the whole matter, she went to bed and dreamed about people pointing fingers, pencils, and other things at her (which I thought was the pointing of the finger of shame—there may be other interpretations). Obviously she was a very guilty person indeed. Figure 4 shows that on the next day she had considerable blood pressure response to the simple step test and enormous difference in her cardiac output and stroke volume. As I said before, this woman is doing her work, she has no complaints, she feels perhaps a little "nervous," as she puts it, but not until the whole story is pieced together do you see

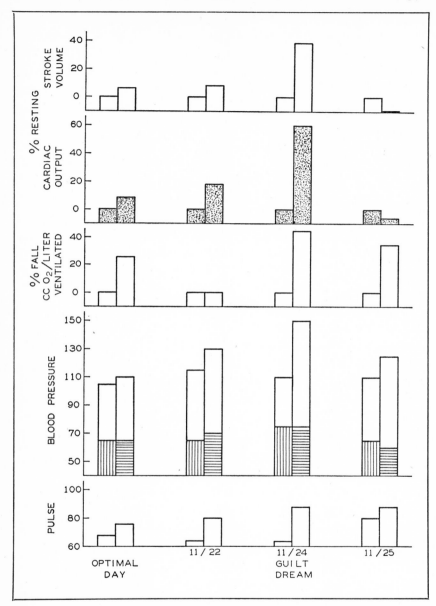

FIGURE 4. CARDIOVASCULAR CHANGES (AFTER EXERCISE) ASSOCIATED WITH CON-
FLICT AND A DREAM OF GUILT*

* From George A. Wolf, Jr., and Harold G. Wolff. Studies on the nature of
certain symptoms associated with cardiovascular disorders. *Psychosomatic Medicine*,
8: 293–319, September–October 1946.

the background and the pressure under which she is operating to perform her daily job. Multiply that by months and years and you can see the load which this individual would carry if this were her usual way of life. Fortunately she is by nature a placid person who accepts her own deficiencies, and pretty soon she is back where she was at first.

These are both what we might call hyperdynamic responses. Some subjects meet tension, anger, or resentment by pressor responses, increased stroke volume, increased cardiac output, or pulse increases, or by all these phenomena together. We have seen these responses in the characteristic premenstrual tension of an unmarried woman; in a woman who, as an unusual experience, went to a night club and stayed up all night; in a doctor scared by symptoms suggesting that his child had polio. In a man following a rather routine sequence of daily duties we find differences between the early and later parts of the week; he works under a bigger strain toward the end of the week than after the week-end.

These measurable differences in response to a given standard test do not take the same form in different people. One is a pulse reactor, another a blood pressure reactor. What makes a person one rather than the other is a question that we have been trying to answer all through this course. Why does the individual pick this organ or that?

Nor is the response to emotional stimulus always on the hyperdynamic side. Figure 5 shows the changes taking place in a person who was pioneering in a field of medicine and research. The first column shows the responses one minute, two minutes, three minutes, and ten minutes after exercise on a maximal day. He was then interviewed by a man who was going to write a general article for a popular magazine on the subject of his investigation. He was in conflict about how much to say, but he was enthusiastic about the importance of the topic and his desire to have his information get in the hands of the public. He allowed the reporter to make statements about his work which, although completely valid and justified in terms of data, was still not in the stage of presentation to the public. He was in conflict as to whether to let the statement go out. His chief, an older person, who usually backed him up completely, added to the burden of his guilt and anxiety about what he did. Our subject felt let down, dejected, beaten, whipped,

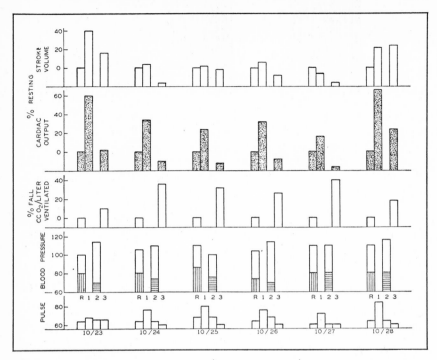

FIGURE 5. CARDIOVASCULAR CHANGES (AFTER EXERCISE) ASSOCIATED WITH A PERIOD OF DEJECTION BEGINNING ON OCTOBER 24. NOTE THE RETURN TO A MORE NORMAL PATTERN ON OCTOBER 28*

unsupported. Note the marked fall in stroke volume and cardiac output. This I think of as a hypodynamic response. It is almost like an opossum reaction, a sham-dead reaction, as though he wished he were done or finished. Figuratively this man had the "heart taken out of him."

I hesitate to make too much of this interesting reaction, or of any specific correlation between mood and the phenomena we have observed. Both the hyperdynamic and the hypodynamic reaction can produce precordial distress. But when you have a displacement in your chest, representing an increased force or cardiac contraction, you complain about it under one set of circumstances and you don't complain

* From George A. Wolf, Jr., and Harold G. Wolff. Studies on the nature of certain symptoms associated with cardiovascular disorders. *Psychosomatic Medicine*, 8: 293–319, September–October 1946.

of it under another set, depending on the general level of apprehension or anxiety in which you live. Let us say only that bodily changes actually occur in company with emotional alterations; they are "real"; and even short of anything we or the patient would call illness, they can add perceptibly to the weight of the physiological load that the body carries.

DISCUSSION

STUDENT. Isn't the psychogenic response to the emotional stimuli a generalized response? Doesn't it have generalized effect on all the tissues of the body?

DR. WOLFF. That is a very interesting question. There seem to be three kinds of reactions. One, I should think, is part of a generalized reaction—that is to say, what is going on in the stomach is probably going on in the hands, in the blood stream, in the heart. That would be akin to Cannon's emergency reaction: the organism in general is set for fight or flight. That is a widespread reaction and seems to involve primarily the sympathetic part of the autonomic nervous system. But these parasympathetic responses—the thing we were talking about this morning—seem to be more local and may be tied up with special patterns. If you put procaine in the stellate ganglion you can produce the picture of vasomotor rhinitis on one side of the nose (on the side procainized): secretion is increased and the turbinates swell. So it looks as if when the sympathetic drops out you are getting a local picture in the nose just like that in weeping and depressed patients. In other words, you can have a generalized response which seems to affect one organ rather nonspecifically and which may not have any special purpose except as part of the total plan of getting away from or getting at the enemy. A second type of reaction is a rather local thing that has some special functions; here in the nose you are closing out the noxious environment by shutting off all the possibilities of taking air or gas in. And, third, you have an individual reacting to change in various degrees, depending on his general state. Minor deviations from the normal may become of major significance if there is some anxiety already present. Little changes in the nose may be the cause of a lot of reaction. About forty per cent of the patients who present themselves with stomach complaints have neither hyperacidity nor hypoacidity; they have very slight changes indeed, hardly enough deviation from the normal to enable you to say that any unusual stimuli are coming from that organ, and yet they will complain of distention, gas, or flatulence. Obviously they are overreacting to minor changes in that organ. The headaches of which some patients complain are associated with minor changes in the contractile state of the muscles of the neck and scalp, enough only to give a sensation of some kind, a little tightness, a fullness; yet these will cause a patient to complain of headache for many years.* The individual is reacting to some defect which, added to all her other troubles, makes life difficult. I am familiar with these three kinds of bodily reactions; there may be a dozen others.

DR. ROMANO.   In our clinical experience with patients with duodenal ulcer the emotional experience is usually much more complex than transitory emotions of disgust or fear or a simple response to external threats.

Many people, clinicians and gastroenterologists and clinical psychiatrists and more lately psychoanalysts, have pointed out that in many instances, particularly in certain social classes, peptic ulcer patients seem to have a need to achieve, to reach out for certain masculine independence goals in a very overdetermined way; they seem to be stepping on the accelerator, riding themselves much more than it seems necessary to do. Further study has revealed that basically one is dealing here with a conflictual area that had to do with dependent-independent need and that actually these people do have dependent needs which are repressed, with a tremendous compensatory overdetermined need to achieve. However, when one works in a municipal hospital as I do, one sees peptic ulcer in patients who have never been successful economically.

DR. WOLFF.   My beggar is an example of such.

DR. ROMANO.   And many of them are psychopaths; many are chronic alcoholics. But in those patients, just as in the more successful group with respect to economic achievement, the conflict situation seems to be the same. Ulcer symptoms often appear to begin when there is a break in the compensatory factor, either when there is frustration of the over-

* For a fuller presentation of Dr. Wolff's conception of headache, see the last five references in the bibliography at the end of the chapter.

compensatory need to achieve or where there is a further block of dependent needs.

DR. BAUER. Some years ago we, too, with the help of Dr. Stanley Cobb, using methods very similar to those of Dr. Wolff, tried to establish some temporal relationship between the onset of arthritis and its exacerbations and remissions. In a large percentage of cases we were able to establish seemingly good temporal relationships between these events and situations of the sort cited by Dr. Wolff. We hope that some day we shall be able to get a better understanding of what actual mechanisms are involved, how these things actually operate in terms of personality.

BIBLIOGRAPHY

1. Bela Mittelmann and Harold G. Wolff. Affective states and skin temperature: Experimental study of subjects with "cold hands" and Raynaud's syndrome. *Psychosomatic Medicine*, 1:271–292, April 1939
2. Charles H. Richards, Stewart G. Wolf, and Harold G. Wolff. The measurement and recording of gastroduodenal blood flow in a man by means of a thermal gradientometer. *Journal of Clinical Investigation*, 21:551–558, September 1942
3. Stewart G. Wolf and Harold G. Wolff. Human Gastric Function: An Experimental Study of a Man and His Stomach. New York, Oxford University Press, 2nd ed., 1947
4. Stewart G. Wolf and Harold G. Wolff. Evidence on the genesis of peptic ulcer in man. *Journal of the American Medical Association*, 120:670–675, October 31, 1942
5. Bela Mittelmann and Harold G. Wolff. Emotions and gastroduodenal function: Experimental studies on patients with gastritis, duodenitis, and peptic ulcer. *Psychosomatic Medicine*, 4:5–61, January 1942
6. Thomas Holmes, Helen Goodell, Stewart G. Wolf, and Harold G. Wolff. The Nose: Experimental Study of Reactions within the Nose in Human Subjects during Varying Life Experiences. Springfield, Charles C. Thomas. In press
7. George A. Wolf, Jr., and Harold G. Wolff. Studies on the nature of certain symptoms associated with cardiovascular disorders. *Psychosomatic Medicine*, 8:293–319, September–October 1946

8. Harold G. Wolff. Personality features and reactions of subjects with migraine. *Archives of Neurology and Psychiatry*, 37:895–921, April 1937

9. Harold G. Wolff. Migraine. *In* Modern Medical Therapy in General Practice, edited by David Barr. Baltimore, William Wood & Company, 1940, page 2068

10. Stewart G. Wolf and Harold G. Wolff. Intermittent fever of unknown origin: Recurrent high fever with benign outcome in a patient with migraine and notes on "neurogenic" fever. *Archives of Internal Medicine*, 70: 293–302, August 1942

11. Donald J. Simons and Harold G. Wolff. Studies on headache: Mechanisms of chronic post-traumatic headache. *Psychosomatic Medicine*, 8:227–242, July–August 1946

12. Harold G. Wolff. Headache and Other Head Pain. New York, Oxford University Press. In press

Case Presentation

I

A PATIENT IN FEAR OF LOSING HER MIND

DR. BAUER. Most of the patients we have seen here have been coming to the clinic for years. They have long clinical records. They may have come originally because of an organic disease, or they may have come because of a neurotic illness. Most of them have been treated on the assumption that they have organic disease, and in such manner as to bring into play many iatrogenic factors—those factors which the physician is responsible for. This we have seen repeatedly in the last two weeks. In some instances treatment had caused either accentuation or fixation of their symptomatology or both. I am sure that you can all look back in your practice and think of patients whom you regret having treated in like manner. You now know that if you had proceeded differently the handling of many of these patients would have been much easier and more satisfactory to both of you.

When a patient comes to you thinking he may have an ulcer (because of what he has read in the health column or what he's been told by a physician) and yet, in taking the history, you feel that he is a neurotic and have evidence for such a diagnosis, your next problem is to inform the patient that many, if not all, of his symptoms are due to the neurosis and not an ulcer. If you think an x-ray examination or other diagnostic studies are needed, you should have no hesitancy in ordering them. If, however, you feel quite certain that the x-ray examination is going to be negative, I think you should tell the patient in advance. Even if an ulcer should be found, you have already indicated to the patient that he has other problems which must be corrected and that the treatment for ulcers which the average textbook recommends will not solve his problems.

With these general comments, then, we'll go on to our first case, which Dr. R. will present.

DR. R. Mrs. Richards* is a thirty-two-year-old married farm woman, mother of three children, who was first seen in the hospital about six months ago. Her presenting complaint at that time was marked fatigue and weakness, from which she had suffered for more than one year. Associated with this were some headaches, pains in the legs, dizziness, and what the patient describes as fogginess and faintness. These symptoms had been present about nine months. Her illness began a year before she came to the hospital, at which time she first noticed increasing weakness and fatigue. She was unable to carry on her ordinary duties on the farm, which included taking care of two children under three years of age. She felt she had to take time off, let the housework slide, make visits to the city to get rest. Each time, on coming back, she felt a little better. This continued for about six months. One day, the date of which she remembers rather well because she was nursing her infant, she and her husband were discussing an episode that had happened a week before when a woman she knew and was distantly related to had been apprehended and taken to a state institution for mental illness. This woman was apprehended by the sheriff as she was patrolling the road in front of her house with a hatchet. She had developed her mental illness after an operation. She lost weight and began to do queer things and say queer things about the house. Eventually she got to the point where she didn't want to see anyone and chased her relatives out of the house when they came to visit her.

While Mrs. Richards was discussing this episode with her husband, she suddenly felt some strange sensations, fogginess, faintness, and dizziness, and she had to stop nursing the child. She became a bit panicky and for the first time wondered if maybe she was losing her mind. She decided she'd better see her doctor, and did so the next day. Her doctor told her that she had a little nervousness that wasn't very serious but suggested that, since it bothered her so much, she come to the city and see a psychiatrist. Coming home from the doctor's office, she had a slight automobile accident. Somebody made a bad turn and she sideswiped another car, apparently due to no fault of her own. The driver of the other car got out and gave her a severe tongue-

* See footnote at page 107.

lashing that she said bothered her quite a bit, but she didn't develop any marked nervous reaction that she could recollect and she was able to drive her car home. On the next day or two she did a little driving, but since that time, up until very recently, she has not driven her car, mainly because, as she says, she's been too weak.

She went to the city and saw a psychiatrist. He assured her that her trouble wasn't very great—that she was a little bit nervous but she'd get over it all right and there was nothing to worry about. In fact, he could hardly see why she was even concerned about it, it was so slight. She went home somewhat reassured, but her weakness and the dizziness and fogginess that came on her in sudden spells continued and she had increasing anxiety about losing her mind.

During this period the woman became increasingly disabled. She didn't want to take care of her children. She felt she couldn't take care of them and was even a bit afraid, as it later developed, that she might possibly do some damage to them. A few months later she returned to her doctor, who treated her for anemia. He continued this treatment when, a few months later, she again returned. All during this period the symptoms I've mentioned became progressively worse. In addition, she had some elevation of temperature, a mild elevation of one or two degrees, and she occasionally noticed a little chilliness but no outright chills.

Six months after her first visit she went back to see the psychiatrist who, on a report from the local physician regarding the anemia she'd been treated for, took a blood count and discovered that her red count was up to seven million. Whether any other tests were made at that time we don't know. The diagnosis of polycythemia was made and she was given some medication for a two-week period. I assume the medicine was phenylhydrazine. She went home with this medication and wasn't seen again during the two-week period. She became progressively and rapidly worse. Finally her doctor went to see her and, finding her remarkably weak and pale, decided she'd better go to the hospital and have another blood test taken. This was done, and her blood count was found to be two million. At this time the phenylhydrazine, or whatever the medication was, was stopped, and the patient was again treated for anemia.

After the red blood cell count was nearly normal, the psychiatrist expressed the desire to resume the phenylhydrazine. The patient was a little bit skeptical about this, saying that she preferred instead to be sent to the hospital. When she finally got into the hospital, two months later, a diagnosis was made of brucellosis, confirmed by blood culture and agglutination titer of about 1 to 1200. She was treated for about three weeks with sulfadiazine, the blood cultures became negative, and the agglutination titers dropped to a level of 1 to 100. In the hospital she had one episode of nervous tension that we know of. She was in the ward with an older woman who was seen in consultation by a member of the psychiatric service. This interview caused Mrs. Richards to become remarkably upset, particularly so when after the interview the other patient expressed disgust and said, "Why don't these people mind their own business and stay away from me?" This seemed to bother Mrs. Richards quite a bit until she was transferred to another room, where she felt a bit more comfortable.

Mrs. Richards was discharged from the hospital after about three months. She went home feeling a little better, but her fear of losing her mind was still quite marked and her weakness persisted. She'd make an attempt for a day or two to take care of her children and the house, and then she'd have to send them back to her mother, although she was rather anxious about the care they would have there. It was a matter of last resort, however, for the patient could not do any work herself.

Another cause of anxiety for the patient during this whole period of illness was the fact that everyone assured her that there was very little wrong with her. Her friends and her relatives, as well as her doctor, said there was nothing wrong and told her she always looked in excellent condition. She did present a rather favorable appearance, and the relatives always criticized her more or less for complaining all the time. Since her discharge from the hospital she's been back on several occasions for checks by the medical service. They've always found her to be in excellent condition. At no time have any physical abnormalities been discovered, except the temperature elevation in the early part of the disease. The medical outpatient department decided to have her come in for a psychiatric consultation. This accounts for her presence in our clinic.

I saw her for the first time on the first day of the course, and I've seen her about four or five times since then. In attempting to elicit etiology for these persistent symptoms I did a moderate amount of probing, some of which was quite disturbing to the patient. She's the type of person who is very placid, very cooperative, quiet, attempts to answer everything as carefully and as truthfully as she can, never expresses resentment for any of the situations that have been detrimental to her, such as the treatment she's had by various doctors and so forth. She has never expressed any direct or implied criticism of the doctors, always excuses them, and says they did the best they could and she's appreciative of that. In my interview with her it was very difficult to get any concrete information, but I'll tell you the history that I got on the first interview.

This woman's past medical history is essentially negative. She had mumps and measles in childhood, not severe. A few years ago she had something that was called arthritis or neuritis and was given some "shots" for that and recovered. Shortly after the onset of the present illness she was injured—kicked rather severely by a cow in the region where she has many of her present aches and pains.

Her family history does not reveal anything significant as far as I could learn. She is the oldest of three, the others being a sister and a brother. She had much of the responsibility of caring for these younger children when she was a child. Her father died when she was twenty-one. Her mother is living and well and has remarried. The patient finished the eighth grade in school, at about the usual age. She was married when she was eighteen years old and has had three children, the oldest of whom is thirteen and the others under three. The reason for the large gap between the oldest child and the second one the patient explains as due to the exigencies of the depression years, when she and her husband decided not to have any more children and used contraceptive devices.

On superficial questioning the patient did not express any difficulties associated with her marital life except those due to her present illness. Their financial situation was poor during the depression years, but during and since the war they have gotten along rather well. While they have a moderate amount of debts they have no great worries over financial matters. Socially this woman seems to be rather well accepted by the community. She has friends. She has gone to church regularly except during the present illness, when she was too weak. She seems to be fairly well adjusted. She's been a very active person, very vigorous. She likes hunting, fishing, trapping. For recreation, aside from visiting her friends, she does a little reading in magazines like *True Story*.

Those are most of the facts that I gained during the first interview. In subsequent interviews, when I asked her what she thought about the interviews and our whole procedure, she was her usual courteous self, but she freely admitted that she didn't feel nearly so comfortable now and was a little bit more anxious than she had been in the past. At least the other doctors who had talked to her had always been able to re-assure her and make her feel a little bit better for a while, but I only made her feel worse. In each visit she felt a little bit worse, depending on how far I probed.

On her next-to-last visit—the day before yesterday—I was able, just before the end, to pick up something that I thought was a very im-portant clue. I asked her if she had any sexual relations before she was married. After being just a little taken aback she said, well, yes, that's why she got married. She'd been engaged to the man for some time and it was just one of those things that happened. She was rather up-set about telling me that. During our most recent interview, yesterday, she expressed the idea that if a certain thing hadn't happened the day before she had definitely planned to make this her last visit to me, for I'd been making her so uncomfortable that her complacency had been disturbed. Rather straightforwardly and accurately she said that she had a fairly good notion about what kind of person she was. She had led a pretty good life aside from this one mistake. But the probing that I had done had made her begin to question whether she was such a nice person. She had talked it over with her husband, and he couldn't see the sense of all this questioning and advised her not to come back even for this last interview. She thought, however, that in all justice and fairness to me she should come back and tell me it was going to be her last visit.

One other point that should be brought out is this. During one of the earlier interviews Dr. Schiele asked her a rather innocent question,

"Why did you get married?" She was rather upset about that and began to cry. This question was asked at about the same time that she had made a reply to another question about not being able to take care of her children. "It's not as though I don't want to take care of them, as though I don't like them," she had said. The two questions came so close together that I think both sides got a little bit confused about which was which and why she began to cry. When I questioned her later as to why she cried she said she thought that Dr. Schiele and I thought that she was a poor mother who didn't like her children. This was the only time she expressed any emotion during any of the interviews.

Now one of the reasons I thought I was hot on the trail of something was that during the first interview all these things that had happened—the whole story that had involved her so much and her whole family and her children—was so terribly important to her that she spoke for nearly the whole hour, and yet she never once mentioned her husband. He was so conspicuous by his absence that I thought surely there was something pertinent there and that's why after one or two more visits I decided to probe along that line. Yesterday when Dr. Romano and Dr. E. joined me in conference with her, I again became the bull in the china shop and tore this thing out into the open, even though Dr. Romano tried to put the soft pedal on it and stop me from doing it. I sort of insisted on bringing it out, and she was a little upset by that. Yesterday Dr. Romano was able to bring out several things during the interview that hadn't come to light before.

I might say also that several days ago I felt that she had been improving somewhat and didn't quite realize it. So I recommended that she try to drive the automobile again as a step toward doing something positive. Yesterday she told me she had driven her automobile at the challenge of her thirteen-year-old daughter, who said, "Why don't you take the car into the garage, mother?" So she drove it down to the mailbox, turned around, drove it back, and put it in the garage. She felt mighty proud of that and pleased to see her daughter's amazement. She was very proud of that accomplishment. I, perhaps, didn't appreciate how much this action meant to her. When she told me about it, I said very calmly, "Well, that's nice. You've done very well." But

Dr. Romano and Dr. E. picked up the ball and threw it back and forth and had her feeling that she had done the most wonderful thing in the world right there and that it was the turning point of her life. Immediately there was more rapport between them and the patient than there had been between her and me during the whole time.

One other point that Dr. Romano stressed and brought out was her attitude toward the woman friend who had become insane. In addition, he asked her whether she'd had such a feeling or experience in childhood. Yes, as a matter of fact, she said, when she was about thirteen years old or a little bit younger there was a woman in the next county who'd gone berserk and had taken her little child and chopped him up into little pieces, buried him under a pile of leaves, and then brought her husband over to see the child. She's always had that memory and has always associated mental illness with that kind of behavior. Well, in the first place, Dr. Romano was able to sympathize with her in a much more active, positive way than I was. I could sit there and say, "That's pretty tough—you had a tough time." But his heart bled for her. It made all the difference in the world, and she could see that at last she had found someone who really knew how she felt. All this time the doctors and her friends had been telling her that there was nothing wrong with her, and that had aroused doubts in her mind about her own mental stability. Then I had come along. I hadn't even reassured her; I had just made her feel miserable. Then she found Dr. Romano and was happy. I don't mean to be facetious; it was a very striking thing to me.

Before I go on to the second thing Dr. Romano was able to do, I must go back one step. The year before she became ill, she had had considerable trouble. Her second child developed an acute intestinal disorder at an early age. The local physician diagnosed it as a kidney disease and said the child would surely die. She wanted to bring the child to the city, but the doctor said, "Well, you can if you want to, but I don't see any sense to it. The child's going to die anyway." For about five days the child had apparently been doing a lot of vomiting and had become markedly dehydrated and was exceedingly sick. As a last resort, she took the child to the city, where a diagnosis was made, the child was operated on, and he made a satisfactory recovery. This was another one of her numerous unpleasant associations with the medical profession, and a time of great stress for her. Shortly after this her husband was temporarily disabled and that threw another burden on the woman. Then some months later another child was sick for quite a long while. This kept her up for days and nights on end. She got to a point where things were so bad that on one occasion (the only time she's ever expressed such an idea) she actually felt she'd like to take that child and shake him, even though she knew he was sick. That was the first time she ever expressed to me any open hostility.

To get back to yesterday's interview—Dr. Romano was able to tie all these things together and to show her that as a child, when this traumatic episode occurred, she had been conditioned to believe that when people go crazy they murder their children. Then there was this woman of her acquaintance who became mentally ill. She couldn't help but get doubts in her mind about her own sanity, for though she felt physically ill people were telling her there was nothing the matter with her. At the time, too, she was much weakened, and was trying to do things she was physically unable to do. Tying all these things in with all the other troubles that she was having with her two young children, Dr. Romano was able to show her they provided a proper setting for the reaction she had had. Dr. Romano was able to reassure her that the feelings she had were perfectly normal for a woman who had been under so much stress. Then he again emphasized this automobile-driving episode and showed her that she was already on the road back. The woman seemed markedly reassured.

After Dr. Romano left, there was one point of significance where I finally got my lick in. The patient told me that yesterday or the day before she had spanked her child—the first time in many, many months or in the past several years that she had been able to do it. She was greatly concerned about such behavior on her part, thinking that maybe she was losing the control she'd been fighting so hard to maintain all this time. I pointed out to her (I hope I did) that actually this was the second point on her road back. Now she was able to spank her child— in other words, to exert some outward aggressiveness without fear that she was going to lose control and perhaps do her child some serious harm.

DISCUSSION

DR. BAUER. When did the undulant fever come into play, do you think?

DR. R. Well, the first symptoms of weakness began nearly two years ago, and I suspect that, as is so often the case with undulant fever, she'd had it a long time before that, although she didn't complain.

DR. BAUER. What role do you think her undulant fever played in her total illness?

DR. ROMANO. I feel that it was a powerful precipitating factor. If she hadn't had the undulant fever, the chances are she could have weathered all these other storms satisfactorily.

DR. BAUER. If you had seen this woman at the time of her hospital entry, would you have been willing to account for all of her symptomatology on the basis of undulant fever?

DR. R. It's quite possible.

DR. BAUER. Any other questions?

DR. ROMANO. I'd like to tie this up before we go on to further discussion. The points that Dr. R. made were the most important ones. We're dealing with a number of variables: first, the nature of the person, who she is, her capacity to deal with daily sources of anxiety, the nature of the emotional defenses she could and did utilize; second, her preparation for illness—which factors were operating shortly before she became sick and during the initial phase of her illness. Essentially these included the birth of two children in a period of two years, the care of the infants, the repetitive and serious illnesses of the children, and her husband's illness. The third set of variables revolved about the onset of undulant fever. Weakness and fogginess probably were indicative of minor and episodic disturbances of consciousness resulting from the effect of undulant fever on cerebral metabolism. A fourth and final set of variables resulted from the patient's witnessing the dramatic acute onset of psychotic behavior in a relative. She and others about her were disturbed about this. The experience mobilized not only the conventional type of anxiety and misinformation concerning insanity and mental hospitals but, more specifically, affected the patient directly.

In this setting this woman began to have difficulty in taking care of her children and of her daily household tasks. They presented serious problems to her. She went for advice not only to her husband but to various doctors who minimized her difficulties. (At least in her opinion they did so; whether they actually minimized them or not we don't know.) She felt they did not recognize her problems. In the face of repetitive inadequacies in dealing with tasks which other people wouldn't recognize, she began to feel, "What's wrong with me? I can't meet these problems and if no one recognizes it but myself, maybe I'm losing my mind, just as these other women lost their minds." Then there was the further fact of that childhood memory of a psychotic woman who had killed her child and buried him under a pile of leaves.

One has, then, the person herself, her preparation for the illness as related to these burdens on her, and then the illness which brought about her inadequacy to meet situations, and with it the feeling of "If this is so, if everyone says I am all right and I can't meet these things, I may lose my mind, and if I lose my mind I may do something to my children such as other people who lose their minds do to children." In that setting a number of fears had their onset—about how she should handle the children, what she should do lest she harm them. Then, of course, further elaboration occurred with the car accident, being scolded, eventually becoming phobic and not driving the car.

One has certain other presumptive data which may relate to this woman's problems, such as what her basic attitude was toward children. For these data, of course, we have little direct evidence. There is the fact, however, that she was the oldest of three children in a family where, at an early age, she had to take care of her younger siblings. What responsibilities she had, how much freedom she had as a child, how many gratifications she had as a child, how quickly she had to grow up and relinquish her childhood, we don't know. But that's one possible set of factors. A second set is, of course, her premarital experience. A mother may have ambivalent feelings in accepting a child who is taboo. A possible third factor is that a long period of contraception, whether dictated by economic factors or not, usually indicates that there are some ambivalent feelings or mixed feelings toward children. Then, of course, there was the birth of two children in a short period of time, and the responsibilities that came with them.

In treating this woman no manipulative program could be followed out. We had no data concerning the environment. We did not speak to the husband or to other members of the family, such as her mother, and we didn't plan any particular regimen for the woman. We were, however, able to operate in three areas with her. We explained some of the normal experiences of sick people; the normal and useful anxiety experienced in illness; its use of preparing the patient to meet the adversity of illness; of the need to withdraw, to become more dependent upon the people who are your friends and helpers, the family, the nurse and doctor. We were also able to tell her about some misconceptions concerning psychotic behavior. Second, as supportive treatment, we were able to reassure her about her illness. The hospital study, reports of examinations, and laboratory tests were used to point out to her that she did have a type of illness which provoked anxiety and weakness. In this case there was no need to use drugs or hydrotherapy, but they are sometimes used as ancillary aids. Third, considerable suggestion was used regarding her present achievement. With our help she was able to release some of the emotional tension of unresolved feelings concerning her past memory and her confusion concerning psychotic patients. We told her that her experiences were normal, that it is possible at times to become somewhat angry or annoyed at a loved person—a husband or child—without feeling that by so doing you may destroy him or be destroyed yourself. Such feelings are not taboo; by feeling anger or hatred one does not destroy or harm the other person. I think those were the chief points we made in our interview with her.

DR. R.   I should add that another part of this woman's phobic reaction was that she refused to read the newspapers or listen to the radio, because every time that she read anything that had to do with destruction, murder, rape, or some such thing, she became exceedingly anxious. I'd also like to say that after Dr. Romano finished explaining all of these things to her and reassured her, she showed a tremendous amount of relief. It was the first time in all the interviews that I saw her show very much reaction; even when she cried, she didn't show as much as here. And in her quiet way one could almost see all this misery melting away. She seemed to feel exceedingly gratified and her reaction seemed to be simple, "I had a problem before, but it is gone now."

DR. BAUER. I'm sure you'll all agree that in this case we're dealing with a patient who obviously had an infectious disease but that treatment of it alone would have been inadequate for the symptoms from which the patient was seeking relief. She apparently received adequate treatment for the undulant fever, the best evidence we have being the fall in agglutination titer. A situation we have all encountered is that of a neurotic patient with multiple symptoms, with or without a slight fever, bearing a diagnosis of undulant fever. In such instances the undulant fever is thought to be the cause of the patient's symptomatology and great effort is made to prove the point. If the blood cultures and agglutination tests are negative, then the physician resorts to doing skin tests. When using the straight vaccine, it is important to keep in mind that you're dealing with an organism which is extremely irritating and capable of causing as marked an intradermal reaction as that obtained with any dead organism, with the possible exception of $E. coli$. Unless one does a control, he's very apt to be misled by the skin tests. Recently we have had available brucellergin, a less irritating agent, and also a protein fraction. The latter gives fewer false positives than any preparation that's been employed to date.

Before doing skin tests on patients suspected of having undulant fever, one should think twice. If you can establish the diagnosis by other means, it is wise to do so for several reasons. First, one can attach no diagnostic significance to agglutination tests that become positive during the ensuing twelve weeks. Such positive tests represent the immunological response to the intradermal injection of the antigen. Unless you are aware of this fact, you may attach diagnostic significance to the positive agglutination test. Second, some patients during the febrile phase of the disease experience extremely marked skin reaction, comparable to the Arthus phenomenon. In such instances sloughing recurs and a chronic ulcer may persist for some months, occasionally as long as a year, so that in those cases where you feel reasonably certain about the diagnosis, especially in the active phase of the disease, it is just as well to forego skin tests. If you do use them, you'd better warn your patients of this possible complication.

STUDENT. Will you say a word or two about the termination of an interview—about ending it in such a way that when the patient leaves you he is not thinking only of his destructive past, but also has some awareness of his assets and real accomplishments to carry him over until the next visit and to assure his return even though his bad dreams and irritability and tension drop off? Will you say a word about that?

DR. ROMANO. With the patient we've been talking about today we emphasized several positive points. We tried to make her realize that the experiences she had had were understandable and were natural phenomena. These experiences were not related to mental disease in any way. We went over her experiences and explained what they were and what had happened. Then we went on to explain that it is natural to have feelings of annoyance toward one's family or one's friends, that it is natural and healthy to have such feelings at times, and even at times to express them without feeling too guilty about it. Next we praised her for what she had accomplished, assuring her that she had already come to the turning point. When she spoke of her achievements in answering her daughter's challenge to drive the car, she added, smiling weakly, "I was tempted to drive the car to town." She felt she could do that; she had no anxiety about doing it. So we used it as a focal point in bringing out the positive factor. "That was excellent," we said. "That means that you are now able to do things, and that in the future you will be able to reach out for more and more of the things you could do before."

We did touch on a number of very sensitive areas. One was her feeling about the child's being born too soon. This was something which had mobilized anxiety and disturbed her delicate equilibrium. Another was indicated by the fact that in reply to questioning she had to make a defensive statement: namely, she had to say, "I want to assure you that I do love my children." That, too, touched on a focal point. I mean, her essential problem was her ambivalent feeling toward her children, which was mobilized and brought out in caricatured form by the illness. That illness made it impossible for her to take care of the children and made her fear she might lose control of herself, which to her was equivalent to going berserk and killing her children.

As to techniques, we have stressed over and over again that as a rule the general physician should stay in the field of reassuring techniques. Even with these techniques the anxiety is sometimes localized. One should try, for the most part, to keep to conscious material. In the interview described today, no material was used which the woman herself did not present. All the interpretations were made on matters which she was able to bring up. In all techniques of medicine, whether surgical intervention or psychotherapy, the principle is that one should never do anything to a person unless one has a reasonably good idea of what one wants to do. In other words, you don't unwrap a person and take away certain defensive covers unless you know what is to be uncovered, what you're going to meet when you unwrap him and how you are going to wrap him up again.

We have stressed that; perhaps we have stressed it too much and have intimidated you. If we have, I think we should not leave it at that. Now there are two fundamental principles in all psychotherapy, in fact in the whole of therapy. First, it is better at times to err in omission rather than in commission. Second, don't reassure a patient or use Pollyanna techniques (don't say, "You are going to be all right; everything is going to be fine," and so on) when you really haven't any understanding of what he is experiencing. If you do, the patient thinks, "How can he say this? I myself don't know what's wrong with me. I don't see what evidence he has to decide what's wrong with me." This is the error in premature or uncritical Pollyanna techniques.

STUDENT. We see quite a bit of brucellosis here, and many times it occurs with the added complication of neurosis. Will you discuss that in more detail?

DR. ROMANO. I think that many times, in brucellosis particularly, the error is made in thinking that the evidence of a positive titer of various dilutions explains the total behavior of the patient. It is important to realize that life is much more complicated than that. In the present case the undulant fever acted principally as a provocative factor. With the illness the patient's defenses crumbled, and this was analogous to what happens in serious emotional problems. The capacity to control forces either within or without the body is lessened or weakened, and the person then feels anxious because he is not able to handle the situation. In this case the undulant fever played the same role as the repetitive traumatic experiences of Dr. Murray's patient. The undulant fever was a provocative agent in that it weakened the controlling or equilibrating forces of the personality.

DR. BAUER. Do you think that what will have been done by tomorrow, when you see this patient for the last time, will be adequate?

DR. ROMANO. I think she'll probably need further help. I don't think she was dragged through a long history of turmoil. I think she gave many of these data in a kind of historical way, and we did not, in explaining things, touch on all her difficulties. We used the knowledge of them but in treatment we kept to the current situation. We didn't discuss the difficulties she had experienced as a mother or her mixed feelings toward marriage and toward her children. No, we didn't go into that at all. We kept to the current situation.

This is another technical point for general practitioners. It may be wise at times to keep to the patient's current problem and not wander too far away. I have a feeling that the woman wasn't too upset by the interviews and that tomorrow we'll see what kind of care and how much care she should have from this point on. Since her husband will come with her tomorrow, we'll try to allay his perplexities and confusions, too. That is another thing a general practitioner can do.

DR. MURRAY. I just want to reinforce the importance of Dr. Romano's point on not trying to counter the symptoms of a patient with Pollyanna reassurances, which may make the patient feel that the thing that is going on in him must be such a bizarre and strange thing that nobody else can meet him on that ground at all. So I think this point is very well taken: be the sympathetic listener until you yourself can formulate the problem and then do something constructive about it.

Case Presentation

II

A PATIENT FACING OLD AGE

DR. BAUER. A member of the class, Dr. P., will tell us about a patient he and Dr. Brosin have interviewed in the clinic during the past week.

DR. P. This patient is a housewife, fifty-six years old. She has been observed at the clinic for the past ten years. She comes in complaining of soreness in the epigastrium, soreness throughout her whole abdominal cavity. She tells me that she has difficulty with her bowels, that they don't seem to empty properly. She has attacks of loose stools about twice a month. They come on for no particular reason. But she also tells me that she does not have digestive distress and that she is able to eat any kind of food and that she has a good appetite. Occasionally she notices little flecks of blood in her stool. I asked her how long she had observed this symptom, and she told me that she had had it from five to fifteen years. In addition to this complaint of bowel distress, she also has had palpitation of the heart for the past four or five years. She says that she has slight shortness of breath on exertion. She also notices that when she worries or feels nervously upset her heart pounds and the trouble with her bowels becomes aggravated.

This woman is a great worrier. She worries about financial matters; she worries about her children; she worries about her husband. She has attacks of feeling blue. She tells me that she has had nothing but trouble all her life. She tells me, too, that she has been nervous all her life. She has had disturbed sleep for the past ten years and she requires some sedative to help her.

As regards her past illnesses, twenty years ago she had an operation for an ectopic pregnancy, at which time a bilateral oophorectomy was performed. Eight years ago she was seen in the clinic because of a small cyst in her right breast. She has returned to the tumor clinic at about

six- to eight-month intervals ever since. Ten years ago she had an operation for hemorrhoids and a fissure.

The history shows considerable disturbance in this woman's family
and home life. When the patient was two years of age her father left
the family and she hasn't heard anything of him since. Four years later
her mother remarried, and after two years this man also left. Her
mother died at fifty-eight. The patient has two brothers and a half
sister. As regards her schooling, she attended school until she was in the
seventh grade and then had to stop and help to support the family. She
did domestic work, had jobs in hotels and restaurants, clerked in stores,
and worked in offices and factories.

At about thirty she married a man many years older than herself,
who is now past seventy. They have three children. She tells me that
she doesn't get along with this husband, that there is considerable friction and always has been. Shortly after they were married her husband
began drinking; he became very irritable at this time and he has remained so during all their married life. She sums this up by saying that
he is "ornery." She further tells me that shortly after she was married
her sex organs went dead on her. They were removed twenty years ago.
In addition, she has always had financial difficulties. At the present
time she is worried about the future, for her husband is soon to be pen-
sioned at $55 a month and she doesn't see how they can get along on
such a small amount. She probably worries more than the average individual would about this.

The patient has attacks of moodiness, attacks of feeling low and blue.
She tells me that at times she has temper outbursts, which do not sub-
side rapidly but hang on for several days. In the second interview she
told me (I asked her if she had any particular worries) that she has
deep fear of cancer. She thinks she has cancer of the bowel. I asked her
why she had picked cancer. She said she doesn't have any particular
reason except that she has noticed these flecks of blood in her stools, she
has discomfort in her abdomen, she has friends that have had cancer.
There is no history of cancer in the immediate family and relatives. The
positive findings on physical examination were an enlarged heart and
an elevation of her blood pressure; one reading was recorded as 200/
130. There was no evidence of congestive failure. The PSP renal func-

tion test was 25 per cent the first hour and 5 per cent the second hour; the concentration tests revealed specific gravities of 1.010, 20, 10, 21, 10, 21. The x-ray of her gastrointestinal tract was normal except for multiple diverticula of the colon. The electrocardiogram showed left axis deviation.

All in all, the main findings regarding this patient are as follows. We have an individual who is fifty-six years of age, who has had a stormy family life. She married a man she didn't like. He has not been kind to her. He is irritable. He has memory defects that are becoming quite prominent and she worries about the possibility that this old fellow is going to be a burden to her someday, that maybe she will have to take care of him. She presents the picture of an individual who is very much depressed; that is probably her main complaint. She has some palpitation of the heart but she tells me that it is aggravated by worry, unhappiness, and these "low feelings." After several talks with this woman, I feel sure that she would not be aware of her hypertension if someone hadn't told her of its presence. As to her bowels, if she had genuine dysfunction I dare say that she would not be able to eat the variety of food that she does. I think those are the main points in this woman's story.

DR. BAUER. Are there any questions anyone wants to ask Dr. P. about the patient before we go on?

STUDENT. I'd like to know how much emphasis the doctor put on diverticulosis?

DR. P. She has not been informed.

DR. BAUER. Any other questions?

DR. P. Her menstrual history—she has had her menopause, had it at thirty-six.

STUDENT. How does she feel toward her children?

DR. P. She loves them very much. A factor I forgot to mention is that her husband insisted that the children be brought up in his faith rather than hers.

STUDENT. Has she ever had any ideas of suicide?

DR. P. Not that I am aware of.

STUDENT. Have there been any difficult situations with the children?

DR. P. No. She says that she is very proud of her children. She has had no difficulty with them. She says they are fine children and co-operative.

DR. BAUER. Her symptoms go back about thirty years?

DR. P. She doesn't set a definite date when this bowel dysfunction commenced. She says, "Oh, five to fifteen years."

STUDENT. How old was she when her sex organs went dead?

DR. P. She was thirty-one.

STUDENT. How much did she talk about her somatic complaint in your interviews with her?

DR. P. These facts that I have told you are what she volunteered without my prodding. She comes in and I ask her what is her difficulty in life, why is she here, and she tells me (and I quote her), "I have soreness in the abdomen." Then she tells me she has so much trouble with her bowels; it seems as though her bowels do not empty right, there is a fullness in the rectum. Those were the main complaints.

STUDENT. She kept coming back to those all the time?

DR. P. That was her main complaint. The only thing of any consequence that I found out in the second interview was that she has this fear of cancer, which she told about on her own initiative and which I think is a paramount issue with her.

STUDENT. Has she ever felt well?

DR. P. Yes. She tells me that she has accomplished a lot of work but has always been moody. She has always had these low spells, but in the last few years, she tells me, they are more or less constant.

DR. MURRAY. Has she ever been able to express resentment against her husband? Has she externalized her frustrations and disappointments?

DR. P. I think so. At least my impression is that there has been constant incompatibility in the family from the time of the marriage, though she didn't say so.

STUDENT. Who seems to get his way most often, she or her husband?

DR. P. It is my impression that the husband is the dominant person. Stubborn, she said he is, and irritable. He has drunk excessively —not so much in recent years but shortly after they were married. And through most of their married life she has had to combat his irritableness. She said that he would become intoxicated, and the intoxication, instead of making him happy, would make his irritability increase. He would come home and wouldn't go to sleep at night, insisting instead on lying awake and arguing about trivialities.

DR. BAUER. What was your first impression?

DR. P. Frankly, the first impression that I had of this patient—she was one of my first—was that she was depressed. She was depressed and dejected and she didn't have much to say, just sat in a slumped position.

DR. BAUER. Are there any other questions? If not, I shall ask Dr. Brosin to discuss this interesting human being.

DR. BROSIN. In contrast to yesterday's beautiful case presentation by Dr. R. and Dr. Romano, the aim this afternoon is not to devote the entire time to the psychological movement of this case but rather to use a patient or two as springboards from which to discuss certain major areas of medical care with emphasis upon the therapeutic possibilities and diagnostic problems. This woman was one of a number that are available.

Probably all of you have patients of advanced age with problems of chronic disease. This case will give you a chance to introduce questions you may have about such cases. It is also an excellent case for discussion here because it involves the problem of estimating the importance of undoubted organic disease, which is the presenting complaint. This woman has had hypertension for at least ten years. The laboratory findings must also be taken into account, as well as the other findings. But that isn't my part of the job. My part, I think, begins with the point that in addition to the chief complaint (soreness of the abdomen, loose stools, palpitation, and slight dyspnea on exertion) we have something added—a cancer phobia. Now what is the meaning of this, how did it start, why should it develop, what does it represent in the woman's economy?

From just a brief acquaintance (I saw this woman only once) I think one can say this is not a true phobia at all. Here is an anxious woman who because of her long acquaintance with physicians, hospitals, and hospital procedure naturally gravitates toward doctors. She focalizes a generalized anxiety, which has a specific social basis not so easy to handle, into a legitimate fear to which people will pay attention —namely, cancer.

During the first week of this course a good many points were made regarding the so-called iatrogenic trauma. Now many of you will review your own history with a clean conscience and say, "Not I. Maybe somebody else did it (the familiar mechanism of projection), but I never scared a patient into an operation because of my own need, and I surely don't encourage belief in the possibility of cancer because my own uncertainties and anxieties are transmitted to the patient." Perhaps you are suave and bland when you intimate to patients the possible presence of a carcinoma, but as members of the medical profession we have a responsibility for the advertising and propagandizing that is going on. I don't mean to decry true medical education in the field of preventive therapy of the carcinomas. But I have heard, even years ago, experts argue whether they were really doing any good, whether they really get many more people into the clinics because of advertising.

I was saying, in a brief and highly oversimplified explanation, that this woman doesn't have a real phobic symptom but does have a generalized anxiety which finds some release through her expression, "I might have a cancer." A further element in this rumination is that it betrays her fear of death. As we talked together, she expressed a good deal of hostility about her husband. I don't think there is any doubt that this depressed woman illustrates the principle we have repeatedly tried to exhibit here—that many depressions (possibly not all but certainly many, if not most) have in them an obvious factor of hostility and anger and aggression turned inward. Some of this woman's hostility is against her husband. She has had a frustrated life; there is really very little for her to have been happy about in her fifty-six years. She made an undesirable marriage in which the husband is a dominating figure. She didn't even have the right to choose her children's religion. Her husband has been periodically drunk and abusive and is chronically irritable; now with the aging process that I have mentioned before he is becoming obviously senile, and she knows that. As we got the story, he is definitely on his way to a psychosis. He is not merely an irritable old gentleman; he is a practically psychotic old gentleman and very hard to live with.

STUDENT. Is the history in accord with that?

DR. BROSIN. Yes. Furthermore, she is keen enough to know this. He has an older brother who is psychotic, so bad that no one can live with him, and our patient verbalizes readily that she can see her husband's future in this brother. You can see that her spot is a bad one. At the age of fifty-six, standing, so to speak, on a mountain peak looking forward to the future at the sundown of her existence, what does she have to face? A psychotic man who has given her endless trouble since her marriage to him twenty-six years ago, children whom she is insecure about, a pension of $55 a month, and no relief in sight. I think that is the general basis for her difficulty; it's the social basis certainly.

Now the specific components on which I think a good deal of therapy can be done are her insecurity about her children (on which we didn't get much significant history), her outright aggression and hostility toward this irritable and senile alcoholic husband, and her feeling of guilt, for she knows it isn't right to hate your husband, especially when he is about to die, even though he has caused you a lot of trouble. Her ruminations about death can be hooked up to this fear of cancer, for which the medical profession may be partly responsible. This is an acute reactive depression. It doesn't have the major components of the true melancholia, the agitated depression, and so on. In therapeutic interviews you can give her guidance, support, catharsis, sympathetic understanding, and perhaps her three youngsters can give her verbal guarantees that they will support her in the event of difficulty. Perhaps the old gentleman can be manipulated around a bit so that he won't be a nuisance to her twenty-four hours a day. Perhaps through the usual types of social relief something can be done for this quite stable woman.

DR. BAUER. Well, here we have an excellent instance of a person who comes to the clinic with obvious organic disease—hypertension which has been present for a long time, for she now has obvious renal impairment. In addition, she has multiple diverticula. Yet it is obvious that the problem that concerns this woman most is not related to the organic disease that she displays. I am sure you wouldn't have to look at this woman very long in order to realize that she is depressed. We would be making a very serious mistake if we told her that her difficulties were due to her hypertension and her diverticulosis. If we prescribed treatment aimed at correcting these two conditions, we'd accomplish very little that would be of help to her. The diverticula represent congenital anomalies which have been present for years. Like all diverticula in the intestinal tract, these are symptomless. They never require treatment unless there is associated inflammation. Many doctors, on finding a duodenal or other intestinal diverticulum, have thought it to be the cause of the patient's symptoms, when in reality they were actually dealing with a neurotic individual who incidentally had a diverticulum. That's a very important point to remember.

This woman does have hypertension, a benign hypertension of probably much longer duration than is recorded. There is little in the way of therapy that we could offer her that will alter the course of the hypertension. Furthermore, she has no symptoms referable to it. If I remember correctly, when we asked her about her shortness of breath we found it was experienced only after going up several flights of stairs—no more than might be experienced by some of us. As far as treatment of her hypertension is concerned, I am sure that if anything can be accomplished psychotherapeutically it will do her more good than would the administration of any drug.

So much for the treatment of her organic disease. The important problem here is the treatment of what is so obvious when you see this woman, a reactive depression. It would be interesting to speculate as to what this woman's life problems represent in the causation of her hypertension: they may have played a very important role.

This woman of fifty-six looks older than her age. Her skin shows a certain amount of atrophy, and she has a dorsal kyphosis of the type seen in older people, which in her case may be related to menopausal osteoporosis. This problem of aging will become an increasing responsibility of all physicians. People now reach the sixties as compared to the average of fifty some years ago. The incidence of old people in our offices is going to increase. We must take into account what aging represents to them in the way of insecurity, as well as the individual's reaction to the aging process. When doing a physical examination or prescribing for older people, we must be mindful of what is normal for the individual's age, and be mindful of it when advising the patient.

As an individual gets older we expect to see certain degenerative changes. The first and most obvious one is in the general appearance of the person, due in part to changes in the skin. You can oftentimes demonstrate abnormalities of the skin by testing its elasticity, its ability to retract promptly. We know that older people are prone to diminution of hearing and vision. They may have dentures which may or may not be satisfactory. The absence of teeth may very greatly govern the patient's dietary intake and must be taken into account. Obvious changes take place in the cardiovascular system. The heart pumps less well, and the inelastic aorta no longer responds to exercise as it did. Circulation to many parts of the body may be impaired in consequence of arteriosclerosis; this may be evidenced peripherally in the form of intermittent claudication, and in other organs depending upon their reaction to a diminution in blood supply.

Unless we always relate these changes in terms of aging, we are bound to make serious mistakes. We may lay far too much emphasis on structural changes that cannot be corrected. One's attitude and interest in the problem of geriatrics will reflect the care given such patients. Many physicians react to the aged as they do to neurotics and to patients with chronic diseases. Unless we are mindful of our reactions to these therapeutic situations, it stands to reason that we shall not do a very good job in caring for these people.

I will ask Dr. Romano to say a few words about the psychological reactions to aging. He works in a large general hospital where he sees a lot of people in this age group and has also encountered these problems in his practice of psychiatry.

DR. ROMANO. I don't think there is very much to add to what you have said so well. I might point out that there is a distinction between dotage and dementia, that in the normal aging process there are certain psychological changes that take place in all of us, and one of them certainly is an increase in inflexibility. So I think an immediate application of this fact to the practice of medicine is that doctors should take into consideration the elderly patient's inability to meet strange or new demands upon him too quickly. I think that is particularly true in drug therapy. Both the introduction of certain drugs without adequate preparation and the changing of the life habits of old people too suddenly may be quite distressing to them; it may be impossible for an elderly person to adapt quickly to such prescriptions.

I think most of the psychological changes of old age occur because of the decreasing capacity of the biological organism to meet new situations and its increasing need to borrow from past experiences. As a result, new situations, new demands, present added hazards, added burdens that are carried with considerable difficulty. With increasing age the distinction between dotage and dementia is quantitative to a certain degree. For instance, in the seventies reminiscing and utilizing past experiences, repetition, economic speech, all these are part and parcel of the aging processes intellectually and emotionally. In dementia there is increasing disturbance of memory, certain compensatory reminiscing, and a confabulatory trend; actually the problem assumes greatest proportions when the person is no longer able to adjust to society.

This morning we spoke briefly of the differential diagnosis of dementia occurring in late middle life. Dementia, impairment or loss of intellectual function, is the result of structural brain disease. By far the most common cause of dementia is cerebral arteriosclerosis. Cerebral arteriosclerosis is not senile dementia. Histologically and clinically they are quite different. Cerebral arteriosclerosis occurs much earlier and is apt to be episodic in course; there is irritability, much less loss of intellectual function than in senile dementia, neurologic signs, aphasia, amnesia, with or without arterial hypertension. Dementia may result from trauma. In patients with chronic alcoholism, subdural hematoma and other head injuries must be kept in mind. Dementia may occur as the result of inflammatory processes, both nonspecific and specific. It may result from primary or secondary neoplastic involvement of the brain. Certain presenile dementias are quite rare. They occur in the late fifties, in women more than in men, and are characterized by a rapid and marked dementia.

Drug intoxications may simulate dementia; if prolonged, they may result in dementia. Chronic metabolic derangements, such as in chronic cardiac failure, uremia, Addison's disease, and carcinoma, may result in irreversible brain damage.

Certain degenerative and possibly familial diseases such as Huntington's chorea may be accompanied by dementia.

Finally, there is a pseudo dementia, sometimes seen in prisons or in compensation cases, called Ganser's syndrome or hysterical psychosis.

DR. WOLFF. May I say just a word about the threat or the occurrence of anxiety in persons with structural brain disease? Take, for instance, an individual with cerebral arteriosclerosis, a man, let's say, of sixty-five or seventy. If that person is precipitated into an anxiety state which lasts for days or weeks or into a depression, very often one is confused about his diagnosis or convinced that one is dealing with a demented old man. Yet with the clearance of the tension and anxiety state, the very serious defect in retention, concentration, recent memory clears up, and you find him functioning about as well, perhaps, as before. Often one is led to make a serious prognosis on the basis of bad performance when one doesn't recognize anxiety and depression in an elderly person.

DR. BAUER. I am sure we have all made the mistake of saying this is just a senile old crock, only to have someone bring back a blood bromide report of 600 milligrams per cent or have someone demonstrate that you are dealing with a very severe vitamin deficiency in an elderly person. All such factors must be considered. The number of mistakes that are made in the treatment of the aged we could go on enumerating indefinitely. We not infrequently tell older people that a little drink now and then won't hurt them; perhaps they ought to have a little whiskey or a cocktail before dinner. Before giving that advice it is wise to find out how the person feels about alcohol, otherwise we may make a bad situation worse.

The important thing is to appreciate the total situation as it concerns the human being in question. There are times when what the textbook or the authorities say just can't be done; it is just poor medicine, absolutely contraindicated. Treatment must be individualized, otherwise we make too many mistakes, such as needlessly subjecting our aged patients to the hazards of prolonged bed rest or exposing them to the ever-lurking infections of hospitals during the winter months. We must always weigh the pros and cons of each diagnostic and therapeutic procedure in terms of ultimate accomplishment and the patient's total welfare and happiness, otherwise we are guilty of poor medical practice.

DR. BROSIN. Any more questions about the patient described today?

STUDENT. Well, I can't see where more interviews are going to help this woman. I want to find out what you think about it. She has some insight into her condition. It seems to me that these external problems have to be dealt with before she is going to be any better.

DR. BAUER. I think this woman can be helped by additional interviews because of the improvement noted to date. It was obvious that the opportunity to discuss her problems frankly and with ease had done her a lot of good. If some of the other things Dr. Brosin suggested could be brought into play, she would certainly be a much happier person than before.

DR. BROSIN. I would agree. At this point perhaps a restatement of what we have been saying all week is called for. The physician is an instrument, a vehicle. You are the medicine. You can do some good in the acute reactive depression because you lend support, you help to bolster the patient's prestige, values, and his self-esteem. The patient gets a chance to unload—what we call catharsis. We shouldn't underrate that element in the therapy. For various reasons there is a tendency to do that—perhaps because of lack of full knowledge of how important supportive care is or because of our own resistance to doing that kind of work. As long as a patient is acutely depressed, you can automatically say to yourself, "I am of value," even though external manipulation is also valuable.

STUDENT. The point I was making is this. I could see somewhat how interviews would be valuable if the person didn't have insight and you brought out that insight. But this patient already has insight. She has already told us that her trouble is due to her husband and her financial situation, and so in this case it is kind of hard for me to understand how interviews would help.

DR. BROSIN. You will forgive us, doctor, if we take a few moments to open up a difficult aspect of this question? In order to make the major treatment problems clear and comprehensible we have, by and large, strictly limited our discussion to factors which are concrete, external, and manipulative at the level at which the general practitioner works. Those are the factors in this case that you can see easily. But we also mentioned this woman's twenty-six-year marriage to a husband who has been giving her a lot of trouble and about whom she is insecure; also her thoughts of death, her own and her husband's. On the one hand, because of her hostility to her husband, she would like to see him dead; on the other, if she loses him, she loses her income and her companion, even in misery, of twenty-six years.

Now here is where interpretative therapy helps a good deal. We don't advocate for a moment that you should apply the microscopy of the psychoanalytic technique and try to explain to her these unconscious ideas. But by talking to her you give her a chance to unload and get rid of the "return of the repressed," which we talked about the other day. Her symptoms then diminish because the force back of them is gone, there is no motor there. You give her a chance to unload her anger and in that way do her a world of good, for in the last analysis her repressed anger may be even more important than her environmental situation. Of course she senses this. She can't handle it. She feels guilty about her anger against an aging man for whom she is responsible.

Then you recall that in one of the section meetings some of you expressed the feeling that psychotherapy has no real market value, for it seems vague, indefinite, perhaps rather thin, and equated to the function of the priest at one end and the quack at the other. This attitude has dual origins and is reinforced by those of your brethren who feel that only surgical intervention really has good market value. The fact is that your time is all you have, and in cases like these it has the highest possible market value.

DR. JENSEN. I'd like to emphasize just one point that was brought out so well by Dr. Bauer in the matter of managing these elderly people, namely, that of truly evaluating the situation that the individual faces and then trying to help him get satisfaction and pleasure out of living. I would like to emphasize the importance of that with respect to children, too.

DR. BAUER. I think we doctors should occasionally try the therapy we prescribe. Take, for example, a purine-free diet. I defy any man in this room—unless he is more abnormal than I think he is—to stay on it a month. Yet we prescribe it. We do other things that are equally foolish. We subject a lot of our patients to other unnecessary measures. I am sure we shall all get a lot further if we really pay more attention to the fellow who comes to us and his real reason for coming to our office. Are there any other questions?

STUDENT.   How about cathartics?

DR. MURRAY.   I told you the first day, in talking about the development of children, that constipation is apt to come along in the life of the child following his thumb-sucking episode and that it often proves a very adequate substitute, an actual pleasure to the child. And here the parents can't defeat the child. We also learned in Dr. Brosin's lecture on the compulsive character that an individual may be preoccupied with that particular part of his body, may endow it with a great deal of his interest, concern, and fantasy life. It symbolizes a great deal to him. You remember in the *Forsyte Saga* how Galsworthy describes the Man of Property: his whole relationship to the things in his environment was to grasp and to hold. We can see that in many instances people have not sublimated, shall we say, that tendency as well as Soames Forsyte had, and are tremendously preoccupied with the nether end of their G.I. tract.

DR. BAUER.   I am sure that in the case of the adult most of us have failed to consider the many problems of constipation and have sometimes missed their significance. There is considerable folklore as well as medical literature pertaining to the difficulties individuals will encounter unless it is controlled. Treatment will depend in large part upon the individual you are dealing with. I know an old minister, seventy-seven, who has one bowel movement every eight days, yet is very healthy. Relating such case records will not be of much help to many of the people who consult you because of the complaint of constipation. It can be a very involved problem and one in which the advice ordinarily given will not remedy the situation. There are a lot of people whom it is reasonably simple to convince that it doesn't matter whether or not their bowels move every day or whether they move once or three times a day. It is important for us to appreciate that it isn't always as simple a problem as would appear at first glance; it may be much more deep seated; it may have a significance which unfortunately the best of the average textbooks of medicine don't even hint at. Unless you look at the problem in that light you will not treat the symptom of constipation very successfully.

I think the important thing is to get away from routine treatment. You must individualize. Some elderly women come in saying that they take one senna leaf in a half cup of water at night and their bowels move perfectly well and have for the past thirty years. Don't interfere with things like that—they accomplish their purpose and keep your patient happy. You aren't going to take one senna leaf away from a poor lady, are you?

STUDENT. Dr. Bauer, one thing that occurs to me is the question how often old people should have a physical examination. I realize that each old individual or aged person is a problem unto himself, but in pediatrics the routine examination is important during the period of growth and development. In geriatrics, where you have the stage of regression, do you have any recommendation? Do you think it is desirable yearly, or at certain periods in one's life?

DR. BAUER. Yearly physical examinations are very worth while provided the physician is fully aware of his responsibility to his patient. This is a threefold responsibility—to apply simultaneously the best principles of preventive, diagnostic, and curative medicine in furthering the health and happiness of an individual. It takes time to adhere to this simple rule, but if you don't adhere to it you defeat the purpose of yearly physical examinations.

Case Presentations

III

1. A PATIENT WITH "FIBROSITIS"

DR. BAUER. In general practice one sees many patients like the first case to be described today.

DR. F. The patient is a man, thirty-five years old, single, who lives with his parents. His chief complaint is soreness of the thighs, legs, and arms that started six and a half years ago. The onset was characterized by painful red spots on the extensor surfaces of the lower legs. They were not accompanied by fever. He was told he had an infection and was treated with sulfa drugs and hot packs. When the lesions disappeared, there was still some swelling above the left knee. He was totally disabled for about ten weeks because of pain in the legs and arms. He then went to a clinic, where a diagnosis of fibrositis was made. He was given vaccines and vitamins, but there was very little or no improvement. It was four months before he went back to his work in a telephone construction gang, and then he was unable to continue with it because of the pain. He next obtained a leave and went to Jacksonville, Florida, in the hope that the warm weather would relieve his pain. He chose that city because a sister and a cousin lived there. After six weeks' schooling he went into a factory in that city and liked his work very well. But he had no relief from his pain and he came back to his work at home. This Florida experiment was repeated, but three years ago he was back again at home, still unable to work for the telephone company.

Since then he has only worked fourteen months. The soreness in his muscles prevents him from doing physical labor. Treatment with vaccines, vitamins, light, and pills has been without effect. Biopsies from each of the deltoid muscles were "negative for fibrositis." Recently he's been advised to take streptococcic vaccine intravenously for his fibrositis. His tonsils were removed at the onset. He said they weren't bad but the doctor said, "We ought to take 'em out anyhow.

They might be the trouble." A series of prostatic massages didn't help either.

The patient told me that at the age of twenty-one he began going with a girl. This continued for two years, but another man stepped in and the affair was broken up. He was somewhat depressed. At the age of twenty-five he started going with another girl, and after some time another fellow stepped in and broke that up, too. The patient, however, had made no advances that would have indicated his desire to marry in either case. This last affair was quite a shock; he felt depressed for at least a year. He felt very insecure and had a definite sense of inferiority. Approximately a year after his depression had disappeared he developed his present trouble.

Sex? He states his reaction is normal. He's never had intercourse. I asked him about these women that he had gone with and he said, "They weren't that kind of girl." He continued masturbation until about two and a half years ago, when he thought that probably he should stop because he felt a sense of guilt.

This man finished the second year of high school; he was an average student, who managed to get along. He liked to play baseball and enjoyed watching other sports. He was very shy, however, and said it was difficult for him to break the ice; somebody would have to talk to him first and then he'd warm up all right.

Children's illnesses: he had only mumps and measles. He had no serious illnesses, but he had a ringworm on the back of his neck and an injury to the right frontal area that resulted in a scar, concerning which he is still very sensitive. It is so slight that I didn't notice it until he blushed. He really was very conscious of the scar and said it had kept him away from his playmates.

This man's father is a farmer, about sixty years of age, in good health. The patient said his dad was domineering; in fact, none of the children got along with him. They just worked on the farm and did what he said. His mother is about the same age and also well. The patient said she's a very ideal person. Everyone gets along with her, and she does everything that her husband wants her to do. He has two brothers and two sisters living and well. There has been no death in the family.

There's always been an excellent relationship between the siblings and the mother.

The patient had to quit school at the age of seventeen to help his father on the farm. He hated farming. He worked for his father until he was twenty-one, and then he was able to leave home. He worked for another farmer for two and a half years and then he was on the CCC. I didn't ask why he wasn't in the Army, for obviously it wasn't necessary to embarrass him any further; this fibrositis was enough to keep him out. He always had good relations with his employer and his fellow workers.

He said that except for the present difficulty his health had been very good but that he's always been quite nervous. Now he's afraid he may be crippled by this illness, although there's been no progression of the disease. He wants work so that he can feel secure. He does not want to marry or assume family responsibilities until he can be assured of good health. At times he wishes that he had completed school so that he would not be required to do physical work.

He sometimes has frontal and occipital headaches, especially if he overworks or becomes overheated. Nervousness does not aggravate his skeletal muscle pain. He used to love to dance and play baseball, but quit because they aggravated his symptoms and he needed more rest. His appetite is very good, he sleeps well, he does not drink, he smokes twenty to thirty cigarettes a day, less when he works. He dreams occasionally but cannot remember his dreams. He said there has been some improvement in his relations with his father since his father moved to a small farm and doesn't need his help.

On the physical examination this man was found to be a fairly well developed and preserved individual; he blushes easily, seems uneasy, but does want to talk about his trouble. He has definite graying at the temples and appears older than his age, thirty-five. Blood pressure: the systolic readings varied from 160 to 145; the diastolic was normal. There was no evidence of joint or muscle swelling. This man, who told me he can't go to dances because sitting for fifteen or twenty minutes watching people dance causes almost unbearable soreness in his muscles, sat in my office for two and a half hours without apparent discomfort while telling me his story. He seemingly forgot about his muscle pains. He said that he can walk a couple of miles but can't dance because of soreness of his leg muscles. He doesn't go out at night because he needs ten or twelve hours' sleep.

Dr. Murray, Dr. Bauer, and Dr. Hinckley saw this man and their diagnosis was psychoneurosis. They advised discontinuing drug therapy and instituting psychotherapy. They emphasized that it will be difficult for the patient to understand that his symptoms are psychogenic. It is difficult for him to appreciate that his illness is not disabling.

We had three interviews with him. He is very reluctant to resume responsibility. He does not want to get married because of his disability. He admits that he could take up bookkeeping, as he is very good at figures and loves the work—in fact, he has done some income tax reports. But he says he's too old to go to a commercial school, for the younger people there would wonder why he was in school at his age. When he was assured that there are people as old as he going to school, he said he might go home and attend school there. This is in line with his usual habit—he has never lived anywhere except near his family.

DR. WOLFF. Is there any evidence of disability now?

DR. F. No, no evidence of any disability at all.

DR. BAUER. He doesn't have any focal points of tenderness, as do many of these people. These focal points may persist weeks, months, or years. It is highly probable that his first symptoms were those of erythema nodosum. He had lesions only on the extensor surfaces of the lower legs, and seemingly swelling of one or both knees. The total duration of the disease was difficult to establish; evidently it was only a matter of weeks. Since then the man has had this very persistent set of symptoms referable to the skeletal system. Otherwise he's well.

DR. WOLFF. Does he have a normal sedimentation rate?

DR. BAUER. Yes.

STUDENT. Did the symptoms begin at the time he was having his love affair?

DR. F. Following that. It was pretty closely tied up, although he didn't admit it at first. Following the second love affair, he was definitely depressed and sleepless for a while.

DR. MURRAY. How do you formulate this case in your own mind?

DR. F. Well, here's a man who evidently has a neurotic personality make-up. He is shy and has a sense of inferiority. As a boy he was so sensitive about the scar that he preferred to stay away from the other children because he thought that they would make fun of him. He tried to withdraw into himself. At the age of seventeen he left school and went to work for his father—no doubt because his father requested him to do so, for they needed a lot of help on the farm. He found his father difficult to deal with and his mother evidently didn't take his part, and so at the age of twenty-one he left home. In other words, at twenty-one he tried to make some effort to grow up. He thought he would like to grow up, but he went to work on another farm. He was in a CCC camp and then he had his first love affair, and still he couldn't grow up. After it turned out badly he went back home, into the arms of his father and mother. Then he tried a second time to grow up. He couldn't do it. He went with a girl for two years, and she probably did all that she could do to interest him but he refused to accept that. He kept living at home all the time; he always saw to it that he had a job close to home, close to his father and mother.

Then, six and a half years ago, his illness began. The peculiar thing about this illness was that he felt better as far as his nervousness and so forth went, when he could find an excuse for not growing up. Certainly if a man is disabled and can't work, he can't support a family or grow up. Then he said, "Well, I'll go to Florida for my health; it's good there." But he had to go to Jacksonville, where some of his relatives were living, and he stayed with them. There's another indication that he refused to grow up. Then he came back home again to his parents. He couldn't stay away from them; he had to come back.

Then he tried all kinds of treatment and forgot about women completely. There's one remarkable thing about this: after he had this depression, this pain in the legs and all over, that solved his sexual life; he had solved his problems about growing up. So he was perfectly happy. One of the most disturbing factors in this case was that he would revolt every time I suggested a way in which he could grow up. For instance, I would suggest different work that he could do; if that work would be a solution to his financial problems and he could get married, he wouldn't consider it. He had ample funds to buy in on a cigar store.

He found a cigar store that he could buy, a little store that he said he could handle. He could sit behind the counter and wouldn't have to do much work, but he didn't like that idea. He was always bringing up the fact that he couldn't do this or that because of the pain in his legs and arms and shoulders. Then we reminded him that he had said he would be able to do bookkeeping. He was quite enthusiastic about that when he left. But probably after he'd walked down the street a couple of blocks he decided that he didn't like that solution either. All in all, then, I think you have here a youngster—I say youngster—of thirty-five. I think that's the whole explanation. Here's a fellow who doesn't want to grow up; he likes to be a child and he'll continue to be one, I think.

QUESTION. What was his family's pattern?

DR. F. His mother was very passive; she just sat back and took things as they came. His father dictated to the entire family. The patient said no one could get along with his father, except by giving in. He had to quit school and give in to his father in every way. Of course, the patient never said that he dislikes his father. You can't suggest that he hates his father; you can't get any admission like that out of him. They get along very nicely, he said!

QUESTION. Did he express any outward hostility toward anyone— toward either of the two suitors who took his girls away from him?

DR. F. No, he didn't express any hostility. As to the suitors, he said, "Well, I didn't make the advances, and somebody came in with just a little more pep than I had and just took them away." It seems as if he just couldn't express any hostility. He has an inferiority complex. In fact, I think he invited these friends of his to come in and take the girls away because it would solve a problem for him. What bothered him later was that he began to think that there must be something wrong with him if he couldn't hold the girls. Then this period of depression began, and he found that the easiest solution was to get a few little erythema nodosum bumps. That was the solution to all his troubles and an end to them. He certainly was enjoying his poor health.

DR. MURRAY. I think that the high lights of this case have been covered. All I can do is review them for you. This is a man, a shy, passive character, who demonstrates an almost pathological reaction to a small scar, saying, "I am different because I have this small scar. I am different from other men." Almost as if to tell you, "I can't be a man." This, of course, is a very, very lame·basis for a rationalization of his inner feeling that somehow he is not a man. In his course of development he makes two very desultory efforts toward marriage. He went around with these girls, as near as one can tell, on much the same basis as a fourteen-year-old adolescent would. After the second frustration he was depressed.

It was with difficulty that one dug out this past history. It was fairly evident that in his long medical treatment there had never been any discussion of a possible relationship between the second frustration, the depression which followed it, and this subsequent crippling illness. We really had to ask him to settle down and dig from his memory the pertinent details of what had happened six and a half years ago. He definitely was depressed, however, and sleepless, and, I think, anxious too, following this second frustration. He went from doctor to doctor, getting all kinds of gunshot treatment. Vitamins, vaccines—he was as full of hypodermic needle holes as a pincushion by the time they got through treating him. But none of the treatments had any influence on him. There followed a series of restless events—moving from place to place, changing jobs, always dissatisfied and restless.

Now one can see, of course, that this illness is the protection against the thing that he thinks he wants but that very obviously he's afraid of —a grown-up relationship with a woman. You get the hint very definitely that his identifications are completely with his passive mother and not with his father. Any active expression of straightforwardness or directness, even a diluted form of the aggressiveness his father shows—all that is completely absent. One definitely sees in him, as he describes his parents, a replica of his passive, long-suffering mother. I think that completes the background of this man's illness. The role his illness plays in supporting his shyness and his rejection of maturity is quite clear.

DR. BAUER. Dr. Brosin, would you want to say anything about people with this type of symptomatology? Has it been your experience that all people who have skeletal symptoms of this sort fall into the same pattern?

DR. BROSIN. Oh, no! I would say absolutely and unconditionally that I don't believe I could equate any personality type with skeletal disease. Since you've motivated me to such denial, may I add here something I'm sure many of you have met? The most painful type of psychosomatic disorder that I know of, for the physician, is that of the highly sadistic, verbally expert individual—the artist, often, or literary person, very high in the field of academic accomplishment, much above the level of the medical department—who has backaches. I hope that will spur others to mention that the backache is the last psychosomatic stronghold of the sadistic intellectual. He spins his rationalizations very thin, and, because his verbal defenses are so good, he foils the therapeutic processes at the level we are speaking of.

DR. ROMANO. I'd like to say a word about the management of this type of person—not in respect to a specific personality type or a specific type of somatic expression—but rather the problem of a person, such as the one here described, who has had considerable difficulty in reaching mature goals, socially, sexually, economically, and so on. In most such instances it is dangerous to use interpretive technique, but it is often possible to help the person supportively. At times, by manipulating certain external factors, you may find certain types of support in the environment. I have in mind a few instances in which a relationship was secured to an employer who acted essentially as a father and a mother. Sometimes certain types of friendship give support to such people. Essentially many of them are what we might call "unweaned sucklings"; they can be helped only when they have some means of compensatory support from without.

You spoke with some surprise of the fact that in spite of the intensity of this man's symptoms he could sit comfortably for two or three hours talking to you. It seems to me that the explanation of that lies in his relationship to you; the gain he secured from that relationship substituted for his symptoms. By means of his symptoms he is able to gain certain ends; for the time being his relationship to you took the place of the symptoms. So it was not strange or incomprehensible.

I think this instance also helps us to see more clearly why so much attention has been paid to the problem of sexuality in living. Modern psychology has often been indicted for what is thought to be its exaggeration of the importance of sexuality. In this case you see that, probably more than any other factor in experience, sexuality is the criterion of normality, the criterion of being mature. Sexuality in its most mature state is the capacity to love someone besides one's self—being able to give to someone else, show tenderness, expend energy not for one's own utilitarian needs but for other people. In speaking of childhood, one of the characters in a play by Bernard Shaw uses the analogy of the receptacle which is not full and which has to be filled—that is, the child's emotional needs have to be met from outside; he has to be secure, protected, loved by others. In maturity this receptacle overflows, and one is able to direct and to channel the overflow to the people one loves and helps. Then in old age the vessel becomes less full, and again one has to be loved and cared for very much as in childhood. I think that in the case described here so clearly we see a person who is essentially a child and therefore needs support. In caring for people like this one of the things that physicians can do is to guard against promoting and entrenching invalidism by too many unnecessary diagnostic tests. They should look at the situation as realistically as possible, come to certain decisions, and help the person reach out again for as mature a goal as is possible for him to achieve. Such an individual's preparation for invalidism, his threshold for it, is much, much lower than a healthier person's.

DR. F. We did assure this man, and he did seem to understand, that there had been no progression in his disease for six and a half years; if anything, there had been some improvement in spite of what he had done and in spite of the lapse of time. We explained to him that he would not be disabled or crippled or deformed or anything like that. He had that pretty well in mind when he left the office—the fact that he didn't have to worry about such a possibility. He said, "Well, I don't think I'll take any more treatment." He felt that he was going to try our suggestions. Of course, I don't know that it's going to work, unless we get another mother for him. That's possible—that he can get a woman who will take the place of his mother. When he gets older, when he doesn't have to worry about family responsibilities, he might marry, say, at the age of fifty. He'll probably solve his problems as he grows older.

DR. MURRAY. Yes, doctor, that's very true but instead of getting married he might well develop an involutional melancholia.

DR. F. Well, I meant to say if you could get him interested in someone who would mother him. If you could bring a mother in there, you might help him. I'd hate to be the mother!

STUDENT. I wonder if there's any analogy or difference to be brought out between this case and the case of a spinster.

DR. MURRAY. Well, yes, of course; a woman is a different problem because the vicissitudes through which her emotions go in her growth and development to normal heterosexuality are different from those of a man. Her ambivalence tends to be toward her mother, upon whom she is dependent. This dependency keeps her fixed and unable to reach out and make a healthy and satisfactory relationship with a male.

In the clinic we've had an excellent case illustrative of this in a young married woman. We've had two very interesting and somewhat stormy days going over the development of this girl's hostility to her husband because she is frigid and childless. What was earlier a capacity to experience at least some pleasant sensations in intercourse has been lost, and with that loss has come a lot of irritability and aggression toward her partner. The nature and character of the childhood emotional patterns which persist in these people are very evident. This girl had shown a marked tomboyishness, and, on the other hand, an equally strong pleasure in playing with dolls. Nevertheless, she completely lacked the real maturity of motherhood, the desire to create and give. In her desire for maternity, one feels, she needed a child for what the child meant to her; it was not the beautiful thing that motherhood is so often pictured as—an opportunity to create and to give to other human beings outside one's self. Very definitely not. This girl is a frightened, driven person—driven by her inner emotions—and she has developed a protective shell of hardness around herself to keep from being hurt. She is the type of girl who has had a number of unhappy experiences with men.

I pointed out to my students that very frequently this type of woman does do just that thing. Fate almost seems to put them into the situation where men hurt them, so that they have a well-rationalized and justifiable hostility to men as the basis for their inability to make an adequate relationship with them. There's a shell around these individuals that prevents them from reaching out warmly to other people and creating natural healthy, friendly relationships with them—relationships which go on to the wonderful happinesses of a true love life. They may go through the motions but their love life has nothing of deep, inner, spontaneous warmth. Coming to the mid-life period, they have missed the meaning of the active biological phase of love-making, and involutional depressive reactions of varied degrees are apt to appear.

This is particularly true of people who harbor deep resentment and hostilities against their mates for their failure to achieve the important inner releases found in a healthy relationship. In the practice of medicine it is important to recognize these things early and do what we can to keep these hostilities from mounting. It has been shown in the cases of the last two days that it is best to make some interpretation regarding the hostility and to develop in these people a little evener, more natural relationship with life and a greater capacity to see their own failings in the misspent relationship, so that they don't project or blame the other party so severely. For this is a very noxious situation if allowed to grow and develop along the lines I've outlined; it may become a background for mid-life depression.

DR. BAUER. This subject of fibrositis is a very interesting one. There's no doubt that we see people with fibrositis; it is part and parcel of any number of the arthritides that we encounter. In fact, in some of our rheumatoid arthritics the symptomatology may be of this nature for months or years prior to the appearance of the objective joint finding. We also see something akin to it in aged people, but that is quite different from what we have seen in the patient described today. In the aged it is associated with loss of elasticity and certain degenerative changes that take place in the tendons and periarticular tissues. Older people often complain that they feel stiffness after sitting for any period of time, only to have it disappear as soon as they move about. This is quite a different story from the case presented this morning, and many others that we see.

The case described today could be duplicated time and time again in the experience of any one of us. The patient is representative of a large group of people whose complaints have long been labelled fibrositis. A considerable body of literature has been written about it by the English, and there are physicians in this country who frequently use this term as a diagnostic label—I'm sure the organicists welcomed its introduction. It serves as a convenient diagnostic compartment in which to place all these people. The diagnosis having been rendered, a very ardent search is made for foci of infection, and then resort is made to vaccine, various forms of physiotherapy, and many other therapeutic measures. These measures serve to promote fixation of the patient's symptoms and continuing disability. It's a diagnostic and therapeutic trap that many of us have been caught in, and it isn't a very comfortable one. In handling this group of people one might better face the facts.

The symptomatology of so-called fibrositis varies greatly. Some patients will tell you that their symptoms are always worse after exercise, or after they have sat in one position for any period of time; others will tell you quite the reverse. The symptoms persist for years—ten, fifteen, twenty, thirty years—and rarely does the individual ever develop any evidence of arthritis. They have the same disability through a major portion of their lives.

The use of the term "fibrositis" is very unfortunate. So far as I can determine from the literature, there is very little evidence that there is an "itis" in these cases. We have done biopsies on a number of these patients. The biopsy specimens, including skin, subcutaneous tissue, fascia and muscle, excised from areas exhibiting focal tenderness showed no evidence of inflammation. I think the suffix "itis" is incorrect.

When some of my medical colleagues who had long tried to convince me that these patients suffer from an organic disease entity went into the Army, they were struck with the fact that such symptoms were extremely prevalent. It was disturbing to them to have to make the diagnosis of fibrositis as frequently as they did. Many of them became more conscious of the problems of the psychoneurotic and what they entail. This experience caused these same physicians to separate off a second group which they call "psychogenic rheumatism."

So far as I'm concerned, most cases of so-called fibrositis and psychogenic rheumatism are one and the same thing. The attempt to differentiate the two is extremely difficult and in most instances is just begging the point. When one sees these people, it's much more to the point to recognize what one is dealing with, decide to proceed in the manner that you have been taught here, and then stand your ground. Do not lean on a false diagnostic crutch.

I'd be the first to admit that curing these people is a very difficult job. I'm sure, however, if you proceed along psychotherapeutic lines, whether they be manipulative or supportive, you can carry a lot of these people year in and year out with a much higher degree of satisfaction on your part and with the patients delivering as well as or better than they did prior to seeing you. Once you take refuge in a diagnosis which implies the presence of organic disease and commit yourself further by employing diagnostic and therapeutic measures of the type such patients have been exposed to, you end with a situation which is much more difficult to deal with than at the onset.

STUDENT.   Unless you make some of these tests, like the sedimentation tests and so on, how can you be sure that organic disease isn't present?

DR. BAUER.   You can't be certain without doing so, particularly in individuals suffering from symptoms similar to the prodromata of rheumatoid arthritis. If, however, you tell the patient that you feel reasonably certain the tests are going to be negative and give him some idea as to the nature of his symptoms, you will be in a much better position, therapeutically speaking. If you always proceed in the same manner as you have in these past two weeks, even when you're dealing with a patient with rheumatoid arthritis, you'll frequently make a diagnosis of neurosis *and* rheumatoid arthritis. That's the important thing.

Just because the sedimentation rate comes back 1.2 millimeters per minute don't say, "Well, the patient has organic disease and my thoughts about explaining certain of his symptoms on the basis of his neurosis were wrong. I'll throw that idea out of the window." That's a point of view medical men exhibit all too frequently.

You've all seen patients who, you felt certain, had a gastric neurosis; you've treated them for years, and they finally turn up with cancer of the stomach. Then one of your colleagues says, "Yeah, see! Cancer of the stomach all the time. Never did have a neurosis." Well, you know as well as I do that that's a very erroneous, very foolish conclusion. A neurotic has to die just like the rest of us. A neurotic has a right to have an organic disease. Some organic diseases we have reason to believe are very intimately related to the underlying neurosis. The exact mechanism involved is, of course, difficult to explain.

STUDENT. Don't you think that the making of certain tests, even though you're pretty sure they're going to be negative, has value in showing the patient that you have objective evidence that he does not have the disease?

DR. BAUER. Yes, but I think it's even more important to be reasonably decisive at the time you do your history and your physical. Tell the patient then that you feel reasonably certain that he doesn't have a beginning rheumatoid arthritis, that you are going to make certain tests but you think they will be negative. Then you're in a much better position therapeutically than if you had proceeded in the other manner. Many of my medical colleagues say they proceed in much the same way as I'm suggesting, only they spend one to three weeks doing diagnostic studies before they come to a decision. I think many of them make a diagnosis of neurosis by exclusion. They must find themselves in an extremely difficult position when they confront the patient with sheaves of paper bearing negative reports, not to mention the patient's reaction. One must establish the diagnosis of neurosis on the basis of the history and also remember that organic disease and neurosis frequently exist together. It is important for practitioners to remember the need to be decisive. Indecision on the part of doctors is very serious and often harmful to patients.

This carrying through of forms of therapy which are aimed at correcting something which doesn't exist is equally serious. It usually means a desire to get rid of the poor patient or refusal on our part to face facts such as our inability to handle the fellow, our fear of handling him, or our rejection of him. These and other possibilities must be taken into consideration in every case.

STUDENT. What do you think about the amount of pain that is actually produced in some of these people who come in complaining of a backache though the x-ray shows they have only a mild marginal arthritis or a sacralization of the lumbar vertebrae or some such thing?

DR. BAUER. Most patients who show evidence by x-ray of marginal lipping of the vertebral bodies and sacralization of the lumbar vertebrae do not have symptoms. Nevertheless, physicians are very apt to ascribe the incapacitating backaches of neurotics to minor structural abnormalities called to their attention by the radiologist. This, of course, is bad medical practice and leads to situations of the type we have already discussed. We must try to avoid diagnostic pitfalls like this, which may lead to invalidism.

DR. WOLFF. May I say a word about a similar type of relationship between symptoms and underlying structural defect in regard to headache? Take one group, the people who have had a slowly growing meningioma for many years, which ultimately caused a lump to appear on the side of the head, without symptoms, without causing the patient any special disability. Then, for one reason or another, it becomes known to the family or friends that this individual has a lump. Then begins a kind of pressure to do something about it, aroused partly by the person's awareness now of this anomaly and also by the urging of his friends and family. Then begins a headache, and the patient presents himself with headache, associated with brain tumor. The headache, however, is a manifestation of emotional conflict, of the pressure produced by the family and friends long after this thing has been under way and has caused what symptoms it can cause.

Another area in which this is clearly seen is in individuals with structural heart disease, notably those with a thoroughly compensated circulatory system associated with symptoms of breathlessness, precordial pain, palpitation—not due to the underlying structural defect but to the reaction of the individual who is aware of the circulatory defect and the prognosis. These symptoms, therefore, arise from the individual's reactions to his difficulty, rather than from the underlying structural defects.

DR. BAUER. Much of what has been said illustrates the evils that arise from overspecialization. Getting inside the left auricle or a knee joint and never being able to get out is very serious business. During this recent war, a well-known cardiologist wanted to restudy the effort syndrome—the soldier's heart or the irritable heart. Having had considerable experience with it in World War I, he wished to review the subject in World War II. He and his colleagues made use of the soldiers in Army hospitals. The cardiologist, an internist, and a psychiatrist worked as a team in selecting the cases. The cardiologist would frequently say, "This type of patient is ideal; we'll take him." The psychiatrist would linger for five or ten minutes, ask fifteen or twenty questions, then the cardiologist would say, "No, that isn't the type of syndrome we're dealing with in World War II." On one occasion they spent the whole day at a hospital and came back without a patient. Why? Because the cardiologists in the last war didn't ask about symptoms beyond the heart. The patients they saw had a chief complaint referable to the heart and there were few questions aimed at finding out whether or not the patient had any other symptoms; I doubt if the patient had a chance to tell whether he had other complaints. Hence from the descriptions in the literature you are led to believe that these people have a very limited symptomatology. Some of them do. Many of them do not.

STUDENT. Dr. Bauer, what's your approach to the patient who comes in without any special symptoms of cardiac disability or anything to relate to his cardiovascular system but you find altered blood pressure, above 200, say, and you feel that he should have some warning about long hours of work or something of that sort? You feel you can't tell him he's getting older, he's got to take it easy. What's your approach to that type of patient?

DR. BAUER. That's a good question. How much you can and should tell will depend upon your patient. With some of the people you see you can discuss the situation very clearly. Certainly you must be truthful with patients. You can't say to the patient, "You're fine; but I never want you to run, never want you to lift." The patient might very well say, "What's wrong with that, doctor? I'm a perfect specimen, yet I can't do this, I can't do that, I can't even strain at stool any more for fear something will happen. That doesn't make sense." You can't just tell the fellow, "Well, you've got hypertension—I want you to be careful, I want you to work less. Goodby! I'll see you in a week." If you're going to tell him, you've got to tell him the truth. You don't have to sit there and say, "Well, now of course the thing I'm most worried about in you is that you're going to have a cerebral hemorrhage one of these days," or, "You might have a coronary occlusion," or "You're going to die of uremia." There's no need to do that.

What you tell a patient depends upon the individual concerned. What you tell a patient on the first visit as opposed to the sixth visit is quite different, because by that time you've really established some rapport with him. Then you can sit down and explain a lot of things, or tell him a lot of things without doing the damage that you would if you'd tried to do it at the time of the first visit. Our medical training has been such that we think a complete history and physical examination must be done on the first visit. The physician says to himself, "I must be sure and get a yes-or-no answer to everything. I must have a complete physical. I must obtain as much laboratory work as I can on this first visit. I've got to make a diagnosis; I've got to give a prognosis; I've got to give some idea of treatment." Well, most patients are sufficiently intelligent to know that you're not God; they don't expect all of that to happen on the first visit. It's just the tradition in which we've grown that makes us think that we have to do all of those things on the first visit.

STUDENT. Dr. Murray, is there any greater tendency in this particular type of personality toward a break with reality?

DR. MURRAY. I think that's a very good question. I think lots of times such reactions as those Dr. Bauer has been speaking of are substitutes for a break with reality. In other words, the individual comes to a fork in the road where he unconsciously makes a choice between a somatic illness and a psychological illness as an expression of his inner conflict. Sometimes he somaticizes his conflict and sometimes he makes a deeper psychological regression, sometimes going down to the point of psychosis. I think this was evident at the time this patient went through a depression and then developed erythema nodosum. Now, whether the erythema nodosum had a certain psychological element in it or not is something that we can't say. We don't know about that. But certain it is that after a time the individual found a handle which he could take hold of unconsciously to express certain unconscious conflicts.

Over and over we saw this in the Army. We had lads come in with an actual dysentery. It may have been a bacillary dysentery or an amebic dysentery. But before the lad broke down with this disease, he was getting near the end of his tether. Now you can be sure that as that lad recovered from his attack of infectious dysentery he was going to become a colitis problem. Even though his original organic illness was gone, he had found a means of expressing the emotional components of his psychological stress—the conflict he'd been in for a long period of time. By and large, you cannot cure that kind of illness so long as the patient's actual situation is such that this means of expression is the only solution to the conflict. He cannot solve this conflict in reality any longer—he's gone beyond that point and he has to have this illness. When he comes home from the Army, you may be able to get him well —or you may not be able to get him well—depending on the depth of his regression.

I think it is well, too, to keep that in mind when you treat these patients—what the possibilities are for improving their lot. Be sure the patient has somewhere to go when you give him insight, that you just don't slip the poor rags of the neurotic symptoms off and leave him bare to the breezes. Nothing is gained if, by insight, you drive an individual to a more deeply regressive illness or a frank depression when previously he had some defense through his symptoms.

2. A PATIENT WITH GASTRIC DISTRESS

DR. H. This patient was fifty-five years old, a spinster, who came to the clinic complaining primarily of symptoms resembling a gastrointestinal syndrome plus headache. At the first visit she was very voluble. We didn't get a chance to talk at all. She wanted to tell you everything; lots of it relevant, some irrelevant. On the second visit it was brought out that she was the next to the last of eight children and her mother was never well after her birth. She apparently thought something had occurred at her birth that made her mother weak. As a young girl this patient developed bronchitis, but the physician who treated her thought it was tuberculosis. So when she met a young man who, she thought, was pretty nice, the doctor advised her not to marry, because childbirth was difficult even for a normal woman and she was not normal; with this tuberculosis it would be very difficult for her to have a child. She promptly left the community, broke off relations with the young man, and has remained a spinster ever since.

About fourteen years ago this woman developed a facial tic. She had no pain but simply a convulsive twitch of the muscles of the face. She's been to numerous doctors. After many of them had told her they couldn't do anything for her, and she'd probably have the tic the rest of her life, she took the matter to the Lord in prayer. She was a very religious person, and gradually the tic left. For this she gives the Lord credit. About the time the tic left, headaches and gastrointestinal disturbances began—pain and constipation, associated with very severe headaches. She's been studied a great number of times in the various departments of the hospital. She's had numerous gastrointestinal studies, numerous gall bladder tests, and other laboratory procedures, but apparently her symptoms have stayed just about the same as they always were. She is dependent upon codeine and various other analgesic combinations for the relief of her headache and gastrointestinal symptoms. Some time ago the gastroscope revealed an ulcer; five weeks ago an examination showed the stomach and lining very swollen and reddened and areas of bleeding in the mucous membrane. She has had some ulcer therapy.

The first time I saw this woman her symptoms were exactly the same as they had been for a long time, and she wouldn't let you forget about them at all. At the termination of this visit she insisted that some form of therapy be given her at once, so that she could control the headaches and the abdominal pain that occurred in spite of the fact that she was on an ulcer regime. At the next visit she was feeling very much improved. I suppose just the ventilation of her thoughts had helped a great deal. She stated that she had thought that the doctor was now arriving at the source of her difficulty; she felt so firmly convinced of it that she had gone to the secretary of her church and told her about the doctors out here. As it happened, the gastroscopist had ordered a routine check-up last week. At that time none of the previous findings were visible to him, and so he sent her down for a gall bladder picture. We thought that the time had probably come to give her a further chance to ventilate her feelings and to stop some of the examinations that were keeping her attention focused on her gastrointestinal symptoms.

DR. WOLFF. May I ask what those changes were between the first and second gastroscopy? Abnormalities noted the first time and none the second, is that it?

DR. H. At the time of the first visit to us, the gastroscope showed swelling of the mucous membrane and areas of bleeding and this ulcer area. But as to symptoms—the fact was that after five weeks of ulcer therapy the symptoms were the same as before, even though apparently under the medical regime some healing had actually taken place in the ulcer area.

DR. WOLFF. The second examination showed the mucosa pale, without hemorrhages?

DR. H. Yes, it was normal.

DR. BAUER. What about the gastric symptoms?

DR. H. They're much better. She insisted at the first visit that some tablets be given her. We gave her just a plain analgesic—colored. I told her she mustn't use them unless she absolutely had to. At the third visit she said she felt very badly indeed that she had forgotten, in the rush of getting here, to bring back the box so that I could count the tablets: she had not taken any of them at all.

*

The course closed with expressions of satisfaction on the part of both the faculty and the student group, and with this statement of its underlying philosophy:

DR. WOLFF. I'm afraid that there may be a growing suspicion that there is a dualism between scientific medicine and the art of medicine; that somehow in becoming interested in a man and his feelings, attitudes, hates, loves, despairs, one is giving up a great tradition on which our discipline is based. It is a fundamental fallacy to look upon man in terms of those things we call scientific, the things we can do with the calorimeter or burette or fluoroscope, and to forget the fact that man is actuated by these very forces we've been talking about. The very fact that he is a man is the thing that isn't measured by these instruments, these simple instruments. I don't think we'll lose our way. We shouldn't be less scientific. The trouble is that we're not too scientific now—we're not scientific enough. We have to become more scientific, we have to become more knowledgeable, we have to know about man, and that means what he's doing in terms of his aims, his purposes, directions, aspirations, frustrations; then we'll get ahead with this subject. Now we're trying to deal with man as though he were an isolated organism. What we need to do is to deal with man in terms of where he wants to go.

List of Suggested Readings

SUGGESTED FOR READING IN CONNECTION
WITH THE COURSE

Bernard Hart. Psychology of Insanity. New York, The Macmillan Company, 4th ed., 1931

Annette Garrett. Interviewing: Its Principles and Methods. New York, Family Welfare Association of America, 1942

Maurice Levine. Psychotherapy in Medical Practice. New York, The Macmillan Company, 1942

Carl Binger. The Doctor's Job. New York, W. W. Norton & Company, 1945

Stewart G. Wolf and Harold G. Wolff. Human Gastric Function. New York, Oxford University Press, 2nd ed., 1947

John C. Whitehorn. Guide to interviewing and clinical personality study. *Archives of Neurology and Psychiatry*, 52:197–216, September 1944

John C. Whitehorn. Psychotherapy. *In* Modern Medical Therapy in General Practice, Volume 1, edited by David Barr. Baltimore, William Wood & Company, 1940

John Romano. Emotional components of illness. *Connecticut State Medical Journal*, 7:22–25, January 1943

Louis Hamman. Relationship of psychiatry to internal medicine. *Mental Hygiene*, 23:177–189, April 1939

J. Romano and G. L. Engel. Physiologic and psychologic considerations of delirium. *Medical Clinics of North America*, 28:629–638, May 1944

SUGGESTED FOR SUPPLEMENTARY READING

Anna Freud and Dorothy T. Burlingham. War and Children. New York, International Universities Press, 1944

Karl A. Menninger. The Human Mind. New York, Alfred A. Knopf, 3rd enl. ed., 1945

Ives Hendrick. Facts and Theories of Psychoanalysis. New York, Alfred A. Knopf, 2nd ed., 1939

George H. Preston. The Substance of Mental Health. New York, Farrar & Rinehart, Inc., 1943

Henry B. Richardson. Patients Have Families. New York, The Commonwealth Fund, 1945

Roy R. Grinker and John P. Spiegel. War Neuroses. Philadelphia, Blakiston, 1945, or
Roy R. Grinker and John P. Spiegel. Men under Stress. Philadelphia, Blakiston, 1945

Gregory Zilboorg. Mind, Medicine, and Man. New York, Harcourt, Brace & Co., 1943

B. Spock and M. Huschka. Psychological Aspects of Pediatric Practice. New York State Committee on Mental Hygiene, 1939

M. Ralph Kaufman. Psychotherapy in general medical practice. *Journal of the Maine Medical Association*, 31:235–239, September 1940

Thomas A. C. Rennie. What can the practitioner do in treating the neuroses? *Bulletin of the New York Academy of Medicine*, 22:23–37, January 1946

William C. Menninger. Depressions. *Diseases of the Nervous System*, 2:244–253, August 1941

Franz Alexander. Fundamental concepts of psychosomatic research. *Psychosomatic Medicine*, 5:205–210, July 1943

E. Lindemann. Hysteria as a problem in a general hospital. *Medical Clinics of North America*, 22:591–605, May 1938

The Menninger Clinic Bulletin
Gynecology and Obstetrics, volume 7, January 1943
Pediatrics, volume 8, November 1944
Psychological Testing, volume 7, May 1943

Charlotte Towle. Common Human Needs: An Interpretation for Staff in Public Assistance Agencies. Federal Security Agency, Social Security Board, Bureau of Public Assistance. Public Assistance Report No. 8. Washington, United States Government Printing Office, 1945

Index

Page numbers given in *italics* indicate the fullest or most explicit discussion of a topic.

Hostility (*cont.*)
    in veterans, 368, 369–370
    paranoid, 278–279
    repression and release of, 70–71,
        74–75, 151–152, 189, 243–
        245, 250, 314, 356–357, 360,
        364, 411, 426
    violence induced by, 326–327
    See also Ambivalence; Marital
        tension
Huntington's chorea, 424
Huschka, M., 450
Hydrotherapy, 128, 188, 307–308
Hypertension, 1, 33, 55, 68, 70,
    117, 259, 260, 266, 415, 416,
    418, 420, 421, 423
    what to tell the patient, 444–445
Hypnosis, 178, 179
Hypochondriasis, 36, 341
Hysteria, 34, 37, 115–121, 152–
    153, *160–161*, 166, 167, 173,
    196, 197, 199, 245–246,
    258–260, 315–317, 330,
    355–358
    consciousness in, 171–172
Hysterical psychosis, 424

Iatrogenic disease, 398, 419
Id, 16, 90, 124, 231–232, 335, 346
Identification, 86–87, 94, 96, 97,
    98, 102–103, 104, 106, 186,
    218, 247–248, 251, 263, 278,
    342, 356, 361, 435
Illness, secondary gains from, 111,
    114, 120, 155–156, 362
Impotence, 153, 324
Indigestion. *See* Gastrointestinal
    disturbances

Insanity
    fear of, 398–413
    meaning of term, 345–346
Insight in psychoneurosis, 35, 130–
    132, 149, 169, 171–173, 193,
    264–265, 363–364, 425
Insomnia, 7, 324
Instinct psychology, 89–90, 124
Instructors in the course
    list of, 3–5
    reactions of, 21, 22, 23
Insulin shock therapy, 17, 19, 291,
    302, 346
Interpretation. *See* Interview tech-
    nique
Interview technique, 15–16, 38,
    42–62, 64, 70, 129, 130,
    135–138, 177–178, 194, 214,
    215–216, 218–220, 221–
    223, 264–265, 363–364,
    404–405, 406, 411
Introjection, 325, 328–329
Involutional depression, 337–339
Involutional melancholia, 290, 330,
    438
Involutional period. *See* Middle age,
    problems of
Isolation, as defense against anxiety,
    249–250, 316

Jealousy. *See* Rivalry situations
"Jewish problem," 249
Jews, psychoneurosis in, 110, 112
Johnson, Samuel, 322

Kaufman, M. Ralph, 126, 450
Kleitman, N., 377